Nutrition and Diet Research Progress

Pathways to Obesity and Main Roads to Recovery

NUTRITION AND DIET RESEARCH PROGRESS

Additional books in this series can be found on Nova's website under the Series tab.

Additional E-books in this series can be found on Nova's website under the E-books tab.

NUTRITION AND DIET RESEARCH PROGRESS

PATHWAYS TO OBESITY AND MAIN ROADS TO RECOVERY

PIERGIUSEPPE VINAI
EDITOR

Nova Science Publishers, Inc.
New York

For permission to use material from this book please contact us:
Telephone 631-231-7269; Fax 631-231-8175
Web Site: http://www.novapublishers.com

LIBRARY OF CONGRESS CATALOGING-IN-PUBLICATION DATA

Pathways to obesity and main roads to recovery / editor, Piergiuseppe Vinai.
p. ; cm.
Includes bibliographical references and index.
ISBN 978-1-61122-740-6 (hardcover)
1. Obesity--Treatment. I. Vinai, Piergiuseppe.
[DNLM: 1. Obesity--etiology. 2. Obesity--therapy. 3. Eating Disorders--etiology. 4. Eating Disorders--therapy. WD 210]
RC628.P325 2011
616.3'98--dc22
2010043932

Published by Nova Science Publishers, Inc. † New York

To Natalia. the love of my life

Contents

Preface		**xi**
Acknowledgments		**xv**
Chapter I	Dealing with an Overfed World *Giovanni Maria Ruggiero*	**1**
Chapter II	The Genetics of Obesity *Federica Tozzi and Andréa Poyastro Pinheiro*	**5**
Chapter III	Neuroendocrine Influences on Appetite and Obesity *Susan Carnell, Charlisa D. Gibson, Leora Benson, Marci E. Gluck and Allan Geliebter*	**21**
Chapter IV	Psychiatric, Psychological, and Familial Parameters in Childhood Obesity *Daniel Stein, Yael Latzer, Laurel Edmunds, Silvana Fennig, Moria Golan, Eitan Gur, Ze'ev Hochberg, Diane Levin-Zamir, Eynat Zubery and Phyllis Speiser*	**59**
Chapter V	Emotions Becoming Food: The Binge Eating Disorder *Piergiuseppe Vinai and Patrizia Todisco*	**83**
Chapter VI	The Night Eating Syndrome *Piergiuseppe Vinai, Gabriella Carpegna, Paola Vallauri, Silvia Cardetti and Noemi Ferrato*	**95**
Chapter VII	Sleep-related Eating Disorder *Mauro Manconi and Matteo Mario Anelli*	**109**

Chapter VIII	Assessment of Obese Patients *Piergiuseppe Vinai, Silvia Cardetti, Gabriella Carpegna[1], Noemi Ferrato, Loriana Murciano, Elena Ponzio and Paola Vallauri*	**121**
Chapter IX	Selecting and Preparing Patients for Bariatric Surgery: The Preoperative Psychological Consultation *Anthony N. Fabricatore and Joseph A. Giorgio*	**157**
Chapter X	Psychosocial Contribution and Prevention of Childhood Obesity *Yael Latzer and Daniel Stein*	**177**
Chapter XI	Improving Healthy Eating Habits and Daily Physical Activity *Sabrina Guidi*	**203**
Chapter XII	Dieting *Anna Tagliabue*	**215**
Chapter XIII	Self-help *Ilyse Dobrow DiMarco*	**223**
Chapter XIV	Cognitive-behavioral Treatment (CBT) for Obesity *Jennifer R. Shapiro and Cynthia M. Bulik*	**237**
Chapter XV	Pharmacotherapy *Roberta Situlin*	**251**
Chapter XVI	Bariatric Surgery: Indications and Procedures *Luca Busetto*	**267**
Chapter XVII	Treatment of Binge Eating Disorder *James E. Mitchell and Kristine Steffen*	**279**
Chapter XVIII	Treatment of Night Eating Syndrome *Kelly C. Allison and Amy Sgrenci Langsam*	**289**
Chapter XIX	Sleep-related Eating Disorder: Relationship to Amnesia and a Review of its Treatment *Michael J. Howell and Carlos H. Schenck*	**299**
Chapter XX	Obesity and its Treatment in Persons with Mental Illness *Jennifer D. Lundgren and Melisa V. Rempfer*	**309**

Chapter XXI Neurosurgery in the Treatment of Obesity **321**
Casey H. Halpern, Ephraim Church, John A. Wolf, Tracy L. Bale, Albert J. Stunkard, Jurg L. Jaggi, M. Sean Grady, Thomas Wadden and Gordon H. Baltuch

Index **335**

Preface

The similar body images of obese patients frequently hide psychopathological and medical differences that need different therapeutic approaches. A group of experts in the field focuses on different factors inducing weight gain and different strategies to lose weight. The aim is to highlight the role that genetic, neuro-endocrinologic and psychological factors play in the onset and maintenance of obesity and how to deal with them. The book is thought for young researchers and clinicians who are beginning to deal with the matter. It focuses on recent findings and future perspectives on onset mechanisms and therapeutic strategies for obesity treatment from well-stated data. The text is divided into four parts:

1. Pathways to obesity,
2. Untying the obesity knot,
3. Main roads to recovery,
4. Future perspectives.

Pathways to Obesity

The body weight excess is a complex disease, caused by biological psychological and social reasons. The aim of this section is to inform on well-stated data regarding, genetic, endocrinological psychological and familial factors that can induce obesity.

In the first chapter, Giovanni Maria Ruggiero discusses the different meanings of excessive weight across various historical periods and cultures and in the second, Federica Tozzi and Andréa Poyastro Pinheiro highlight the recent data on genetic pathways underlying the susceptibility to obesity. In the third chapter, Susan Carnell, Charlisa D. Gibson, Leora Benson, Marci E. Gluck & Allan Geliebter widely discuss the role of appetite and obesity-related hormones in the development, maintenance and co-morbidities of excessive weight.

To be overweight during childhood and adolescence is a risk factor for obesity in adulthood and may be associated with psychological and social problems such as reduced school and social performance, less favorable quality of life, societal victimization and peer teasing, lower self-and body-esteem, and neuropsychological dysfunctioning. These topics are analyzed in the fourth chapter by Daniel Stein, Yael Latzer, Laurel Edmunds, Silvana Fennig, Moria Golan, Eitan Gur, Ze'ev Hochberg, Diane Levin-Zamir, Eynat Zubery & Phyllis Speiser.

In the fifth chapter, Piergiuseppe Vinai and Patrizia Todisco discuss the psycho-pathological and clinical characteristics of Binge Eating Disorder (BED) and the influence of this diagnosis on the outcome of obesity treatments.

Usually, food intake is suppressed during the night but several patients eat at nighttime. The subsection "The dark side of food", including chapters six and seven, focuses on nocturnal eaters. In the sixth chapter, Gabriella Carpegna, Paola Vallauri, Silvia Cardetti, Noemi Ferrato and Piergiuseppe Vinai focus on recent findings and new suggested diagnostic criteria for Night Eating Syndrome (NES), while in the seventh, Mauro Manconi and Matteo Anelli inform on clinical and polysomnographic data of patients affected by Sleep -Related Eating Disorder (SRED).

Untying the Obesity Knot

This part of the book is dedicated to medical and psychological assessment of obese patients. In Chapter Eight, Piergiuseppe Vinai, Gabriella Carpegna, Silvia Cardetti, Noemi Ferrato Loriana Murciano, Elena Ponzio and Paola Vallauri suggest a sort of flow chart useful in discriminating different "obesities," including a list of instruments useful to find out medical and psychological diseases frequently related to obesity.

Anthony N. Fabricatore and Joseph A. Giorgio, in the nineteenth chapter, discuss the needing of a psychological assessment for patients seeking surgical treatment. Bariatric surgery is the treatment of choice for extremely obese individuals, but the complexity of surgical procedures, as well as the associated risks, warrant careful selection and preparation of candidates.

Main Roads to Recovery

This section focuses on different approaches to obesity. The general idea is that overweight/obese patients are not all similar. Different "obesities" need different therapeutic approaches. Each chapter underlines the core characteristics of each specific treatment, including indications, contraindications, positive effects and limits.

In Chapter Ten, Yael Latzer & Daniel Stein highlight the need of promoting health-generated strategies to reduce the risk of child and adolescent obesity. They emphasize that prevention programs should be multidisciplinary and carried out on a public policy level, taking into consideration the important role of the family and of the school.

Sabrina Guidi, in Chapter Eleven, reports the available data regarding influence of changing lifestyle on the Metabolic Syndrome (MS), a combination of medical disorders increasing the risk of cardiovascular disease, and Anna Tagliabue, in Chapter Twelve, focuses on the importance of an healthy diet in prevention and management of obesity.

In Chapter Thirteen, Ilyse Dobrow DiMarco describes the specific features of self-help programs for obesity treatment.

Jennifer R. Shapiro & Cynthia M. Bulik (in Chapter Fourteen) review the history and advancement of Cognitive Behavioral Therapy (CBT) for obesity treatment, describe how it is applied to weight management and discuss benefits and limitations of this approach.

Roberta Situlin, in Chapter Fifteen, focuses on characteristics, mechanism of action, side effects and contraindications of different drugs used in pharmacotherapy of weight excess.

In Chapter Sixteen, Luca Busetto highlights different techniques of bariatric surgery, evidencing the risk/benefit profile of any procedure such as indications and contraindications among adults and adolescent patients.

The subsection: "Treatments of specific disorders inducing obesity" includes the last four chapters of this part of the book. It focuses on treatments of Binge Eating Disorder, Night Eating Syndrome, Sleep Related Eating Disorder and on therapy of obesity in persons with a serious mental illness. James E. Mitchell and Kristine Steffen summarize the therapeutic strategies useful to deal with BED, Kelly C. Allison. & Amy Sgrenci Langsam those for NES and Michael J Howell & Carlos H Schenck show recent data on therapy of the SRED. Jennifer D. Lundgren, & Melisa V. Rempfer discuss the therapy of obesity in persons with serious mental illness and individuals in treatment with atypical antipsychotic medications.

Future Perspectives

In the last part of the book, a group of experts (Casey H. Halpern, Ephraim Church, John A. Wolf, Tracy L. Bale, Albert J. Stunkard, Jurg L. Jaggi,. Sean Grady, Thomas Wadden, and Gordon H. Baltuch), highlights recent research on deep brain stimulation in obesity treatment.

Acknowledgments

I am grateful to all the outstanding colleagues for their fundamental contributions to this project; it has been a great honor for me to collaborate with them. I would like also to acknowledge my sons: Luisa for drawing the tables of Chapter XVI, and Paolo for his help in the translation of the text. Last, but not least, my sincere thanks goes to my wife, Natalia, for her great support to my work.

In: Pathways to Obesity and Main Roads to Recovery
Editor: Piergiuseppe Vinai
ISBN: 978-1-61122-740-6

Chapter I

Dealing with an Overfed World

Giovanni Maria Ruggiero
Studi Cognitivi Post Graduate Psychotherapy School, Milan, Italy

Abstract

Obesity has different meanings across various historical periods and cultures. In pre-historic cultures and societies, obesity was associated with attractiveness, strength, and fertility. For most of human history, mankind struggled with food scarcity; it has been viewed as a sign of wealth and prosperity. During the twentieth century, the prevalence of obesity in general population skyrocketed; the weight that is viewed as an ideal has become lower, and people's views concerning healthy weight have changed in the opposite direction. These changes are believed to be due to increasing rates of adiposity leading to increased acceptance of extra body fat as being normal.

Historical Notes

When dealing with the historical development of the societal views regarding eating, we must remember that in many cultures, there has been the conflict between the two poles of the eating dilemma: dieting and bingeing. For example, ancient Rome had both sumptuary laws and disparagement for excess at table. We can find in Petronius the glorious Cena Thrimalchionis and how can we forget that Latin literature is full of descriptions of so-called Lucullan repasts? Here, Cicero inveighs against degenerate dining while in other places, Horace celebrates bingeing.

Focusing on the overeating pole of the dilemma, we know that obesity has different meanings across various historical periods and cultures. For most of human history, mankind struggled with food scarcity (Mazzone and Fantuzzi, 2006); thus, obesity has historically been viewed as a sign of wealth and prosperity. It was common among wealthy people in Europe in the Middle Ages and the Renaissance (Bloomgarden, 2003), as well as in Ancient East Asian civilizations.

In pre-modern human cultures and societies, obesity is associated with attractiveness, strength, and fertility. Some of the more ancient cultural products, known as Venuses, are statuettes representing an obese female figure. Their widespread use throughout pre-historic Mediterranean and European cultures suggests a central role for the obese female form in magical rituals and suggests cultural approval of the obese body form.

With the onset of the industrial revolution, height and weight thus both increased through the 19th century in the developed world. During the 20th century, as populations reached their genetic potential for height, weight began increasing much more than height, resulting in obesity (Caballero, 2007)

The Modern Age

During the twentieth century, the prevalence of obesity in general population skyrocketed, so that in 1997, the World Health Organization (WHO) recognized obesity as a global epidemic. In 2005, the WHO estimates that at least 400 million adults (9.8% of world population) are obese.

Obviously enough, this phenomenon is related to the increase of the amount of food available. The United States had the highest availability, with 3,754 calories per person in 2003. Most of these extra calories came from an increase in carbohydrate consumption rather than fat consumption. The primary source of these extra carbohydrates are sweetened beverages, which now account for almost 25 percent of daily calories in young adults in America (Caballero, 2007).

During the late 1990s, Europeans had 3,394 calories per person; in the developing areas of Asia, there were 2,648 calories per person; and in sub-Saharan Africa, people had 2,176 calories per person. Total calorie consumption has been found to be related to obesity (Marantz, Bird, and Alderman, 2008).

Current rates of being overweight and obesity in the United States are 61% and 14% in adults and children, respectively. Obesity in adults has nearly doubled since 1980, from 15% in 1980, to 27% by 1999 (Wellman and Friedberg, 2002). Childhood overweight issues are rapidly rising in the U.S., particularly among African Americans and Hispanics (Strauss and Pollack, 2001). In the Far East, Japan (Matsushita et al., 2004) and even China (Yu, 2006) show rapid increases in the prevalence of the problem.

In addition, a sedentary lifestyle plays a significant role in obesity. Worldwide, there has been a large shift towards less physically demanding work. This is due to increasing availability of mechanized transportation and of labor-saving technology in the home. In children, there appears to be declines in levels of physical activity due to less walking and physical education (Ness-Abramof and Apovian, 2006). The widespread availability of nutritional guidelines has accomplished little to address the problems of overeating.

However, while calorie consumption in excess is an important factor for understanding obesity, it cannot explain the current dramatic increase seen within specific countries or globally (Yach, Stuckler, and Brownell, 2006). There are other social and cultural factors.

The correlation between social class and BMI varies globally. A review in 1989 found that in developed countries, women of a high social class were less likely to be obese. No significant differences were seen among men of different social classes. In the developing world, women, men, and children from high social classes had greater rates of obesity (Sobal and Stunkard, 1989; McLaren, 2007). It is plausible that in affluent societies, wealthy people are under greater social pressure to remain slim and have greater expectations for physical fitness. In addition, the Western preference for thinness is increasingly being exported worldwide as part of the process of globalization.

This increase of overweight and obese people is accompanied, in modern Western Culture, by the dissemination of a popular belief that a more slender body aspect is more desirable. Weight reduction through manipulation of diet is a general preoccupation, while weight gain is accelerating. In contemporary American culture, Puritan roots and modern consumerism are in conflict with each other.

On the other hand, it is true that not only modern Western culture regards excess weight as unattractive. Also, past cultures viewed obesity as the result of a character flaw. The obese or fat character in Greek comedy was a figure of mockery. During Christian times, food was viewed as a gateway to the sins of sloth and lust. People of all ages can face social stigmatization and may be targeted by bullies. Various stereotypes of obese people have found their way into expressions of popular culture. A common stereotype is the obese character who has a warm and dependable personality, presumably in compensation for social exclusion, but equally common is the obese vicious bully. It can be argued that depiction in popular culture adds to and maintains commonly perceived stereotypes, in turn harming self esteem of obese people. A charge of discrimination on the basis of appearance could be leveled against these depictions.

Public perceptions in Western society regarding healthy body weight differ from those regarding the weight that is considered ideal, and both have changed since the beginning of the 20th century. The weight that is viewed as an ideal has become lower since the 1920s. This is illustrated by the fact that the average height of Miss America winners increased by 2% from 1922 to 1999, while their average weight decreased by 12% (Rubinstein and Caballero, 2000). On the other hand, people's views concerning healthy weight have changed in the opposite direction. In Britain, the weight at which people considered themselves to be overweight was significantly higher in 2007 than in 1999. These changes are believed to be due to increasing rates of adiposity leading to increased acceptance of extra body fat as being normal (Johnson et al., 2008).

Conclusion

In conclusion, acceptable body shape is culturally constructed. In "western" societies, a strong cultural value is placed on thinness, especially for women, but there are still differences in interpretation among subcultures. In the U.S., Davidson and Knafl (2006) found that Black Americans evaluated obesity to be positively related to attractiveness and sexual desirability, while Caucasian Americans viewed obesity in a negative way.

References

Bloomgarden, Z. (2003). Prevention of Obesity and Diabetes. *Diabetes Care, 26*, 3172–3178.

Caballero, B. (2007). The global epidemic of obesity: An overview. *Epidemiol Rev, 29*, 1–5.

Marantz, P.R., Bird, E.D. & Alderman, M.H. (2008). A call for higher standards of evidence for dietary guidelines. *American Journal of Preventive Medicine, 34,* 234–40.

Davidson, M. & Knafl, K. (2006). A Dimensional analysis of the concept of obesity. *Journal of advanced nursing, 54,* 342-50.

Johnson, F., Cooke, L., Croker, H., Wardle, J. (2008). Changing perceptions of weight in Great Britain: comparison of two population surveys. *British Medical Journal, 3,* 3-7.

Matsushita, Y., Yoshiike, N., Kaneda, F., Yoshita, K., Takimoto, M H. (2004). Trends in Childhood Obesity in Japan over the Last 25 Years from the National Nutrition Survey. *Obesity Research, 12*, 205–214.

Mazzone, T. & Fantuzzi, G. (2006) *Adipose Tissue and Adipokines in Health And Disease.* Totowa NJ: Humana Press,

McLaren, L. (2007). Socio-economic status and obesity. *Epidemiol Review, 29,* 29–48.

Ness-Abramo, F. R. & Apovian, C. M. (2006). Diet modification for treatment and prevention of obesity. *Endocrine, 29,* 5–9.

Rubinstein, S. & Caballero, B. (2000). Is Miss America an undernourished role model? *Journal of the American Medical Association, 283,* 1569-1623.

Sobal, J. & Stunkard, A. J. (1989). Socio-economic status and obesity: A review of the literature. *Psychological Bulletin, 105,* 260–75.

Strauss, R. S. & Pollack, H. A. (2001). Epidemic increase in childhood overweight, 1986-1998. *Journal of the American Medical Association, 286,* 2845-2848.

Wellman, N.S. and Friedberg, B. (2002). Causes and consequences of adult obesity: health, social and economic impacts in the United States. *Asia Pacific Journal of Clinical Nutrition, 11*,705-709.

Yach, D. Stuckler, D. and Brownell, K.D. (2006). Epidemiologic and economic consequences of the global epidemics of obesity and diabetes. *Nature Medicine, 12,* 62–6.

Yoshiike, N. Seino, F. Tajima, S. Mendelson, R. Dollard, D. Hall, P. Zarrabi, S. Y. Desjardin, E. (2002). Twenty-year changes in the prevalence of overweight in Japanese adults: *the National Nutrition Survey. Obes Rev,* 3, 183–190.

Yu, C. K. H. Teoh, T. G. & Robinson, S. (2006). Obesity in Pregnancy. *An International Journal of Obstetrics & Gynecology, 113,* 1117-1125.

In: Pathways to Obesity and Main Roads to Recovery
Editor: Piergiuseppe Vinai
ISBN: 978-1-61122-740-6

Chapter II

The Genetics of Obesity

Federica Tozzi and Andréa Poyastro Pinheiro

Federica Tozzi University of North Carolina at Chapel Hill, Department of Psychiatry, Chapel Hill, North Carolina, USA

Andréa Poyastro Pinheiro Graduate Program in Epidemiology, Department of Social Medicine, Federal University of Rio Grande do Sul, Brazil

Abstract

The increased prevalence of obesity has been fuelled by lifestyle changes in recent decades that encourage overfeeding and a sedentary way of life. Although the percentage of overweight and obese individuals is worryingly high, especially in Western countries (International Association for the Study of Obesity, 2009), not all individuals are affected by this obesogenic environment. Wide inter-individual variation exists in the predisposition to gain weight; thus factors other than environment play a role in the development of obesity. Several lines of evidence indicate genetic factors may explain at least part of this variability.

Common obesity is a complex disease, caused by several genetic and non-genetic risk factors, and the vast majority of obesity cases do not segregate with a Mendelian pattern of inheritance. Until recently, progress in the search for susceptibility genes has been slow and offered limited success. However, the recent availability of novel technologies and approaches has led to the identification of a number of loci associated with obesity. Such discoveries in the field of obesity genetics were made possible mostly by means of large-scale meta-analysis of candidate gene and genome-wide association studies, through international collaborative data sharing of samples. In this rapidly changing field, investigators still face challenges of unraveling the specific contributions of each identified locus and understanding the biological pathways underlying the susceptibility to obesity. These discoveries will be helpful for the development of more effective and tailored treatments.

Introduction

Obesity is a widely heterogeneous condition. Although no diagnostic tools distinguish obese patients into subtypes, several useful categorizations could be proposed, based on BMI, age of onset, fat distribution, and behavioral features, such as the presence or absence of binge eating.

A classification of obesity according to genetic etiology includes three main categories: monogenic, syndromic, and polygenic obesity. Clear evidence indicates obesity runs in families; however, the vast majority of obesity cases do not segregate with a Mendelian pattern of inheritance. Common obesity is a complex disease caused by several genetic (polygenic) and non-genetic (environmental) risk factors. Monogenic forms are rare. In this chapter, we illustrate the state of the art of obesity genetics, with particular focus on polygenic obesity and the most recent advances in the field.

Family and Twin Studies

Numerous studies have indicated the contribution of genetic factors to the susceptibility of obesity (Rankinen et al., 2006). The determination of familial resemblance is often the first step in exploring whether genes play a role in the etiology of a disease. When familial predisposition to a disease exists, resemblance for the disorder is observed amongst blood relatives of affected individuals. Family studies on obesity clearly indicate an increased risk of developing obesity in children with an obese parent (Reilly et al., 2005); this risk becomes even higher if both parents are obese (Whitaker et al., 1994). Unfortunately, family studies cannot establish whether the predictive value of parental obesity is due to genetic factors, environmental factors, or a combination of both. However, twin and adoption studies can unravel the question further by determining the extent observed familiality is explained by genetic factors. Twin studies enable the decomposition of variance in liability into genetic and environmental factors, and they provide estimations of the magnitude of these effects (Neale and Cardon, 1992). Because monozygotic (MZ) twins are assumed to be fundamentally genetically identical, discordance in MZ twins likely results from environmental influences. Conversely, differences between dizygotic (DZ) twins who share roughly 50% of the genome could be due to either genetic or environmental influences. By comparing the similarity of monozygotic twins and dizygotic twins for a given trait, an estimate of the relative contribution of genes and environment to trait liability can be derived. Twin studies have provided evidence for a moderate to high heritability, indicating that 40% to70% of the interindividual variation in common obesity is explained by genetic factors (Maes et al., 1997; Stunkard et al., 1986; Stunkard et al., 1990).

Monogenic Obesity

Monogenic forms of obesity are caused by a mutation in a single gene, and the genetic mutation alone is sufficient to cause the condition.

Table 2.1. Main features of monogenic obesity

Mutations	Locus	Notes
Leptin gene	7q31.3	Defect in leptin production Early-onset obesity, hyperphagia Impaired immunity and fertility Clinical response to leptin administration (leptin normalizes food intake)
Leptin receptor gene	1p31	Early onset obesity, lack of pubertal development, reduced secretion of growth hormone and thyrotropin. Impaired fertility
Melanocortin 4 receptor gene (MC4R)	18q22	Severe obesity with variable clinical expression. High levels of fasting insulin. Symptoms tend to partially ameliorate in adult life.
Proopiomelanocortin gene (POMC)	2p23	Hyperphagia and severe early onset obesity, hypocortisolaemia and adrenocorticotropic hormone deficiency, pale skin and red hair pigmentation
Prohormone convertase 1 gene (PC1)	5q15-q21	Extreme childhood obesity, abnormal glucose homeostasis, hypogonadotropic hypogonadism, hypocortisolism, elevated plasma proinsulin, POMC concentrations, and low insulin levels. Impaired fertility

Monogenic forms are rare in humans, but frequently constitute the most severe types of obesity. These forms are characterized by an early onset and often are associated with additional phenotypic manifestations; however, they lack the developmental delay and brain dysfunction that complicate clinical presentations of pleiotropic (or syndromic) forms. Autosomal recessive and autosomal dominant are the modes of inheritance of most of these obesity forms. To date, at least 20 single-gene defects have been identified as responsible for autosomal forms of human obesity, including congenital leptin and leptin receptor deficiency as well as defects in the proopiomalanocortin and melanocortin receptor 4 genes. Table 2.1 summarizes main features of monogenic obesity.

Syndromic Obesity

This category includes forms in which obesity is one of the clinical features of the syndrome. It might be associated with mental retardation, abnormalities of organs, or characteristic dysmorphic features. Currently, 20 to 30 different syndromes have been identified. The genetic causes of these forms are chromosomal abnormalities or other discrete genetic defects. The genetic alteration could be either autosomal or X-linked. Among others, Prader-Willi, Bardet-Biedl, and Cohen are pleiotropic obesity syndromes.

Prader-Willi Syndrome, the most common syndromal cause of obesity, provides an illustrative example. This syndrome has an estimated prevalence of 1 in 25,000 and is characterized by severe obesity beginning very early in life. Weight at birth may be within normal range, but usually is followed by mild prenatal growth retardation. Diminished fetal activity during the pregnancy is another common feature. After feeding difficulties that characterize the very first months of life (due to diminished swallowing and sucking reflexes), these patients start to present very severe hyperphagia around age 12 to 18 months. Other symptoms are hyporeflexia, hypotonia, short stature, hypogonadism, and mental retardation. Prader-Willi syndrome is caused by the lack of the paternal segment 15q11.2-q12 (Cassidy and Driscoll, 2009), but the specific gene responsible for the development of this syndrome is yet to be identified. Several candidate genes within the 15q region have been studied, and their expression has been reported as absent in the brains of patients with Prader-Willi syndrome (Cassidy and Driscoll, 2009).

Table 2.2 summarizes main characteristics of the most frequent pleiotropic obesity syndromes. All are characterized by childhood-onset obesity. A complete list may be found in OMIM [http://www.ncbi.nlm.nih.gov].

Polygenic Obesity

Polygenic obesity is the most common type of obesity, and the inheritance pattern is complex. Both environmental and genetic factors contribute to development of the disease, and the genetic component is polygenic and epistatic. In other words, the genetic vulnerability is likely associated with the effects of multiple genes, each with modest effect, and some genes are needed to mediate the effect of others. The search for genetic loci associated with obesity includes molecular genetics' techniques, briefly described below.

Genome-wide Linkage and Candidate Gene Association Studies

Two commonly used genetic analytic approaches are genome-wide linkage analysis and case control association studies. Large samples of families with multiple ill members are required for linkage analysis studies. Genetic markers—spread across the genome—are genotyped to identify chromosomal regions harboring genes that influence the trait of interest.

The principle of a linkage study is that if a disease runs in a family, genetic markers should run the same way in the family. However, linkage studies identify chromosomal regions associated with the disease and not specific genes. Usually, the areas under the linkage include millions of base pairs (and thus many genes). Further studies are needed to identify the specific genes. Candidate genes located under the linkage peaks can be explored using case control association approaches to verify whether they are, in fact, associated with the phenotype of interest.

In case control association studies, cases that display a trait of interest are compared with controls who do not display the trait. If certain genotypes are present more often in cases than controls, then the gene is associated with the disease.

Table 2.2. Main characteristics of the most frequent pleiotropic obesity syndromes

Syndrome	Mode of inheritance	Locus	Additional clinical features
Albright hereditary osteodystrophy (pseudohypoparathyroidism type Ia)	Autosomal dominant	20q13.2	Short stature, round faces, subcutaneous ossifications, brachydactyly, and other skeletal anomalies, impaired olfaction and end-organ resistance to parathyroid and other hormones
Alstrom syndrome	Autosomal recessive	2p13	Small stature, cardiomyopathy, type 2 diabetes, hyperthyroidism, retinal dystrophy, progressive sensori-neural hearing loss. No mental retardation
Bardet-Biedel syndrome	Autosomal recessive	Defects at various chromosomal loci	Finger abnormalities, dyslexia and learning disabilities, progressive retinal dystrophy and renal disease
Borjeson-Forssman-Lehmann syndrome	X-linked dominant disease	Xq26	Microcephaly, severe mental retardation, epilepsy, short stature and large ears, hypogonadism and gynecomastia.
Cohen syndrome	Autosomal recessive	8q22-q23	Short stature, microcephaly, opthalmopathy, thin extremities and characteristic facial features (overrepresented in the Finnish population)
Fragile X syndrome	X-linked dominant with decreased penetrance	Xq27.3	Moderate to severe mental retardation, macro-orchidism, and distinct facial features, including long face, large ears, and prominent jaw
Mehmo syndrome	X-linked	X22.13	Mental retardation, epilepsy, hypogonadism and microcephaly
Prader-Willi syndrome	Autosomal dominant	15q11-q13	Diminished fetal activity, mental retardation, short stature, muscular hypotonia, hypogonadotropic hypogonadism, small hands and feet
Simpson-Golabi-Behmel, type 2	X-linked	Xp22	Craniofacial defects, skeletal and visceral abnormalities
Ulnar-mammary syndrome (also called Schinzel syndrome)	Autosomal dominant	12q24.1	Hypoplasia or aplasia of upper limbs on the ulnar side, hypoplastic nipples, delayed puberty, dental abnormalities, genital anomalies, and alterations of gastrointestinal tract The range and severity of physical abnormalities varies greatly among affected individuals; some cases may be very mild, while others may be more severe.
Wilson-Turner syndrome	X-linked	Xp21.1-q22	Mental retardation, gynecomastia, speech difficulties, tapering fingers, and small feet

Usually, genetic markers within candidate gene or genes are genotyped. Those genetic markers are single nucleotide polymorphisms (SNPs): DNA sequence variations that occur when a single nucleotide (A, T, C, or G) in the genome sequence is altered. The genes to be studied—candidate genes—are selected based on prior hypotheses that implicate the genes in the pathogenesis of the disorder. Statistical analyses contrast genotype frequencies in cases versus controls (Balding, 2006). The case control association approach is suitable when considerable prior knowledge of the pathophysiology of a trait could implicate specific genetic variants.

Genome-wide Association Studies (GWAS)

With the completion of the Human Genome Project in 2003, the International Hap Map Project in 2005, and the development of new technologies that can assay more than one million variants rapidly and accurately, it is now possible to genotype the entire genome (i.e., all the chromosomes). A genome-wide association study involves a comprehensive coverage of common genetic variation across the genome to find genetic markers associated with a particular disease. Thus, GWAS do not require a focus on biological candidate genes or a prior knowledge of the pathophysiology of the disease (Hirschhorn and Daly, 2005), potentially enabling discovery of previously unsuspected candidate genes and new etiological pathways. Similar to all complex diseases, multiple testing in GWAS (several hundred thousand to million SNPs are genotyped and tested) requires very large samples to detect genes with small effect sizes. Over the past few years, GWAS have produced many highly significant findings. Notably, some of these findings may be false positives (i.e., due to chance) or may be the result of genotyping or analytical errors. Thus, genetic variants that initially are associated with a disease or trait (discovery stage) have to be replicated in independent samples (replication stage) to be considered "true hits" (Cichon et al., 2009; Vimaleswaran and Loos, 2010).

Research Findings in Common Obesity

The last several years have yielded substantial progress in identifying susceptibility genes for common (or polygenic) obesity, mainly through large-scale candidate gene case control and GWAS.

Genome-wide linkage studies, on the other hand, have not proved to be successful in identifying genetic variations implicated in common obesity (Vimaleswaran and Loos, 2010). More than 250 loci from 61 genome-wide linkage scans were originally detected, with only 15 of these loci being replicated (Rankinen et al., 2006). However, none of these replicated loci could be narrowed down enough to identify the genes or mutations under the linkage peak, including a meta-analysis of 37 genome-wide linkage studies comprising data on more than 31,000 Europeans from 10,000 families (Saunders et al., 2007).

Many candidate genes studies have been published. Candidate genes have been selected based on their physiological roles in metabolic pathways, evidence from animal models, and monogenic types of obesity. Candidate gene studies often yield conflicting results with a dearth of replicated findings. Small sample sizes lack statistical power to identify small effects for a complex disorder like common obesity, and sample size may be responsible for the limitation of this method. Testing associations in larger populations (around 5,000 cases and 5,000 controls) and using a meta-analytic approach have mitigated some limitations of the candidate gene approach. Large-scale studies have demonstrated compelling evidence of association with obesity and related traits for variants within several genes: melanocortin 4 receptor (MC4R), adrenergic b3 receptor gene (ADRB3), prohormone convertase 1/3

(PCSK1), brain-derived neurotrophic factor (BDNF), and endocannabinoid receptor 1 (CNR1) (Vimaleswaran and Loos, 2010). Below, a summary of the most robust findings for each identified variant is included.

Melanocortin 4 Receptor Gene (MC4R)

Pathogenic mutations in the MC4R gene have been found in about 5% of obese children (Farooqi et al., 2003). MC4R is implicated in the regulation of food intake and energy balance (Huszar et al., 1997). A population-based study (N =7,937) showed a significant protective effect of the I103 allele (frequency: ~3.6%) on obesity risk (Heid et al., 2005). In addition, three meta-analyses indicated that carriers of the I103 allele have a 20% lower risk of obesity than V103V homozygotes (Geller et al., 2004; Stutzmann et al., 2007; Young et al., 2007). Also, analysis on another MC4R mutation (the I251L variant) indicated a nearly 50% reduced risk of obesity for carriers of the L251 allele (frequency: ~0.41–1.21%) (Stutzmann et al., 2007).

Adrenergic b3 Receptor Gene (ADRB3)

ADRB3 is involved in the regulation of lipolysis and thermo genesis. The W64R ADRB3 variant association with obesity has been reported in three studies (Clement et al., 1995; Walston et al., 1995; Widen et al., 1995). More recently, a meta-analysis with data on 44,833 individuals indicated a significant association of the W64R variant with BMI in East Asians, with carriers of the R64 allele having a 0.24 kg/m2 higher BMI compared with non-carriers. Conversely, this association was not detected in Caucasians (Kurokawa et al., 2008).

Prohormone Convertase 1/3 Gene (PCSK1)

The PCSK1 gene encodes an enzyme that converts prohormones into hormones implicated in the regulation of energy metabolism (Loos, 2009). Rare PCSK1 variants have been identified as causal in monogenic obesity (Farooqi et al., 2007; Jackson et al., 1997). A study of 13,659 European individuals established an association of PCSK1 variants with common obesity: two common PCSK1 non-synonymous variants, N221D and the Q665E–S690T pair, were associated with obesity risk in adults and children (Benzinou et al., 2008).

Brain-derived Neurotrophic Factor Gene (BDNF)

BDNF is involved in body weight regulation, eating behavior, body weight, and hyperactivity (Kernie et al., 2000). BDNF mutations have been reported in severe obesity and hyperphagia (Gray et al., 2006). A population-based study, with a sample of 10,109 women, indicated that individuals homozygous for the M66 allele of the V66M variant have a significantly lower BMI (- 0.76kg/m2) than carriers of the V66 allele (Shugart et al., 2009).

Moreover, another study confirmed the association of the BDNF mutation with BMI through the genome-wide association approach (Thorleifsson et al., 2009).

Endocannabinoid Receptor 1 Gene (CNR1)

A study on 5,750 individuals of European ancestry revealed that the CNR1 SNP rs806381 increased the risk of obesity in children [odds ratio (OR) = 1.39,P = 3×10^{-5}] and adults (OR =1.31, P = 6×10^{-4}) (Benzinou et al., 2008). CNR1 has also been implicated in human obesity due to its role in the regulation of energy metabolism and food intake (Loos, 2009).

Several large GWAS on obesity, involving hundreds of thousands individuals, were published in 2009 and 2010. As expected, results indicated many genes factor in the risk for obesity. These studies provide evidence that each gene contributes to only a slight increase in body weight. Below, a summary of the main findings of GWAS in obesity is presented.

Overall, 19 loci have been identified in GWAS, and two genes have shown the most consistent results: the fat mass-associated (FTO) gene and the melanocortin-4 receptor (MC4R) gene. FTO was the first gene associated with common obesity and related traits in a study where variants in the first intron of the gene showed a highly significant association with type 2 diabetes mediated through BMI (Frayling et al., 2007). The finding was replicated in more than 38,000 individuals from 13 cohorts. Other GWAS yielded associations between FTO gene variants and BMI in samples of different ethnicities (Dina et al., 2007; Scuteri et al., 2007). While consistent findings have been encouraging to researchers, actual effect sizes have been small, and all FTO variants explain a very small percentage of the population variance in BMI (i.e., <1%) (Frayling et al., 2007). The FTO protein is involved in energy balance and is widely expressed in peripheral and brain tissues (Fredriksson et al., 2008; Gerken et al., 2007; Stratigopoulos et al., 2008). FTO plays an important role in adipocyte lipolysis, and the association with obesity may occur, at least in part, through altered activity of this biochemical pathway (Wahlen et al., 2008). Additionally, the loss of FTO in mice leads to a significant reduction in adipose tissue and lean body mass, as a consequence of increased energy expenditure, indicating that FTO is functionally involved in energy homeostasis by the control of energy expenditure (Fischer et al., 2009).

Another locus, "near-MC4R" (188 kb downstream of MC4R) has been identified along with FTO in large collaborative studies. A large meta-analysis by the Genomic Investigation of Anthropometric Traits (GIANT) consortium combined seven GWAS for BMI including a total of 16,876 individuals. Although 10 loci were investigated for replication, only FTO and "near-MC4R" were confirmed in individuals from Europe and USA (Loos et al., 2008). Another study also identified the "near-MC4R" locus in 2,684 Asian Indians, and replication was verified in 11,955 individuals of Asian-Indian and European ancestry (Chambers et al., 2008). Following this study, six new loci were identified and replicated in a very large collaborative study, including 32,387 adults of European ancestry from 15 cohorts and a replication sample of 59,082 individuals (Willer et al., 2009). Besides the previously established "true hits" within the FTO and near-MC4R loci, the other loci were: near-NEGR1 (neuronal growth regulator 1), near-TMEM18 (transmembrane protein 18), in SH2B1 (SH2B adaptor protein 1), near-KCTD15 (potassium channel tetramerisation domain containing 15), near-GNPDA2 (glucosamine-6- phosphate deaminase 2), and in MTCH2 (mitochondrial carrier homologue 2).

Table 2.3. Genes in which loci associated with obesity from candidate gene and genome wide association studies have been identified

Location in chromosome	Gene name	Gene symbol
1p31.1	Neuronal growth regulator 1	NEGR1
1q41	Lysophospholipase-like 1	LYPLAL1
1q25.2	SEC16 homologue B *(Saccharomyces cerevisiae)* RAS protein activator like 2	SEC16B, RASAL2
2p25.2	Transmembrane protein 18	TMEM18
3q27	Ets variant gene 5	ETV5
4p13	Glucosamine-6-phosphate deaminase 2	GNPDA2
5q15-q21	Prohormone convertase 1/3	PCSK1
6p12	Transcription factor AP-2 β	TFAP2B
6q14-q15	Endocannabinoid receptor 1	CNR1
8p12-p11.2	Adrenergic β3 receptor	ADRB3
8p23.1	Methionine sulfoxide reductase A	MSRA
10p12	Phosphotriesterase related	PTER
11p13	Brain-derived neurotrophic factor	BDNF
11p11.2	Mitochondrial carrier homologue 2 *(Caenorhabditis elegans)*	MTCH2
12q13	BCDIN3-domain-containing, FAS apoptotic inhibitory molecule 2	BCDIN3D, FAIM2
14q31	Neurexin 3	NRXN3
16p11.2	SH2B adaptor protein 1, ATPase, Ca^{2+} transporting, cardiac muscle, fast twitch 1	SH2B1, ATP2A1
16q22-q23	v-Maf musculoaponeurotic fibrosarcoma oncogene homologue	MAF
16q12.2	Fat-mass and obesity associated gene	FTO
18q11-q12	Niemann-Pick disease, type C1	NPC1
18q22	Melanocortin 4 receptor	MC4R
19q13.11	Potassium channel tetramerisation domain containing 15	KCTD15

Four genome-wide association studies for BMI were meta-analyzed by deCODE Genetics, including 34,416 Europeans and African Americans. (Thorleifsson et al., 2009). Replication of 43 SNPs was carried forward in 5,586 Danish individuals and for confirmation in discovery stage data of the GIANT consortium. In addition to the FTO and near-MC4R loci, and four loci (near-NEGR1, near-TMEM18, in SH2B1, near-KCTD15) identified by the GIANT consortium previously, four loci were discovered: SEC16B (SEC16 homologue B), between ETV5 (Ets variant gene 5) and DGKG (diacylglycerol kinase), in BDNF, and between BCDIN3D (BCDIN3-domain- containing) and FAIM2 (FAS apoptotic inhibitory molecule 2). Nevertheless, together, these 12 obesity-susceptibility loci explain less than 1% of the variation in BMI and have limited predictive value of obesity (Li et al., 2010)

Additionally, genetic analysis of obesity-related phenotypes (early-onset and morbid adult obesity, adult waist circumference and waist:hip ratio) in large-scale samples and meta-analyses led to the identification of seven novel loci (Heard-Costa et al., 2009; Lindgren et al., 2009; Meyre et al., 2009): NPC1 (Niemann–Pick disease, type C1), near-MAF (v-Maf musculoaponeurotic fibrosarcoma oncogene homologue), near-PTER (phosphotriesterase related), TFAP2B (transcription factor AP-2 b) and MSRA (methionine sulfoxide reductase A), LYPLAL1 (lysophospholipase-like 1), and NRXN3 (neurexin 3). The role of some of the newly identified loci (e.g., KCTD15, GNPDA2, etc.) in adiposity and energy balance regulation is not yet or is poorly known; others have a known effect (e.g., FTO, MC4R, SH2B1, etc.); and for many genes (BDNF, TMEM18, FTO, SH2B1), evidence shows they are expressed in the brain, indicating the relevance of centrally mediated mechanisms in the regulation of food intake and energy expenditure.

Table 2.3 contains a list of the genes in which loci associated with obesity from candidate gene and genome wide association studies have been identified.

Research Findings on Binge Eating Disorder

Binge Eating Disorder (BED) deserves special attention. This eating disorder is so frequently associated with obesity that it could be considered a subtype of obesity. However, patients with BED may also be overweight or within a normal weight range, especially at the beginning of the disorder.

Studies showing evidence for the genetic influence in the development of BED indicate heritability estimates between 41 and 57% (Javaras et al., 2008; Reichborn-Kjennerud et al., 2004). The disorder aggregates in families, partially independently of obesity, although relatives of patients with BED display a markedly higher prevalence of severe obesity in adulthood compared to relatives of patients without BED (Hudson et al., 2006).

Only a few molecular genetic studies have examined BED. Mutations within the MC4R gene have been associated with BED in obese individuals (Branson et al., 2003). However, two subsequent studies failed to replicate this finding (Hebebrand et al., 2004; Lubrano-Berthelier et al., 2006). Polymorphisms within the endocannabinoid degrading enzyme fatty acid amide hydrolase (FAAH) and the circadian locomotor output cycles kaput (CLOCK) genes were assessed in overweight/obese individuals with and without BED: only an association between the FAAH gene and overweight/obesity without BED was detected (Monteleone et al., 2008a; Monteleone et al., 2008b). Associations with binge eating have also been reported for variants within the ghrelin (Monteleone et al., 2007), serotonine transporter (Monteleone et al., 2006), and glucocorticoid receptor genes (Cellini et al., 2010). None of the aforementioned associations were replicated, and no GWAS of BED have been published yet. Thus, the genetic research of BED is still in its infancy, and large collaborative GWAS are warranted to detect genetic variations associated with the disorder and to determine if common genetic factors underlie obesity with and without binge eating.

Conclusion

The most recent findings and advances in the field of obesity genetics have several implications for future research and for public health. However, the translation of these findings into clinical practice is neither trivial nor immediate.

The identification of the genetic basis of the disease undoubtedly has a major impact in understanding the pathophysiological pathways leading to obesity. Recent progress in obesity genetics provides evidence for a role of the central nervous system on body weight regulation; this occurs through regulation of appetite, energy expenditure and other mechanisms (e.g., food reward mechanisms), indicating the etiology of obesity cannot be restricted solely to peripherally mediated mechanisms.

Although monogenic forms of obesity are rare, the understanding of pathogenetic mechanisms leading to obesity is relevant for understanding the basis of common obesity. The defects identified in these disorders lead to deregulation of centrally mediated mechanisms that control energy balance (O'Rahilly and Farooqi, 2008). GWAS have also identified genetic variations associated with obesity in genes expressed in the brain, pointing toward the centrally mediated mechanism of obesity.

The translation of the genetic findings into clinical practice is complicated by the complex nature of this genetic predisposition. As noted, common obesity is a polygenic disease, and each of the several implicated genes has a small effect in increasing the risk to develop the disease. Recent GWAS of various common medical conditions have identified over 70 common SNPs and showed that each SNP has a small contribution to the increased disease risk: mean odds ratios of these confirmed risk SNP is 1.36 (Bodmer and Bonilla, 2008). In the case of obesity, the FTO gene has the largest effect size, which has been estimated between 1.25 and 1.32 increase in the risk of obesity for each risk allele carried by an individual. All of the other genes associated through recent GWAS have smaller effect sizes. One application of genetic findings is to use known genetic markers to predict the risk of an individual developing the disease. However, based on the current knowledge, it is unlikely that current genetic findings may have this application for common diseases. Recent studies (Lin et al., 2009) indicated that, in presence of good clinical predictors, the additive effect of multiple loci, each with small effect size, does not add information above and beyond the clinical factors in predicting disease risk. Currently, family history of obesity provides a better predictive value than the detected genetic variants. With further advances in the genetics of obesity, the prediction of the disease development based on genetic tests could become more feasible.

Besides the potential for disease development risk prediction, and its application for diagnostic tools and prevention strategies, the knowledge derived from genetic studies may have other clinical implications. The identification of the genetic basis of a disease and understanding the biological pathways involved in its etiology comprise the first step for development of new and more effective treatments.

The emergence of GWAS has revolutionized the field of genetics, investigating complex diseases and traits, including those related to obesity. Candidate gene studies, however, will continue to be a valuable method, because they allow a more comprehensive analysis of biologically relevant candidates in interaction with other genes and environmental factors. Large-scale studies and meta-analyses of the detected gene-disease associations will remain imperative in reliably validating or disproving the findings. Still, genetic analysis has revealed only a very small part of the expected genetic variation.

The initial analytical effort in the new human genetic era of high-definition whole-genome scans has concentrated its effort in testing the common disease-common variant hypothesis. However, several lines of recent evidence from analysis of copy number variation (CNV) in common obesity suggest rare and penetrant gene variants may account for some of the genetic risk factors. Also, studies on gene-gene interactions will need to be performed, and more accurate measures of adiposity besides BMI might further improve power. Moreover, associations should be examined in populations with different ancestries and distinct environments, because absence of association in one ancestry or environment does not exclude association in another. Finally, the contribution of environmental factors to obesity needs to be considered together with genetic risk factors and represents some of the future challenges to capturing the real impact of genetic risk factors for obesity.

References

Balding, D. J. (2006). A tutorial on statistical methods for population association studies. *Nat. Rev. Genet. 7*, 781-791.

Benzinou, M., Creemers, J. W., Choquet, H., Lobbens, S., Dina, C., Durand, E., Guerardel, A., Boutin, P., Jouret, B., Heude, B., et al., (2008). Common nonsynonymous variants in PCSK1 confer risk of obesity. *Nat. Genet. 40*, 943-945.

Bodmer, W. & Bonilla, C. (2008). Common and rare variants in multi factorial susceptibility to common diseases. *Nat. Genet. 40*, 695-701.

Branson, R., Potoczna, N., Kral, J. G., Lentes, K. U., Hoehe, M. R. & Horber, F. F. (2003). Binge eating as a major phenotype of melanocortin 4 receptor gene mutations. *N. Engl. J. Med. 348*, 1096-1103.

Cassidy, S. B. & Driscoll, D. J. (2009). Prader-Willi syndrome. *Eur. J. Hum. Genet. 17*, 3-13.

Cellini, E., Castellini, G., Ricca, V., Bagnoli, S., Tedde, A., Rotella, C. M., Faravelli, C., Sorbi, S. & Nacmias, B. (2010). Glucocorticoid receptor gene polymorphisms in Italian patients with eating disorders and obesity. *Psychiatr. Genet,* 20(6), 282-8.

Chambers, J. C., Elliott, P., Zabaneh, D., Zhang, W., Li, Y., Froguel, P., Balding, D., Scott, J. & Kooner, J. S. (2008). Common genetic variation near MC4R is associated with waist circumference and insulin resistance. *Nat. Genet. 40*, 716-718.

Cichon, S., Craddock, N., Daly, M., Faraone, S. V., Gejman, P. V., Kelsoe, J., Lehner, T., Levinson, D. F., Moran, A., Sklar, P., et al., (2009). Genomewide association studies: history, rationale, and prospects for psychiatric disorders. *Am. J. Psychiatry 166*, 540-556.

Clement, K., Vaisse, C., Manning, B. S., Basdevant, A., Guy-Grand, B., Ruiz, J., Silver, K. D., Shuldiner, A. R., Froguel, P. & Strosberg, A. D. (1995). Genetic variation in the beta 3-adrenergic receptor and an increased capacity to gain weight in patients with morbid obesity. *N. Engl. J. Med. 333,* 352-354.

de Zwaan, M. (2001). Binge eating disorder and obesity. *Int. J. Obes. Relat Metab Disord. 25* Suppl 1, S51-S55.

Dina, C., Meyre, D., Gallina, S., Durand, E., Korner, A., Jacobson, P., Carlsson, L. M., Kiess, W., Vatin, V., Lecoeur, C., et al., (2007). Variation in FTO contributes to childhood obesity and severe adult obesity. *Nat. Genet. 39*, 724-726.

Farooqi, I. S., Keogh, J. M., Yeo, G. S., Lank, E. J., Cheetham, T. & O'Rahilly, S. (2003). Clinical spectrum of obesity and mutations in the melanocortin 4 receptor gene. *N. Engl. J. Med. 348*, 1085-1095.

Farooqi, I. S., Volders, K., Stanhope, R., Heuschkel, R., White, A., Lank, E., Keogh, J., O'Rahilly, S. & Creemers, J. W. (2007). Hyperphagia and early-onset obesity due to a novel homozygous missense mutation in prohormone convertase 1/3. *J. Clin. Endocrinol. Metab 92*, 3369-3373.

Fischer, J., Koch, L., Emmerling, C., Vierkotten, J., Peters, T., Bruning, J. C. & Ruther, U. (2009). Inactivation of the Fto gene protects from obesity. *Nature 458,* 894-898.

Frayling, T. M., Timpson, N. J., Weedon, M. N., Zeggini, E., Freathy, R. M., Lindgren, C. M., Perry, J. R., Elliott, K. S., Lango, H., Rayner, N. W., et al., (2007). A common variant in the FTO gene is associated with body mass index and predisposes to childhood and adult obesity. *Science 316*, 889-894.

Fredriksson, R., Hagglund, M., Olszewski, P. K., Stephansson, O., Jacobsson, J. A., Olszewska, A. M., Levine, A. S., Lindblom, J. & Schioth, H. B. (2008). The obesity gene, FTO, is of ancient origin, up-regulated during food deprivation and expressed in neurons of feeding-related nuclei of the brain. *Endocrinology 149*, 2062-2071.

Geller, F., Reichwald, K., Dempfle, A., Illig, T., Vollmert, C., Herpertz, S., Siffert, W., Platzer, M., Hess, C., Gudermann, T., et al., (2004). Melanocortin-4 receptor gene variant I103 is negatively associated with obesity. *Am. J. Hum. Genet. 74*, 572-581.

Gerken, T., Girard, C. A., Tung, Y. C., Webby, C. J., Saudek, V., Hewitson, K. S., Yeo, G. S., McDonough, M. A., Cunliffe, S., McNeill, L. A., et al., (2007). The obesity-associated FTO gene encodes a 2-oxoglutarate-dependent nucleic acid demethylase. *Science 318*, 1469-1472.

Gray, J., Yeo, G. S., Cox, J. J., Morton, J., Adlam, A. L., Keogh, J. M., Yanovski, J. A., El, G. A., Han, J. C., Tung, Y. C., et al., (2006). Hyperphagia, severe obesity, impaired cognitive function, and hyperactivity associated with functional loss of one copy of the brain-derived neurotrophic factor (BDNF) gene. *Diabetes, 55*, 3366-3371.

Grilo, C. M. (2002). Binge eating disorder. In C. G. Fairburn and K. D. Brownell, *Eating disorders and obesity—A comprehensive handbook* (pp. 1178-1182. ed.). New York, Guilford Press.

Heard-Costa, N. L., Zillikens, M. C., Monda, K. L., Johansson, A., Harris, T. B., Fu, M., Haritunians, T., Feitosa, M. F., Aspelund, T., Eiriksdottir, G., et al., (2009). NRXN3 is a novel locus for waist circumference: a genome-wide association study from the CHARGE Consortium. *PLoS. Genet. 5*, e1000539.

Hebebrand, J., Geller, F., Dempfle, A., Heinzel-Gutenbrunner, M., Raab, M., Gerber, G., Wermter, A. K., Horro, F. F., Blundell, J., Schafer, H., et al., (2004). Binge-eating episodes are not characteristic of carriers of melanocortin-4 receptor gene mutations. *Mol. Psychiatry, 9*, 796-800.

Heid, I. M., Vollmert, C., Hinney, A., Doring, A., Geller, F., Lowel, H., Wichmann, H. E., Illig, T., Hebebrand, J. & Kronenberg, F. (2005). Association of the 103I MC4R allele with decreased body mass in 7937 participants of two population based surveys. *J. Med. Genet. 42,* e21.

Hirschhorn, J. N. & Daly, M. J. (2005). Genome-wide association studies for common diseases and complex traits. *Nat. Rev. Genet. 6*, 95-108.

Hudson, J. I., Hiripi, E., Pope, H. G., Jr. & Kessler, R. C. (2007). The prevalence and correlates of eating disorders in the National Comorbidity Survey Replication. *Biol. Psychiatry*, *61*, 348-358.

Hudson, J. I., Lalonde, J. K., Berry, J. M., Pindyck, L. J., Bulik, C. M., Crow, S. J., McElroy, S. L., Laird, N. M., Tsuang, M. T., Walsh, B. T., et al., (2006). Binge-eating disorder as a distinct familial phenotype in obese individuals. *Arch. Gen. Psychiatry 63*, 313-319.

Huszar, D., Lynch, C. A., Fairchild-Huntress, V., Dunmore, J. H., Fang, Q., Berkemeier, L. R., Gu, W., Kesterson, R. A., Boston, B. A., Cone, R. D., et al., (1997). Targeted disruption of the melanocortin-4 receptor results in obesity in mice. *Cell 88*, 131-141.

International Association for the Study of Obesity (2009). (http://www.iotf.org/).

Jackson, R. S., Creemers, J. W., Ohagi, S., Raffin-Sanson, M. L., Sanders, L., Montague, C. T., Hutton, J. C. & O'Rahilly, S. (1997). Obesity and impaired prohormone processing associated with mutations in the human prohormone convertase 1 gene. *Nat. Genet.* 16, 303-306.

Javaras, K. N., Laird, N. M., Reichborn-Kjennerud, T., Bulik, C. M., Pope, H. G., Jr. & Hudson, J. I. (2008). Familiarity and heritability of binge eating disorder: results of a case-control family study and a twin study. *International Journal of Eating Disorders 41*, 174-179.

Kernie, S. G., Liebl, D. J. & Parada, L. F. (2000). BDNF regulates eating behavior and locomotor activity in mice. *EMBO J. 19*, 1290-1300.

Kurokawa, N., Young, E. H., Oka, Y., Satoh, H., Wareham, N. J., Sandhu, M. S. & Loos, R. J. (2008). The ADRB3 Trp64Arg variant and BMI: a meta-analysis of 44 833 individuals. *Int. J. Obes. (Lond) 32*, 1240-1249.

Li, S., Zhao, J. H., Luan, J., Luben, R. N., Rodwell, S. A., Khaw, K. T., Ong, K. K., Wareham, N. J. & Loos, R. J. (2010). Cumulative effects and predictive value of common obesity-susceptibility variants identified by genome-wide association studies. *Am. J. Clin. Nutr. 91*, 184-190.

Lin, X., Song, K., Lim, N., Yuan, X., Johnson, T., Abderrahmani, A., Vollenweider, P., Stirnadel, H., Sundseth, S. S., Lai, E., et al., (2009). Risk prediction of prevalent diabetes in a Swiss population using a weighted genetic score—the CoLaus Study. *Diabetologia 52*, 600-608.

Lindgren, C. M., Heid, I. M., Randall, J. C., Lamina, C., Steinthorsdottir, V., Qi, L., Speliotes, E. K., Thorleifsson, G., Willer, C. J., Herrera, B. M., et al., (2009). Genome-wide association scan meta-analysis identifies three Loci influencing adiposity and fat distribution. *PLoS. Genet.* 5, e1000508.

Loos, R. J. (2009). Recent progress in the genetics of common obesity. *Br. J. Clin. Pharmacol. 68*, 811-829.

Loos, R. J., Lindgren, C. M., Li, S., Wheeler, E., Zhao, J. H., Prokopenko, I., Inouye, M., Freathy, R. M., Attwood, A. P., Beckmann, J. S., et al., (2008). Common variants near MC4R are associated with fat mass, weight and risk of obesity. *Nat. Genet. 40,* 768-775.

Lubrano-Berthelier, C., Dubern, B., Lacorte, J. M., Picard, F., Shapiro, A., Zhang, S., Bertrais, S., Hercberg, S., Basdevant, A., Clement, K., et al., (2006). Melanocortin 4 receptor mutations in a large cohort of severely obese adults: prevalence, functional classification, genotype-phenotype relationship, and lack of association with binge eating. *J. Clin. Endocrinol. Metab 91*, 1811-1818.

Maes, H. H., Neale, M. C. & Eaves, L. J. (1997). Genetic and environmental factors in relative body weight and human adiposity. *Behav. Genet. 27*, 325-351.

Meyre, D., Delplanque, J., Chevre, J. C., Lecoeur, C., Lobbens, S., Gallina, S., Durand, E., Vatin, V., Degraeve, F., Proenca, C., et al., (2009). Genome-wide association study for early-onset and morbid adult obesity identifies three new risk loci in European populations. *Nat. Genet. 41*, 157-159.

Monteleone, P., Tortorella, A., Castaldo, E., Di, F. C. & Maj, M. (2007). The Leu72Met polymorphism of the ghrelin gene is significantly associated with binge eating disorder. *Psychiatr. Genet. 17*, 13-16.

Monteleone, P., Tortorella, A., Castaldo, E. & Maj, M. (2006). Association of a functional serotonin transporter gene polymorphism with binge eating disorder. *Am. J. Med. Genet. B Neuropsychiatr. Genet.* 141B, 7-9.

Monteleone, P., Tortorella, A., Docimo, L., Maldonato, M. N., Canestrelli, B., De, L. L. & Maj, M. (2008a). Investigation of 3111T/C polymorphism of the CLOCK gene in obese individuals with or without binge eating disorder: association with higher body mass index. *Neurosci. Lett. 435*, 30-33.

Monteleone, P., Tortorella, A., Martiadis, V., Di, F. C., Canestrelli, B. & Maj, M. (2008b). The cDNA 385C to A missense polymorphism of the endocannabinoid degrading enzyme fatty acid amide hydrolase (FAAH) is associated with overweight/obesity but not with binge eating disorder in overweight/obese women. *Psychoneuroendocrinolog, 33*, 546-550.

Neale, M. & Cardon, L. (1992). *Methodology for the Study of Twins and Families*. Kluwer Academic Publisher Group: Dordrecht, The Netherlands.

O'Rahilly, S. & Farooqi, I. S. (2008). Human obesity as a heritable disorder of the central control of energy balance. *Int. J. Obes. (Lond), 32* Suppl 7, S55-S61.

Rankinen, T., Zuberi, A., Chagnon, Y. C., Weisnagel, S. J., Argyropoulos, G., Walts, B., Perusse, L. & Bouchard, C. (2006). The human obesity gene map: the 2005 update. *Obesity. (Silver. Spring) 14*, 529-644.

Reichborn-Kjennerud, T., Bulik, C. M., Tambs, K. & Harris, J. R. (2004). Genetic and environmental influences on binge eating in the absence of compensatory behaviors: a population-based twin study. *International Journal of Eating Disorders 36*, 307-314.

Reilly, J. J., Armstrong, J., Dorosty, A. R., Emmett, P. M., Ness, A., Rogers, I., Steer, C. & Sherriff, A. (2005). Early life risk factors for obesity in childhood: cohort study. *BMJ 330*, 1357.

Saunders, C. L., Chiodini, B. D., Sham, P., Lewis, C. M., Abkevich, V., Adeyemo, A. A., de, A. M., Arya, R., Berenson, G. S., Blangero, J., et al., (2007). Meta-analysis of genome-wide linkage studies in BMI and obesity. *Obesity. (Silver. Spring) 15*, 2263-2275.

Scuteri, A., Sanna, S., Chen, W. M., Uda, M., Albai, G., Strait, J., Najjar, S., Nagaraja, R., Orru, M., Usala, G., et al., (2007). Genome-wide association scan shows genetic variants in the FTO gene are associated with obesity-related traits. *PLoS. Genet. 3*, e115.

Shugart, Y. Y., Chen, L., Day, I. N., Lewis, S. J., Timpson, N. J., Yuan, W., Abdollahi, M. R., Ring, S. M., Ebrahim, S., Golding, J., et al., (2009). Two British women studies replicated the association between the Val66Met polymorphism in the brain-derived neurotrophic factor (BDNF) and BMI. *Eur. J. Hum. Genet. 17*, 1050-1055.

Stratigopoulos, G., Padilla, S. L., LeDuc, C. A., Watson, E., Hattersley, A. T., McCarthy, M. I., Zeltser, L. M., Chung, W. K. & Leibel, R. L. (2008). Regulation of Fto/Ftm gene expression in mice and humans. *Am. J. Physiol Regul. Integr. Comp Physiol 294*, R1185-R1196.

Striegel-Moore, R. H. & Franko, D. L. (2003). Epidemiology of binge eating disorder. *International Journal of Eating Disorders 34*, 19-29.

Stunkard, A. J., Foch, T. T. & Hrubec, Z. (1986). A twin study of human obesity. *JAMA 256*, 51-54.

Stunkard, A. J., Harris, J. R., Pedersen, N. L. & McClearn, G. E. (1990). The body-mass index of twins who have been reared apart. *N. Engl. J. Med., 322*, 1483-1487.

Stutzmann, F., Vatin, V., Cauchi, S., Morandi, A., Jouret, B., Landt, O., Tounian, P., Levy-Marchal, C., Buzzetti, R., Pinelli, L., et al., (2007). Non-synonymous polymorphisms in melanocortin-4 receptor protect against obesity: the two facets of a Janus obesity gene. *Hum. Mol. Genet., 16*, 1837-1844.

Thorleifsson, G., Walters, G. B., Gudbjartsson, D. F., Steinthorsdottir, V., Sulem, P., Helgadottir, A., Styrkarsdottir, U., Gretarsdottir, S., Thorlacius, S., Jonsdottir, I., et al., (2009). Genome-wide association yields new sequence variants at seven loci that associate with measures of obesity. *Nat. Genet., 41*, 18-24.

Vimaleswaran, K. S. & Loos, R. J. (2010). Progress in the genetics of common obesity and type 2 diabetes. *Expert. Rev. Mol. Med., 12*, e7.

Wahlen, K., Sjolin, E. & Hoffstedt, J. (2008). The common rs9939609 gene variant of the fat mass- and obesity-associated gene FTO is related to fat cell lipolysis. *J. Lipid Res., 49*, 607-611.

Walston, J., Silver, K., Bogardus, C., Knowler, W. C., Celi, F. S., Austin, S., Manning, B., Strosberg, A. D., Stern, M. P., Raben, N., et al., (1995). Time of onset of non-insulin-dependent diabetes mellitus and genetic variation in the beta 3-adrenergic-receptor gene. *N. Engl. J. Med., 333*, 343-347.

Whitaker, R. C., Wright, J. A., Koepsell, T. D., Finch, A. J. & Psaty, B. M. (1994). Characteristics of children selecting low-fat foods in an elementary school lunch program. *Arch. Pediatr. Adolesc. Med., 148*, 1085-1091.

Widen, E., Lehto, M., Kanninen, T., Walston, J., Shuldiner, A. R. & Groop, L. C. (1995). Association of a polymorphism in the beta 3-adrenergic-receptor gene with features of the insulin resistance syndrome in Finns. *N. Engl. J. Med., 333*, 348-351.

Willer, C. J., Speliotes, E. K., Loos, R. J., Li, S., Lindgren, C. M., Heid, I. M., Berndt, S. I., Elliott, A. L., Jackson, A. U., Lamina, C., et al., (2009). Six new loci associated with body mass index highlight a neuronal influence on body weight regulation. *Nat. Genet. 41*, 25-34.

Young, E. H., Wareham, N. J., Farooqi, S., Hinney, A., Hebebrand, J., Scherag, A., O'Rahilly, S., Barroso, I. & Sandhu, M. S. (2007). The V103I polymorphism of the MC4R gene and obesity: population based studies and meta-analysis of 29 563 individuals. *Int. J. Obes. (Lond), 31*, 1437-1441.

In: Pathways to Obesity and Main Roads to Recovery
Editor: Piergiuseppe Vinai
ISBN: 978-1-61122-740-6

Chapter III

Neuroendocrine Influences on Appetite and Obesity

Susan Carnell[1], Charlisa D. Gibson[2], Leora Benson[3], Marci E. Gluck[4] and Allan Geliebter[5]

[1]New York Obesity Research Center, Department of Medicine, St. Luke's-Roosevelt Hospital Center, Columbia University College of Physicians and Surgeons, New York, NY. Institute of Human Nutrition, Columbia University, New York, NY, USA
[2]New York Obesity Research Center, Department of Medicine, St. Luke's-Roosevelt Hospital Center, Columbia University College of Physicians and Surgeons, New York, NY. Institute of Human Nutrition, Columbia University, New York, NY
[3]Institute of Human Nutrition, Columbia University, New York, NY, USA
[4]Obesity and Diabetes Clinical Research Section, National Institute of Diabetes and Digestive and Kidney Diseases, National Institute of Health, Phoenix, AZ, USA
[5]New York Obesity Research Center, Department of Medicine, St. Luke's-Roosevelt Hospital Center, Columbia University College of Physicians and Surgeons, New York, NY. Institute of Human Nutrition, Columbia University, New York, NY Department of Psychiatry, St. Luke's-Roosevelt Hospital Center, Columbia University College of Physicians and Surgeons, New York, NY. Department of Psychology, Tour College, New York, NY, USA

Abstract

This chapter will outline the role of appetite- and obesity-related hormones, including ghrelin, peptide YY, glucagon-like peptide 1, cholecystokinin and leptin, in the development, maintenance and co-morbidities of obesity. The focus will be on literature from clinical studies in obese and normal-weight adult humans, but the smaller number of studies in children will also be reviewed. New evidence from genetic and fMRI studies of appetite and obesity will also be briefly described, and directions for future research will be discussed.

Introduction

Obesity is a highly complex disease. It is complex in terms of its consequences, which include impaired glucose metabolism and abnormal hormonal profiles, as well as numerous psychological impacts. But it is also complex in terms of its causes—apart from the broad environmental factors that work to increase everyone's weight, many biological processes, likely to be genetically influenced, vary between individuals and conspire to make some people develop or maintain obesity while others stay lean.

In this chapter, we focus primarily on two major influences on body weight regulation: hormones affecting appetite and the brain. We begin by summarizing what is currently known about the roles of appetite-related hormones released in the gut and the brain and their relationship to energy intake and weight. We also review the relationship between body weight and cortisol, a stress hormone with demonstrable effects on appetite, and estrogen, a sex hormone related to eating behavior. Following this, we review progress in the functional neuroimaging of obesity, a relatively new field that is helping to reveal brain pathways underpinning appetitive behavior and cover a small number of innovative studies that combine hormone measures and brain imaging data to better understand the mechanisms of interactions between the gut and brain in humans.

Hormones, Appetite and Body Weight

Our food intake and body weight are influenced by a complex set of gut-brain interactions involving a host of hormones, most of them released in the gastrointestinal tract. For example, in the short term, gut peptides such as peptide YY [$PYY_{3\text{-}36}$], glucagon-like peptide 1 [GLP-1], and cholecystokinin [CCK] are released on receipt of nutrients to modulate further food intake (Moran, 2006), while in the longer term, weight gain and fat storage are influenced by other factors, such as release of insulin from the pancreas and leptin from adipose tissue (Strader & Woods, 2005). Other hormones may also be influential, including cortisol, a hormone produced by the adrenal gland in response to stress and involved in appetite regulation (Wolkowitz, Epel, & Reus, 2001) and energy balance via gluconeogenesis and lipolysis (Epel, Lapidus, McEwen, & Brownell, 2001), and estradiol, a form of estrogen that may decrease intake in females.

Gut Hormones

Physiological research in animals and humans has contributed to a basic understanding of how gut hormones communicate with the brain to influence nutrient digestion, absorption, transport, and storage (Chaudhri OB, 2008). More recently, research has focused on how gut hormones influence food intake. Peripheral hormones may signal satiety by passing through the blood-brain barrier to act directly on the brain, by acting indirectly via the vagus nerve, or by slowing gastric emptying, leading to increased gastric distension (Hellstrom et al., 2004), also communicated to the brain. Ghrelin, $PYY_{3\text{-}36}$, GLP-1. Insulin, and leptin can all cross the blood brain barrier, suggesting direct central action (Banks & Kastin, 1998; Banks, Tschop,

Robinson, & Heiman, 2002; Kastin, Akerstrom, & Pan, 2002; Nonaka, Shioda, Niehoff, & Banks, 2003). However, PYY, GLP-1 and CCK seem to signal satiety primarily via the vagus nerve (Wren & Bloom, 2007). Vagal signals related to ingestion are processed by the brainstem (i.e., nucleus tract solitaris) (Berthoud, 2008b), and proceed to the hypothalamus, which integrates the peripheral hormonal signals. In addition to activity in the periphery, a number of appetite-regulating hormones are synthesized in the CNS (Strader & Woods, 2005); these neuropeptides will not be discussed in detail here. Gut hormones involved in appetite control can be divided into those that decline following meals and help initiate food intake (ghrelin) and those that rise following meals and may help to terminate food intake and regulate inter-meal intervals (e.g., CCK, GLP-1, $PYY_{3\text{-}36}$). In concert with the action of these peptides, leptin and insulin are adiposity signals, which send signals to the brain about food surpluses and deficits and help to maintain energy homeostasis.

Ghrelin

Ghrelin, mainly secreted from the stomach, is an endogenous ligand for the growth hormone stimulatory receptor [GHS-R]. Three bioactive molecules are derived from the ghrelin gene: acylated ghrelin, des-acyl ghrelin, and obestatin. Although des-acyl ghrelin composes more than 90% of all ghrelin released (Soares & Leite-Moreira, 2008), the acylated form plays a key role in regulating multiple metabolic processes, including gastric acid secretion and emptying (Bloomgarden, 2007; Levin et al., 2005), insulin secretion (Yada et al., 2008), and glucose metabolism (Sun, Asnicar, & Smith, 2007). Ghrelin passes through the blood brain barrier, and is therefore capable of acting on hypothalamic neurons directly (Korbonits, Goldstone, Gueorguiev, & Grossman, 2004). It also sends information to the brain via vagal afferents containing ghrelin receptors, as well as being directly released within the hypothalamus.

Ghrelin appears to be a potent orexigenic (intake-promoting) peptide (De Vriese & Delporte, 2008; Wren et al., 2001), quite independent of its GH releasing action (Ruter et al., 2003). In a randomized double-blind cross-over study, Wren et al., (Wren, et al., 2001) found a 28% dose-dependent reduction in food intake in nine healthy adults following serial intravenous [IV] ghrelin (vs. saline) infusions. Studies in humans show that plasma ghrelin levels rise prior to meals and decline rapidly postprandially (Carlson, Turpin, Wiebke, Hunt, & Adams, 2009; English, Ghatei, Malik, Bloom, & Wilding, 2002; Zwirska-Korczala et al., 2007), suggesting a role in pre-meal hunger and meal initiation (Cummings et al., 2001). Postprandial suppression may be proportional to the caloric content of the meal, with higher energy values related to larger declines in ghrelin (Callahan et al., 2004).

Central ghrelin administration enhances the secretion of the appetite-stimulating neuropeptides agouti-related peptide [AgRP], and neuropeptide-Y [NPY] in the arcuate nucleus [AN] of the hypothalamus in animals (Olszewski et al., 2003), resulting in an increase in meal number but not meal size (Murphy & Bloom, 2006; H.Y. Chen et al., 2004). Ghrelin also appears to stimulate dopamine neurons in the ventral tegmental area [VTA] and promote dopamine turnover in the nucleus accumbens [NA] of the ventral striatum (Jerlhag et al., 2007). Ghrelin's effect on reward processing in the mesolimbic dopaminergic pathway may be an integral part of its orexigenic action (Abizaid et al., 2006; Malik, McGlone,

Bedrossian, & Dagher, 2008), since blocking VTA ghrelin receptors in mice decreases food intake (Jerlhag, et al., 2007).

Ghrelin levels are higher during periods of fasting, hunger, or under conditions associated with negative energy balance. such as short-term starvation, cancer, or anorexia (Bloomgarden, 2007). In contrast, conditions of positive energy balance (e.g., hyper-glycaemia, insulin resistance, obesity) are associated with lower ghrelin concentrations, such that obese individuals have fasting ghrelin levels 27% lower than their lean counterparts (Garcia-Unzueta et al., 2005). In spite of reduced ghrelin levels in the overweight, obese, and insulin-resistant population, there does not appear to be a dampening in the propensity to gain weight; this may be due to down-regulation of ghrelin release in response to overeating or excess body weight. An initial smaller decline in ghrelin following a meal has been noted in morbidly obese (Carlson, et al., 2009; Sodowski et al., 2007; Zwirska-Korczala, et al., 2007) and obese binge-eating disorder (BED) subjects (Geliebter, Gluck, & Hashim, 2005), that may act to maintain hunger in these individuals.

Given its potent influence on appetite and weight, ghrelin may be a useful target for weight loss therapies. Weight loss by diet or exercise causes ghrelin concentrations to rise in obese individuals (Geloneze et al., 2003), and this may contribute to diet-induced hunger and difficulty maintaining weight loss. In contrast, gastric bypass, currently the only effective long-term treatment for severe obesity (Wadden & Goldstein, 1996), may reduce ghrelin concentrations due to surgical reduction of the stomach (the predominant releaser of ghrelin) (Fruhbeck, Diez Caballero, & Gil, 2004; Garcia de la Torre et al., 2008; Lin et al., 2004; Morinigo et al., 2004; Tritos et al., 2003). This ghrelin decrease may contribute to the greater weight loss in comparison to dietary methods and other surgeries (Cummings, Overduin, Shannon, & Foster-Schubert, 2005; Cummings et al., 2002), and pharmaceutical companies are currently designing ghrelin antagonist drugs (i.e., NOX-B11), as potential obesity treatments (Neary & Batterham, 2009).

Peptide YY [PYY]

PYY is a hormone derived from the lower gut and synthesized from entero-endocrine L cells. It has two molecular forms, $PYY_{1\text{-}36}$ and $PYY_{3\text{-}36}$, of which $PYY_{3\text{-}36}$ appears to be the major anorexigenic agent, acting on the brain either by penetrating the blood brain barrier or by binding to receptors on vagal afferents, leading the arcuate to suppress NPY activation and inhibit food intake (le Roux & Bloom, 2005; Koda et al., 2005). $PYY_{3\text{-}36}$ also acts to delay gastric emptying and increase distension via an ileal brake mechanism, which inhibits appetite and feeding (Adrian et al., 1985).

Animal and human studies have both shown that, in the short term, $PYY_{3\text{-}36}$ increases satiety, potentially acting to reduce meal size and regulate inter-meal intervals (Batterham et al., 2003; Batterham et al., 2002; Challis et al., 2003). Batterham et al., (Batterham, et al., 2003) examined the effects of $PYY_{3\text{-}36}$ infusion on appetite and caloric intake in 12 obese and 12 lean Ss following a 12-h fast in a double-blind, placebo-controlled, crossover study. Compared with an infusion of saline, caloric intake two hours post PYY infusion was decreased by around 30% in both lean and obese Ss. This result persisted in the 12-h post-infusion period, causing further reductions in food intake in both groups. PYY levels appear to rise in response to food ingestion, peaking at one to two hours post-meal (Lin & Chey,

2003). Release is relative to caloric load and different macronutrients (Lomenick, Melguizo, Mitchell, Summar, & Anderson, 2009; Weickert et al., 2006), with the greatest release observed following fat ingestion (Essah, Levy, Sistrun, Kelly, & Nestler, 2007). However, there are also different actions according to site of administration, with suppression of food intake found peripherally (Batterham, et al., 2003), but increases of food intake after central injection (Corp, Melville, Greenberg, Gibbs, & Smith, 1990; Hagan, 2002).

PYY_{3-36} levels may differ with body weight. Batterham et al., (Batterham, et al., 2003) demonstrated both reduced pre-meal (fasting) levels, and a smaller postprandial rise in obese humans, consistent with a PYY_{3-36} deficiency in obesity (le Roux, Batterham et al., 2006). Consistent with this, bariatric surgery, which causes a robust rise in postprandial PYY peripherally, also produces an early sense of satiety and reduced meal size (Garcia-Fuentes et al., 2008; Karamanakos, Vagenas, Kalfarentzos, & Alexandrides, 2008; Korner et al., 2005; Korner et al., 2009; le Roux, Aylwin et al., 2006; Morinigo et al., 2006). Since obese participants remain sensitive to the anorexigenic impact of exogenously administered PYY_{3-36} (Wynne & Bloom, 2006), pharmaceutical companies are trying to develop drug analogs to induce the anorexigenic properties of PYY_{3-36} (Neary & Batterham, 2009).

Glucagon-Like Peptide 1[GLP-1]

GLP-1, a hormone co-released with PYY in the lower gut and produced by the brainstem, is another anorexigenic peptide. Concentrations increase following a meal and plateau one to two hours after meal cessation (Adam & Westerterp-Plantenga, 2005), and peripheral and central GLP-1 administration enhance satiation and reduce subsequent food intake in humans (Gutzwiller, Drewe et al., 1999; Hellstrom, et al., 2004). In a double-blind, placebo-controlled, crossover study Gutzwiller et al., (Gutzwiller, Drewe, et al., 1999) examined the effect of IV infusions (0, 0.375, 0.75, 1.5 pmol/kg/min) of GLP-1 (vs. saline) on appetite and food intake in 12 patients with Type 2 diabetes, and found a 27% reduction in food intake following GLP-1. GLP-1 influences appetite by acting as an ileal brake for the upper GI tract, by sending signals to the hypothalmus via the vagus nerve, brainstem, or by crossing the BBB (Berthoud, 2008a; Naslund & Hellstrom, 2007; Tang-Christensen, et al., 1996). GLP-1's functions also include potentiation of glucose-stimulated insulin secretion (the incretin effect), enhancement of β-cell growth and survival, and inhibition of glucagon release (Lim et al., 2009; Tang-Christensen, Vrang, & Larsen, 2001).

GLP-1 levels are associated with body weight: lean (vs. obese) individuals have higher circulating levels of GLP-1 both prior to and following food consumption (Verdich et al., 2001). Higher levels of GLP-1 have also been consistently reported following gastric bypass and may contribute to sustained post-surgical weight loss and resolution of diabetes (Bose, Olivan, Teixeira, Pi-Sunyer, & Laferrere, 2009), suggesting that it may be possible to treat obesity with GLP-1 analogs currently used to treat diabetes (e.g., exenatide) (Neary & Batterham, 2009).

Cholecystokinin [CCK]

CCK was the first gut hormone to be investigated for its effects on appetite. Synthesized in both the GI tract and the brain, CCK reaches peak levels within 15 to 30 min after food consumption and remains elevated for up to five hours (Liddle, Goldfine, Rosen, Taplitz, & Williams, 1985; S. Suzuki, Ramos, Goncalves, Chen, & Meguid, 2005). Both exogenous and endogenous CCK are capable of reducing meal size and duration (Baile, McLaughlin, & Della-Fera, 1986; Kissileff, Pi-Sunyer, Thornton, & Smith, 1981; Pi-Sunyer, Kissileff, Thornton, & Smith, 1982). In a double-blind study, Pi-Sunyer et al., (Pi-Sunyer, et al., 1982) showed that six of eight obese men consumed significantly less food during a single intravenous infusion of the C-terminal octapeptide of cholecystokinin (4ng/kg/min) compared with a saline infusion. CCK promotes satiety by delaying gastric emptying and facilitates digestion by stimulating the release of pancreatic digestive enzymes and bile from the gall bladder (Arora & Anubhuti, 2006). CCK also activates CCK-1 receptors on the vagus nerve and the dorsomedial hypothalamus to downregulate NPY mRNA expression and reduce food intake (Chen, Scott, Zhao, Moran, & Bi, 2008).

Despite the effect of CCK on short-term appetite, plasma concentrations are not significantly different in obese and lean individuals (Foschi et al., 2004; Sodowski, et al., 2007; Zwirska-Korczala, et al., 2007). Studies of post-bariatric surgery changes in CCK are sparse, and changes are variable (Foschi, et al., 2004; Kellum et al.). Despite CCK's short-lived and predominant action on meal size and duration, meal number tends to increase correspondingly when CCK is administered chronically, resulting in minimal effect on total food intake (West, 1984). Thus, CCK may not be independently involved in the regulation of energy balance and body weight. However, it may work synergistically with adiposity signals (insulin and leptin) to enhance short-term control of intake (Riedy, Chavez, Figlewicz, & Woods, 1995) and thereby influence intake in the long term (Matson, Reid, & Ritter, 2002; Wang, Barachina, Martinez, Wei, & Tache, 2000).

Insulin

Synthesized in the pancreas, insulin is a long-term regulator of glucose, lipid and protein metabolism. Insulin rises postprandially to optimize the use of blood glucose for energy expenditure by promoting storage of glucose in the liver and muscle as glycogen, and in organs and visceral and subcutaneous fat depots as fat. Insulin was the first identified adiposity signal and plays an important role in lipolysis and fatty acid release in the bloodstream, as well as being a potent inhibitor of proteolysis (protein degradation) (Baskin et al., 1999). Insulin penetrates the brain by altering the formation of endothelial cells comprising the BBB (Banks, 2008). It also decreases food intake by activating receptors in the hypothalamus, particularly the arcuate nucleus [ARC] (Baskin, et al., 1999; Woods, Lutz, Geary, & Langhans, 2006) and inhibiting orexigenic NPY expression in the ARC and paraventricular nucleus [PVN] of the hypothalamus during fasting (Baskin, et al., 1999; Schwartz et al., 1992).

Plasma insulin varies directly with adiposity (Baskin, et al., 1999). Basal and postprandial insulin are greater in obese than in lean individuals (Carroll, Kaiser, Franks, Deere, & Caffrey, 2007), and higher visceral fat in the liver is associated with lower insulin sensitivity

(Maffeis et al., 2008). Following the vast majority of restrictive bariatric operations, insulin tends to fall and insulin resistance resolves, sometimes entirely (Ballantyne, Farkas, Laker, & Wasielewski, 2006; DePaula, Macedo, Schraibman, Mota, & Vencio, 2009; Garcia de la Torre, et al., 2008; Korner, et al., 2009; Nijhuis, van Dielen, Buurman, & Greve, 2004). These "metabolic" surgeries are, therefore, being further investigated as a potential alternative to pharmacological treatment for diabetes.

Leptin

Leptin is predominantly a long-term satiety signal released from adipose tissue that generates feedback signals to the brain about the degree of fat storage (Strader & Woods, 2005). However, small amounts are also secreted by the stomach soon after food ingestion, implying a role in short-term satiety (Bado et al., 1998). Leptin helps control adipose metabolism by stimulating lipolysis (lipid breakdown) and suppressing lipogenesis (lipid production) (Kersten, 2001). Recent evidence suggests that, in lean individuals, leptin decreases food intake by permeating the BBB via transporters and transmitting signals about metabolic status from the periphery to the hypothalamus. Once bound to its central receptor, leptin down-regulates appetite stimulating neuropeptides (e.g., NPY, AgRP, galanin), while simultaneously up-regulating the anorexigenic alpha- melanocyte-stimulating hormone, cocaine- and amphetamine- regulated transcript, and corticotropin-releasing hormone (Arora & Anubhuti, 2006; Sahu, 1998). Leptin increases slowly after meals (Cummings, et al., 2001), and differences may not be evident until two hours after eating (Elimam & Marcus, 2002; Taylor, Hubbard, & Anderson, 1999).

The relationship between leptin and obesity is complex. Certainly, fasting leptin is strongly associated with levels of body fat (Calandra, Musso, & Musso, 2003), with higher fasting and postprandial levels of leptin observed in obese (vs. lean) individuals (Carlson, et al., 2009; English, Ghatei, Malik, Bloom, & Wilding; Gil-Campos, Aguilera, Ramirez-Tortosa, Canete, & Gil, 2009). Yet high levels of circulating leptin evidently do not lead to suppression of appetite among obese individuals. This may be because leptin evolved to be a signal of dangerously low levels of body fat rather than unhealthily high levels (Rosenbaum & Leibel, 1999) and therefore does not emit an "upper limit" signal. Consistent with this theory, when leptin concentrations decrease following weight or fat loss (Wolfe, Jimerson, Orlova, & Mantzoros, 2004; Rissanen, Makimattila, Vehmas, Taavitsainen, & Rissanen, 1999), individuals feel hungry suggesting that leptin begins to send signals to the brain to defend existing levels of body fat. Leptin's effects on appetite and feeding behavior have prompted many investigators to study this adipokine as a potential treatment for obesity. However, leptin injections in obese humans have not been nearly as efficacious in reducing food intake and body weight as in short-term animal studies, probably because of the development of leptin resistance at high levels of body fat (Heymsfield et al., 1999; Hukshorn et al., 2002). New evidence on the effects of gastric leptin is also emerging and suggests that meal-related changes in leptin may interact with CCK release to suppress intake (Attele, Shi, & Yuan, 2002; Wang, et al., 2000).

Cortisol

Cortisol secretion is a major component of the stress response (Koo-Loeb, Costello, Light, & Girdler, 2000), aiding in regulation of cardiovascular responses to stressful situations. The key hormonal pathway governing the endocrine response to stress is the hypothalamic-pituitary-adrenal [HPA] axis. Corticotropin-releasing hormone [CRH] is released in response to stress, transported to the pituitary gland, and stimulates the release of adrenocorticotropic hormone [ACTH]. ACTH then travels to the adrenal gland, where it stimulates the release of cortisol in humans (George, Khan, Briggs, & Abelson, 2010). Levels peak around awakening and then decrease steadily throughout the day. During times of stress, cortisol inhibits additional release of CRH and ACTH, creating a negative feedback loop and hypercortisolemia.

Although acute elevation of cortisol plays a protective role during stress, persistently elevated levels promote insulin resistance and abdominal obesity (Bjorntorp & Rosmond, 2000; Jayo, Shively, Kaplan, & Manuck, 1993). Many studies have observed that chronic stress overactivates the HPA axis and fuels insulin release, in turn activating abdominal fat storage (Dallman, Akana, Strack, Hanson, & Sebastian, 1995). Cortisol is involved in appetite regulation (Wolkowitz, et al., 2001), and exogenous administration of glucocorticoids can increase food intake and result in obesity in both humans (Tataranni et al., 1996) and animals (Bray, 1985). Dallman et al., (Dallman et al., 2003) reported greater intake of sucrose in rats after administration of glucocorticoids, leading to greater abdominal fat depots. In healthy females, high cortisol reactors to a laboratory stressor ate more food compared to low cortisol reactors (Epel, et al., 2001). In another recent study, peak cortisol response following CRH infusion was associated with increased caloric intake and total snack consumption (George, et al., 2010).

There have been conflicting reports, of the association between cortisol levels and weight status. Cortisol levels in obese women following a laboratory stress test were significantly correlated with a higher waist-to-hip ratio [WHR] in obese women with binge eating disorder (Gluck, Geliebter, Hung, & Yahav, 2004), which persisted after weight loss treatment (Gluck, Geliebter, & Lorence, 2004). Thus, there is evidence that secretion of cortisol may lead to weight gain and obesity by stimulating appetite and caloric intake while also stimulating increased fat accumulation and preferential deposition of fat in visceral areas. However, for some individuals, weight gain results from the body's attempt to down-regulate cortisol secretion in response to chronic activation of the HPA axis by persistent stress. This would explain the inverse relationship between low morning cortisol levels and obesity (Coutinho, Moreira, Spagnol, & Appolinario, 2007; Roberts, Troop, Connan, Treasure, & Campbell, 2007; Rosmond, Holm, & Bjorntorp, 2000). Additionally, allthough many studies have observed a relationship between increased cortisol levels with increased food intake, it should be noted that some have not (Appelhans, Pagoto, Peters, & Spring, 2010; Raspopow, Abizaid, Matheson, & Anisman, 2010).

Estrogen

Among females, the sex hormone estradiol (the main estrogen in humans) may also affect appetite. Studies have shown that women vary in their food intake throughout the menstrual cycle, with the lowest daily food intake during ovulation, when plasma estradiol levels are highest (Buffenstein, Poppitt, McDevitt, & Prentice, 1995). In addition, post-menopausal women, who are depleted of estrogens, show increased food intake, which can be prevented by estrogen therapy (Lovejoy, 1998, 2003). They are also more prone to weight gain (Lovejoy, 1998, 2003) and have higher obesity prevalence compared with age-matched controls (Butera, 2010). Mechanisms are not yet well defined, but estradiol has been shown to reduce the induced feeding effects of ghrelin (Clegg et al., 2007) and NPY (Santollo & Eckel, 2008), and to increase the eating inhibition effects of CCK (Asarian & Geary, 2006) and leptin (Clegg, Brown, Woods, & Benoit, 2006), suggesting interactions between estradiol and specific appetite-related hormones. Animal studies have also highlighted specific brain regions involved in decreasing food intake in response to estradiol, including the ventromedial hypothalamus [VMH] (Jankowiak & Stern, 1974), the PVN of the hypothalamus (Butera & Beikirch, 1989), and the caudal brainstem (Asarian & Geary, 2006).

Studies in Children

It is clear from the evidence above that there are systematic differences in hormone function between lean adults and those with common (i.e., polygenic) obesity. However, it is not clear whether abnormalities in obese individuals are predictors of weight gain or correlates of long-term overeating and the obese state. Studying obese children does not resolve this but may provide some insight because metabolism is less compromised at the time of assessment. Understanding hormonal contributions to obesity throughout development may also give a clearer perspective on the biology of appetite and inform the development of early interventions to prevent obesity from persisting into adulthood.

PYY

Several studies now suggest that tonic levels of PYY may be lower in obese than lean children (Stock et al., 2005). In one study of 9 to 13 year olds, obese (vs. lean) children demonstrated lower fasting levels of PYY, and lower levels were associated with greater BMI (Roth et al., 2005). Others have found evidence for differences in circadian and meal-related fluctuations. In a study of 7 to 11 year olds, plasma PYY was assessed every hour from 8 am to 4 pm, with a standardized (60% carbohydrate, 30% fat, 10% protein) breakfast meal given at 8 am and lunch meal at 12 pm. Lean children exhibited increases in PYY following breakfast (PYY higher at 9 am vs. 8 am), decreases as the next meal approached (PYY lower at 12 pm vs. 9 am), increases after lunch (PYY higher at 1 pm vs. 12 pm), and decreases through the afternoon (PYY lower at 4 pm vs. 1 pm). In contrast, the obese children showed no changes in PYY following breakfast and no afternoon decline (Lomenick, Clasey, & Anderson, 2008). Since developmental course and duration of obesity were not tracked, it is not possible to surmise whether PYY dysregulation preceded weight gain. However, fasting levels in the first study increased after successful weight loss, implying a secondary effect (Roth et al., 2005). There is also some suggestion that obese children differ in hormonal responses to various macronutrients: there was a smaller PYY response in obese (vs. lean) children in response to a high-carbohydrate or high-fat (vs. high-protein) meal (Lomenick et al., 2009).

Ghrelin

Circulating levels of ghrelin are markedly increased in children with Prader-Willi syndrome (a condition characterized by insatiable appetite and consequent obesity) when compared with controls (Haqq et al., 2003), suggesting a primary effect. However, when ghrelin is assessed in samples of children and infants without genetic syndromes involving obesity, higher weight tends to be associated with lower levels (Bellone et al., 2002; Savino et al., 2005), suggesting that ghrelin concentrations may show early adaptation, with obese children demonstrating down-regulation. However, another group has shown that, although lower levels of ghrelin in cord blood were not associated with milk intake or feed frequency over the first six days of life (James, James, Drewett, & Cheetham, 2007), they did predict slower weight gain over the first three months of life in healthy term infants (James, Drewett, & Cheetham, 2004), suggesting that ghrelin abnormalities could also be predictive.

Insulin and Leptin

As in adults, higher weight in children is associated with higher circulating leptin (Garcia-Mayor et al., 1997; Schoppen et al., 2010), and decreased insulin sensitivity (Eyzaguirre & Mericq, 2009; Weiss & Caprio, 2006), both of which are likely to be caused or maintained by the obese state. However, low cord blood leptin has been associated with lower size at birth and with greater weight gain from birth to 24 months, independent of birth-weight (Ong et al., 1999), consistent with another study finding that lower cord leptin predicted increased weight gain in the first six months of life, and higher BMI and leptin at three years (Mantzoros et al., 2009), even when adjusting for confounding factors such as birth weight for gestational age and maternal or paternal BMI. However, as in the ghrelin literature, leptin levels did not show a relationship to feeding behavior (James, et al., 2007). This suggests that leptin may be correlated with body weight changes determined by other factors (e.g., metabolic factors), and tonic levels merely track the catch-up growth that is demonstrated by children with low birth weight (Osmond & Barker, 2000).

Functional Neuroimaging, Appetite and Body Weight

Since the advent of functional Magnetic Resonance Imaging [fMRI] in the early 1990s, it has become the dominant approach in imaging studies due to the absence of radioactive exposure, the lower cost, and the high spatial and temporal resolution as compared with

Positron Emission Tomography [PET]. Functional MRI works by identifying regionally specific changes in blood oxygen concentrations, which act as indirect markers of local brain activity. Although the neuroimaging approach has been advancing rapidly from the domain of cognition and sensation to major psychiatric disorders, such as schizophrenia and depression, it has only recently been applied to the topics of eating behavior, eating disorders, and obesity (Chowdhury & Lask, 2001).

Regions of Interest

A range of brain areas are implicated in the motivation and control of feeding behavior in humans (Druce & Bloom, 2006). The hypothalamus, already mentioned, is a key site for homeostatic intake regulation (Suzuki, Simpson, Minnion, Shillito, & Bloom, 2010), but a variety of midbrain and cortical areas may also be involved. For example, eating is often driven by hedonic, as well as homeostatic factors, and therefore engages the mesolimbic pathway, a well-defined circuit including the ventral tegmental area [VTA] and the striatum, the dorsal (top) part of which includes the caudate nucleus and putamen, and the ventral (bottom) part of which includes the nucleus accumbens [NA] and olfactory tubercle (Palmiter, 2008) The mesolimbic pathway is highly innervated by dopamine neurons and involved in many different types of reward-related behavior, including drug addiction (Di Chiara et al., 2004; Lenard & Berthoud, 2008; Volkow, Fowler, & Wang, 2004). Connected to the mesolimbic pathway are a number of structures within the limbic system, including the amygdala and hippocampus, both of which are associated with emotion, learning, and memory (Richter-Levin & Akirav, 2000).

Another key region is the prefrontal cortex [PFC], within which there are at least three distinct neural systems, all relevant for eating behavior—the orbitofrontal cortex and ventromedial prefrontal cortex (OFC and vmPFC; associated with affect and reward), the dorsolateral prefrontal cortex (dlPFC; involved in executive or cognitive control and complex goal-directed behavior), and the cingulate cortex (involved in attention and error detection) (Davidson, 2003). The OFC receives projections from areas including the insular cortex (also known as the gustatory cortex, or primary taste cortex) (Pritchard, Schwartz, & Scott, 2007), inferior temporal cortex (visual processing and object memory) (Barbas, 2000) and hypothalamus. OFC activation is associated with innate and learnt taste, odor, and flavor reward (Rolls, 2000). The dlPFC is involved in working memory (Levy & Goldman-Rakic, 2000) and executive functions such as action planning and response inhibition (Heyder, Suchan, & Daum, 2004). The posterior cingulate cortex [PCC] plays a role in attention and memory, while the anterior cingulate cortex [ACC] is involved in cognitive and emotional control (Vogt, Finch, & Olson, 1992), all of which may be important for feeding behavior. Notably, the PFC has extensive structural connections with the mesolimbic pathway, enabling top-down modulation of reward-related areas (Ferry, Ongur, An, & Price, 2000).

Studies in Lean Adults

Visual Food Stimuli

The most common neuroimaging paradigm in appetite research has been to assess brain responses to food pictures. In one study (Killgore et al., 2003), women were shown pictures of high-calorie foods, low-calorie foods, and non-edible food-related objects (e.g., forks) following a 90 min fast. Results revealed more BOLD activity in the posterior cingulate, superior temporal gyrus, amygdala/hippocampus, inferior medial prefrontal cortex and insula when exposed to food (vs. non-food) stimuli, and more bilateral activation in medial and dorsolateral prefrontal cortex and thalamus (sensory processing) when exposed to high-calorie (vs. low-calorie) foods. Another study comparing adults' responses to pictures of foods and control stimuli (Porubska, Veit, Preissl, Fritsche, & Birbaumer, 2006) following a five-hour fast revealed increased bilateral activation in the insular/opercular cortex and OFC, while a more recent study (Passamonti et al., 2009) conducting scans following a shorter, two-hour fast revealed greater activation in the ventral striatum, amygdala, and ventral ACC in response to appetizing (vs. bland) foods.

Other researchers have examined the influence of hunger by varying pre-scan fasting periods. In one study (Fuhrer, Zysset, & Stumvoll, 2008), men viewed pictures of foods and non-foods following a 14-h fast (fasted/hungry) on one day, and a one-hour fast (fed/satiated) on another. In both conditions, the food cues preferentially activated the superior and inferior insula, anterior midprefrontal cortex, striatum and extrastriate cortex, thalamus, and cerebellum (motor control), whereas non-foods triggered greater activity in the parietal lobe (spatial attention) and bilateral middle temporal gyrus. Further, there was an interaction with fasting such that in the fed state, there was increased food-related activity in the posterior middle temporal gyrus (visual processing); while in the fasted state, there were increased responses in the striate, extrastriate cortex, and OFC. Results are consistent with the power of food to recruit a large network of cortical and subcortical structures, including reward areas, and particularly during conditions of caloric need (Cornier, Von Kaenel, Bessesen, & Tregellas, 2007).

Taste and Olfactory Food Stimuli

Other studies have administered small amounts of food as brief taste stimuli. For example, one study measuring PET activation in response to chocolate consumption revealed decreased insular activation and increased OFC activation with successive tastes (Small, Zatorre, Dagher, Evans, & Jones-Gotman, 2001). Using fMRI, another group reported different responses to tastes of chocolate milk and chicken broth depending on fasting status, such that there was greater activation in the anterior insula and inferior occipital-temporal area after a 24-h fast (vs. a normal meal 2.5 to 3 h before) (Uher, Treasure, Heining, Brammer, & Campbell, 2006). A more recent study (Haase, Cerf-Ducastel, & Murphy, 2009) compared adults' responses to tastes of sucrose, caffeine, saccharin, guanosine 5'-monophosphate, sodium chloride and citric acid after a liquid preload (fed) or after a 12-h fast with no preload (fasted). Analysis revealed greatest activation for sucrose and an effect of hunger such that in the fed state, the insula and OFC showed greater activation, while during hunger, there was greater activation in hypothalamus, amygdala, hippocampus, parahippocampus and entorhinal cortex, as well as insula and OFC.

Another approach is to present people with food aromas or olfactory stimuli. In one study, adults underwent PET scans while smelling and tasting their favorite foods (Wang et al., 2004) and showed activation of the superior temporal cortex, insula and OFC, with OFC activation tracking self-reports of hunger and desire for food. Another study presented adults with taste and odor stimuli in varying combinations and revealed significant activation to correctly paired stimuli in the amygdala, insula/frontal operculum, ventral striatum, caudal OFC, and anterior ACC (de Araujo, Rolls, Kringelbach, McGlone, & Phillips, 2003), showing that non-visual food cues activate a similar range of reward-related brain areas as visual food cues.

Food Ingestion

While the studies above address brain responses to food stimuli or cues, which might be considered predictors of forthcoming intake rather than brain responses to food intake itself, other studies have attempted to examine the effect of substantial ingestion. In one PET study, males were scanned following a 36-h fast and again after consuming a satiating liquid meal while in the scanner. Pre-meal (fasted), activation was found to be higher in the hypothalamus, insula, OFC, ACC, parahippocampal and hippocampal formation, thalamus, caudate and putamen, precuneus, and cerebellum, while post-meal (fed), there was greater activation in the ventromedial PFC [vmPFC], dlPFC, and inferior parietal lobule (Tataranni et al., 1999). These results are consistent with a role for the hypothalamus in the fasted state where intake regulation is homeostatic as well as hedonic, but not in the fed state in which initiation of eating is likely to be hedonically mediated. In support, several studies focusing on the hypothalamus have now demonstrated dose-dependent reductions in activity following glucose ingestion (Smeets, de Graaf, Stafleu, van Osch, & van der Grond, 2005; Liu, Gao, Liu, & Fox, 2000; Matsuda et al., 1999).

Dopamine Function

One advantage of PET over fMRI is that it may be used to image changes in brain dopamine activity (Volkow et al., 2003) by injecting [^{11}C] raclopride, a DA D2 receptor radioligand , which competes with endogenous DA, allowing inferences about changes in extracellular DA. This is particularly useful for research on appetite, which involves reward area activation. For example, one PET study found decreased binding potential in the dorsal striatum (caudate and putamen) after (vs. before) consumption of a favorite meal, reflecting increased levels of dopamine receptor occupancy arising either from increased dopamine release or reduced dopamine reuptake during eating. Further, greater decreases in binding potential in these areas were correlated with higher ratings of meal pleasantness, suggesting that dopamine increases may be associated with the experience of reward (Small, Jones-Gotman, & Dagher, 2003).

Studies Comparing Lean and Obese Adults

Visual Food Stimuli

A number of studies have now compared fMRI responses to food cues in obese and lean individuals. In one study, adult women were presented with pictures of high-calorie foods, low-calorie foods, eating-related utensils and neutral images while in a neutral state (neither hungry nor satiated). Analysis revealed that high-calorie foods activated the putamen, caudate, anterior insula, hippocampus, and parietal cortex to a greater degree in obese vs. lean persons (Rothemund et al., 2007). A similar study compared responses to pictures of high-calorie foods, low-calorie foods and cars following a post-breakfast eight- to nine-hour fast and found that obese (vs. lean) women showed greater activation in the insula, amygdala, hippocampus, medial and lateral OFC, nucleus accumbens/ventral striatum, caudate and putamen, medial PFC, and ACC in response to high-calorie foods vs. cars, and greater activation to high-calorie vs. low-calorie foods in the same areas with the exception of the putamen (Stoeckel et al., 2008), suggesting that obese individuals may experience heightened mesolimbic activation on the sight of food, which may correspond to greater perceived reward and ultimately to greater intake.

Taste and Olfactory Stimuli

Obese and lean individuals may also differ in brain responses to the taste and smell of food. For example, Del Parigi et al., (Del Parigi, Chen, Salbe, Reiman, & Tataranni, 2005) measured PET activation in response to a 2 ml taste of a liquid meal following a 36-h fast, and found that obese (vs. lean) individuals showed greater activation in the middle-dorsal insula and midbrain and lesser activation in the posterior cingulate, temporal cortex and OFC. In another study comparing food and non-food odors, following a 24-h fast, all individuals showed responses to food smells in the bilateral insula and opercular cortex, ACC and PCC, and ventral striatum, consistent with the highly appetizing nature of food smells. However, obese (vs. lean) persons showed greater activation the bilateral hippocampus/ parahippocampal gyrus, providing some evidence for heightened responsivity in limbic areas (Bragulat et al., 2010).

Food Ingestion

Other studies have examined responses to the ingestion of larger amounts of food. In one study, PET activation was assessed following a 36-h fast (fasted), and again after administration of liquid meal directly following the fast. Following the liquid meal, obese (vs. lean) men showed greater activation in the ventromedial, dorsomedial, dorsolateral and anterior lateral PFC, together with an attenuated decrease in hypothalamic and thalamic activation, and significantly lower reductions in limbic/paralimbic activity; these results are consistent with sluggish satiety responses and more persistent hedonic responses to food (Gautier et al., 2000). In support of an obese-lean difference in hypothalamic responsivity, one study found reduced activity in obese (vs. lean) persons in response to an oral glucose following a 12-h fast (Matsuda, et al., 1999). However, it is notable that in contrast to the dlPFC result in this study, other studies have found that obese (vs. lean) persons exhibit less activation in the dlPFC following either a fixed or satiating meal (e.g., Le et al., 2006); this suggests that in certain samples, dlPFC activity may relate to inhibition of intake due to satiety or conscious restraint (Coletta et al., 2009; DelParigi, et al., 2005).

Dopamine Function

There are currently two potentially competing theories of dopamine function in obesity: 1) *the hyper-responsivity hypothesis:* obese people experience more dopamine activity in response to food than lean people are hence more motivated to seek it out (Davis, Strachan, & Berkson, 2004) and 2) *the hypo-responsivity hypothesis*: obese people experience less dopamine activity in response to food than lean people (Johnson & Kenny, 2010; Steele et al.; Volkow et al., 2008; Wang et al., 2001) motivating them to seek out food (Geiger et al., 2008), and particularly palatable items high in fat, sugar and salt, which provide a bigger reward (Kelley, 2004; Kelley, Schiltz, & Landry, 2005; Ongur & Price, 2000), and promote weight gain (Berthoud & Morrison, 2008; Kelley, 2004). The hypo-responsivity is plausible, since overloading receptors with extracellular levels of neurotransmitter (e.g., dopamine) in response to food stimulation can lead to down-regulation of release over time. In support of the hyporesponsivity hypothesis (Gainetdinov, 2007), PET data have revealed lower striatal dopamine D_2 receptor availability in obese (vs. lean) individuals either following intravenously administered glucose or at rest, with the lowest binding potential in those with the largest BMI (Haltia et al., 2007; Wang, et al., 2001), while other studies have shown a higher prevalence of the TaqI *A*1 allele of the dopamine D_2 receptor [DRD2] gene (associated with low D2 receptor availability (Pohjalainen et al., 1998) in obese people (Blum et al., 1996; Comings, Gade, MacMurray, Muhleman, & Peters, 1996; Thomas, Critchley, Tomlinson, Cockram, & Chan, 2001). The decreased D2 striatal receptors could affect food intake by acting on cortical pathways involved in inhibitory control and reward: one PET study found that morbidly obese patients had decreased D2 receptor availability in the striatum, which was positively correlated with activation in the dlPFC, OFC, ACC and somato-sensory cortex (Volkow 2008). The "hyper" and "hypo" theories may be reconcilable with consideration of the type of food stimulation. For example, dopamine activity in response to anticipated reward (triggered by exposure to food cues) may be intact or exaggerated, while activation in response to actual food ingestion may be compromised (Stice, Spoor, Bohon, Veldhuizen, & Small, 2008).

Studies of Weight Change

While fMRI studies of obese-lean comparisons provide vital information about the neurobiology of obesity, it is not possible to infer whether neurological abnormalities precede, follow, or simply track the development of obesity. Prospective studies and cross-sectional ones comparing post-obese (i.e., formerly obese, post dietary weight-loss) individuals with currently obese or lean individuals may give clues to the legacy of the obese state and potentially to the neural predictors of weight gain.

For example, a series of studies from the same research group have now reported PET responses in obese, post-obese and always-lean groups following a 2 ml taste or satiating amount of liquid meal, following a 36-h fast. One such study showed that tasting food in the fasted state resulted in greater insula activation in obese and post-obese (vs. always-lean) adults (DelParigi et al., 2004), while an fMRI study from a different lab found that post-obese individuals failed to show the attenuation of insula, visual cortex and hypothalamic responses to palatable food (vs. non-food) cues under conditions of overfeeding that was observed in lean individuals (Cornier et al., 2009). Using a longitudinal design, another study of obese patients experiencing 10% weight loss from a one- to two-month liquid formula diet showed greater activation in areas including the brainstem, parahippocampal gyrus, and inferior frontal gyrus, and lesser activation in areas including the cingulate gyrus, middle frontal gyrus and precentral gyrus (motor planning) (Rosenbaum, Sy, Pavlovich, Leibel, & Hirsch, 2008).

Together, the results above suggest that obese persons and those at high risk of weight (re)gain may show greater reward-related activation in response to food. However, other studies (Le, et al., 2006; Le et al., 2007) have also reported greater post-meal activation in the dlPFC in lean and post-obese (vs. currently obese) females, possibly reflecting enhanced cognitive control of eating and resistance to initial or repeated development of obesity.

Studies in Children

Since developmental changes in fronto-parietal brain networks involved in cognitive (Schweinsburg, Nagel, & Tapert, 2005) and emotional (Burnett & Blakemore, 2009) processing may influence brain activation to food cues, it is essential to test whether findings in adults extend to children and adolescents. Conducting studies in this age group may also help identify predictors of weight gain.

In one of very few fMRI studies in youth with common, polygenic obesity, responses to food images were assessed in 10 to 17 year olds, and overweight (vs. lean) children demonstrated greater pre-meal activation in the PFC and post-meal activation in the OFC to food (vs. non-food), as well as smaller post-meal (vs. pre-meal) decreases in prefrontal, limbic, and nucleus accumbens activation to food (vs. control) (Bruce et al., 2010). These results are consistent with other studies, one reporting greater pre-meal than post-meal activation in amygdala, OFC, medial frontal cortex, operculum/insula, parahippocampal gyrus, cingulate gyrus and fusiform gyrus among lean adolescents (Holsen et al., 2005) and the other reporting post-meal increases in a similar set of reward-related areas in adolescents with Prader-Willi syndrome, compared with decreases among age-matched lean controls (Holsen et al., 2006). Together, these studies suggest that the neural representation of perceived food reward value may be more pronounced among obese children.

In another fMRI study of adolescents, responses to anticipated (conditioned cue) as well as actual tastes of a chocolate milkshake were assessed and revealed that obese (vs. lean) girls had greater activation in the anterior and middle insula and somatosensory brain areas in both conditions, plus decreased activation in the caudate nucleus in the taste condition (Stice, Spoor, Bohon, Veldhuizen, et al., 2008). These results are consistent with the dopamine hyporesponsivity theory (e.g., Wang, et al., 2001), and suggest that, despite seemingly high levels of appetitive reward (generated by anticipation of food before/during a meal and triggered by visual food stimuli), obese persons may show lower levels of ingestive reward (generated by actual ingestion of food), resulting in a net effect of less striatal activation.

Neuroimaging Studies in High-risk Samples

A more direct way to study causal processes is to study those who have never been obese but are at high risk for excessive weight gain due to familial or genetic factors. In one of the first studies to take this approach, Stice et al., (Stice, Spoor, Bohon, & Small, 2008) examined fMRI responses to the ingestion of a milkshake (vs. tasteless solution) in two studies of college students and adolescents and found a stronger inverse relationship between BMI and caudate nucleus activation in those with the DRD2 TaqI A1 (vs. A2) allele, which is related to depressed dopamine function and has been associated with obesity in several studies (Blum, et al., 1996; Comings, et al., 1996; Thomas, et al., 2001). A later study of lean and obese adolescent females looked at fMRI responses to imagined intake of palatable foods, unpalatable foods and glasses of water, cued by pictures, following a four- to six-hour fast. Initial BMI was positively correlated with activation in the putamen and lateral OFC during exposure to appetizing (vs. unappetizing) food cues, and positively correlated with activation in the OFC and frontal operculum during exposure to appetizing food cues (vs. water). However, the presence of the TaqIA1 allele attenuated the relations between BMI and OFC and operculum responses, while the presence of the DRD4-7repeat allele attenuated the relation between BMI and operculum only. One year later, it was found that lesser initial putamen and OFC activation was associated with greater weight gain in those with the Taq1A1 allele, while lesser operculum activation was associated with greater weight gain in those with DRD2 TaqIA1 and DRD4 7-repeat allele. These results suggest that those who show initial hyporesponsivity in food reward circuitry may be at a greater risk of weight gain if they have the DRD2 TaqIA1 or DRD4-7R alleles, although the influence of initial BMI was not considered in this analysis (Stice, Yokum, Bohon, Marti, Smolen, 2010).

Studies of Specific Eating Behaviors

A limitation of studies testing the relationship between brain activation and obesity is that the biological phenotype of body weight is actually the result of expression of a range of diverse, genetically influenced, behavioral phenotypes (Carnell, Haworth, Plomin, & Wardle, 2008; Carnell & Wardle, 2008a, 2008b, 2009). Examining the neurological correlates of these phenotypes may give us a deeper understanding of the bio-behavioral mechanisms of appetite and help to explain inconsistencies in obese vs. lean comparison studies.

Binge Eating

A well-characterized phenotype with relevance to obesity is binge eating, the consumption of excessively large amounts of food in one sitting with an accompanying sense of loss of control. In a study using SPECT, a technique similar to PET, one study demonstrated greater hunger-correlated activation in frontal and prefrontal regions in obese binge-eating (vs. lean non binge-eating) women following exposure to a freshly cooked lunch meal of their own selection, prior to consumption (Karhunen et al., 2000). Using fMRI, another study reported greater activation to highly palatable food stimuli specifically in the frontal premotor area among obese binge-eating women, but not in obese non binge-eating, lean binge-eating or lean non binge-eating women (Geliebter et al., 2006). Although it is unclear how to interpret the activation in these frontal areas, which have been associated with both reward and cognitive control, both studies are consistent in showing greater general responsivity to palatable food cues and enhanced drive to eat in binge eaters (Yanovski, 2003), which may lead to the initiation of a binge meal.

Eating Behavior Questionnaires

Another approach is to link brain imaging data with scores on questionnaire scales of eating behavior. For example, in Del Parigi et al.'s PET study of brain activation to food tastes, obese (vs. lean) individuals showed not only higher self-reported scores of dietary disinhibition (the tendency for dietary restraint to break down when confronted by emotional or external cues to eat) (Stunkard & Messick, 1985), but greater increases in activation in several regions including the middle-dorsal insula and midbrain, and greater decreases in activation in the posterior cingulate, temporal cortex, and OFC (DelParigi, et al., 2005). In a more direct analysis within lean subjects, scores on emotional eating and dietary restraint (Van Strien, 1986) were associated with enhanced dopaminergic activity in the dorsal striatum following food stimulation by presentation of warmed food followed by a small taste (Volkow, et al., 2003), also highlighting a link between responsiveness to external food cues and activity in reward-related brain areas.

The questionnaire approach has also shed light on the meaning of dlPFC activation among lean individuals and successful dieters, with several studies reporting positive associations between indices of dietary restraint and dlPFC activation, one using taste stimuli and showing accompanying negative associations with OFC activation (DelParigi et al., 2007), and one using visual picture stimuli, and finding the dlPFC activation difference only in the sated state (Coletta, et al., 2009). Since the dlPFC is implicated not only in cognitive control but in gut hormone-related satiety (i.e., glucagon-like peptide-1 [GLP-1]) (Pannacciulli et al., 2007) and anticipated reward (Grant et al., 1996; Schur et al., 2009), the exact role of the dlPFC in eating and obesity may not be clear without consideration of network activation in other cortical areas (Hirsch, Moreno, & Kim, 2001; Kim, Relkin, Lee, & Hirsch, 1997). For example, certain eating behaviors may be associated with different patterns of interaction between brain areas: Passamonti et al., found that scores on a measure of sensitivity to external food cues were positively correlated with differences in ventral striatum connectivity to amygdala and premotor cortex when presented with appetizing (vs. bland) foods, and negatively correlated with ventral striatum connectivity to dorsal ACC, and with amygdala connectivity to ventral and dorsal ACC in response to appetizing (vs. bland) foods. These results suggest that external food cue sensitivity may be associated with more reward-related activation in emotion and motor areas and less reward-related activation in areas involved in attention and cognitive control (Passamonti et al., 2009).

Combining Neuroimaging and Hormones in Study of Appetite and Weight

So far, the research we have presented addresses endocrine and neurological factors separately. Combining neuroimaging methods with experimental manipulations of hormone levels via feeding or direct infusions may help create a more nuanced picture of how these two systems interact.

Measuring Hormones

To understand the interaction between hormone levels and brain activation, they both should be measured. In the fmri study by Matsuda et al. the authors (Matsuda, et al., 1999) revealed a positive correlation between the time to reach the maximum response in the hypothalamus and fasting glucose and insulin concentrations after an oral glucose load, following a 12-h fast, among both obese and lean subjects. Another study administered PET scans during satiation via a 25-min liquid meal, following a 36-h fast, and found an association between increases in post-prandial GLP-1 levels and increases in activation in both the hypothalamus and the dLPFC (pannacciulli, et al., 2007). These studies support the existence of close relationships between hormonal responses and activation of brain areas involved in regulation of eating.

Direct Hormone Manipulations

Other studies have utilized direct hormone infusions. In a seminal study by Batterham et al., adult males were infused with physiologically relevant doses of PYY_{3-36} to mimic the hormone profile after satiation, while on another day they received saline infusions, designed to simulate the fasted state. In order to reveal brain areas associated with PYY increases, the authors looked for areas in which activity increased with PYY and decreased with saline infusion, and found the requisite pattern in the OFC, parabrachial nucleus, VTA, insula, ACC, ventral striatum (globus pallidus, putamen), regions of the frontal, parietal, temporal and cerebellar cortices, and posterior hypothalamus. Further, intake at a post-scan buffet was predicted by hypothalamic activation in the saline ("fasted") condition, and by deactivation in OFC in the PYY ("fed") condition, consistent with a switch from homeostatic to hedonic determination of feeding when sated (Batterham et al., 2007). Seeming discrepancies between Matsuda et al.'s hypothalamic deactivation to oral glucose (Matsuda, et al., 1999) and Batterham et al.'s (Batterham, et al., 2007) hypothalamic activation with PYY could reflect either methodological differences or differences in neural responses to glucose vs. PYY.

Another study examined the effect on adult males of 20-min intravenous infusions of ghrelin on fMRI responses following a three-hour fast, and found post-ghrelin infusion increases in response to the food (vs. non-food) pictures in the amygdala, OFC, insula and striatum (Malik, et al., 2008). These findings are consistent with others showing that ghrelin activates dopamine neurons in the VTA and increases dopamine turnover in the nucleus accumbens (Balleine, 2005; Jerlhag, et al., 2007), and suggest that ghrelin's orexigenic effect may involve an up regulation of mesolimbic dopaminergic activity accompanied by increased motivational salience of high-energy foods (Lenard & Berthoud, 2008; Malik, et al., 2008).

Hormone Abnormalities

Another approach is to examine neurological responses to food among those with long-term or genetic alterations of appetite-related hormones. One study of leptin-deficient adults reported reduced fMRI activation during leptin-supplementation (vs. after supplementation was withdrawn) in areas including the insula, and greater activation in regions including the prefrontal cortex in response to food pictures vs. neutral stimuli (Baicy et al., 2007), suggesting strong associations between leptin and brain areas associated with reward and satiety. This finding also generalizes to leptin-deficient adolescents, who initially demonstrate ventral striatum activation in response to food (vs. non-food) images in both the fed and fasted state, but show reductions following one week of leptin administration (Farooqi et al., 2007).

Leptin may also interact with brain responses to food in common polygenic obesity. In one study, obese patients who had lost 10% of initial weight on a liquid diet were given twice-daily subcutaneous injections of leptin or saline for five weeks. Post treatment, the leptin (vs. saline) group showed significantly less activation to food cues in areas including insula, parahippocampal gyrus and middle and superior frontal gyri, consistent with a correction of the heightened appetitive responsivity and drive to eat that accompanies leptin depletion (Rosenbaum, et al., 2008). Taken together, these studies are consistent with a model in which leptin down-regulates "hedonic" activation in reward areas in response to food stimulation, while simultaneously up-regulating homeostatic control by enhancing the central response to peripheral satiety signals (Farooqi, et al., 2007; Hukshorn, et al., 2002).

Bariatric Surgery

Other studies have indirectly examined more comprehensive hormone alterations, such as those following Roux-en-Y Gastric Bypass [RYGB], a bariatric weight loss surgery that appears to work to some degree by increasing "satiety" (anorexigenic) hormones such as PYY and GLP-1, and decreases in "hunger" (orexigenic) hormones such as ghrelin (Ashrafian & le Roux, 2009; Cummings, 2009; Cummings, Overduin, & Foster-Schubert, 2004). Two small pilot studies have reported changes in D2 receptor availability following RYGB, with one reporting increases in post-surgical availability in the ventral striatum, putamen, and caudate nucleus (Steele, et al.), and the other decreases in availability in the same areas plus hypothalamus, substantia nigra, medial thalamus, and amygdala, which were associated with weight loss (Dunn et al., 2010). Further research is needed to resolve this apparent discrepancy, but on the face of it the first findings is consistent with surgical correction of striatal hyporesponsivity, and the second more consistent with correction of hyper-responsivity. Consistent with Dunn et al., We have also found greater post-surgical reductions in activation in VTA, lentiform nucleus, middle frontal gyrus, posterior cingulate, culmen and middle temporal gyrus following exposure to visual cues representing highly palatable high-ED foods vs. Less palatable, low-ED foods (Ochner, Gibson, Carnell, Dambkowski, & Geliebter, 2010).

Conclusion

Our understanding of endocrine aspects of body weight grows deeper, but there is much still to learn about the peripheral and central effects of hormones on appetite. Likewise, the advent of neuroimaging techniques in obesity research has increased our knowledge about the cortical and sub-cortical networks representing appetite in the human brain, and advances in design and analysis promise to expand existing findings. What is currently missing is a comprehensive picture of how hormones and brains work together to influence eating behavior. However, an increasing number of studies are now combining hormone measures or manipulations with neuroimaging techniques to push our understanding to new frontiers.

The implications of these new discoveries and modes of investigation are far-reaching, and studies of gut-brain interactions may assist with drug discovery. To date, orlistat (lipase inhibitor), sibutramine (recently withdrawn in Europe) and phentermine-like sympathomimetics are the only approved anti-obesity agents, while exenatide (GLP-1 analogue) and sitagliptin (DPP-IV inhibitor) are licensed adjuncts to current diabetes treatments (Neary & Batterham, 2009). However, the findings that $PYY_{3\text{-}36}$ and GLP-1 induce changes in OFC and PFC activation (Batterham, et al., 2007; Pannacciulli, et al., 2007), suggest that drug analogues may show promise for obesity treatments by altering the perceived reward value of food. Neuroimaging studies of RYGB could also assist in the development of nonsurgical interventions to mimic its effects (Berthoud, 2004). Leptin is another potential therapeutic agent, although administration in obese humans has not been as effective as in animals, likely due to leptin resistance (Heymsfield, et al., 1999; Hukshorn, et al., 2002). Nevertheless, synthetic forms of leptin, as well as amylin, PP, oxyntomodulin, and ghrelin antagonist drugs are all being tested in clinical trials (Ravussin et al., 2009; Roth et al., 2008).

New research into the neuroendocrine correlates of obesity also raises some scientific, practical and ethical issues. For example, if studies of infants or children at high genetic or early environmental risk for obesity reveal differences in hormone levels or neural responses to food, which turn out to predict later weight gain, it may be desirable to design targeted pharmacological or behavioral interventions to reduce obesity risk. Educational interventions to encourage children to focus on internal (similar to homeostatic) vs. external (similar to hedonic) cues to manage intake have shown some success (Johnson, 2000), as have interventions to slow eating rate (Ford et al., 2010), and non-eating related interventions to regulate striatally mediated reward expectation using cognitive strategies (Delgado, Gillis, & Phelps, 2008). Care must be taken that individuals being informed of innate biological predispositions do not develop fatalistic attitudes that could mitigate against behavioral change (Sanderson, Persky, & Michie, 2009). However, most would agree that expanding our knowledge of all contributions—whether biological or behavioral, genetic or environmental—will ultimately help us tackle the daunting public health problem of obesity.

References

Abizaid, A., Liu, Z. W., Andrews, Z. B., Shanabrough, M., Borok, E., Elsworth, J. D., et al., (2006). Ghrelin modulates the activity and synaptic input organization of midbrain dopamine neurons while promoting appetite. *J Clin Invest, 116*(12), 3229-3239.

Adam, T. C., & Westerterp-Plantenga, M. S. (2005). Glucagon-like peptide-1 release and satiety after a nutrient challenge in normal-weight and obese subjects. *Br J Nutr, 93*(6), 845-851.

Adrian, T. E., Savage, A. P., Sagor, G. R., Allen, J. M., Bacarese-Hamilton, A. J., Tatemoto, K., et al., (1985). Effect of peptide YY on gastric, pancreatic, and biliary function in humans. *Gastroenterology, 89*(3), 494-499.

Appelhans, B. M., Pagoto, S. L., Peters, E. N., & Spring, B. J. (2010). HPA axis response to stress predicts short-term snack intake in obese women. *Appetite, 54*(1), 217-220.

Arora, S., & Anubhuti. (2006). Role of neuropeptides in appetite regulation and obesity—a review. *Neuropeptides, 40*(6), 375-401.

Asarian, L., & Geary, N. (2006). Modulation of appetite by gonadal steroid hormones. *Philos Trans R Soc Lond B Biol Sci, 361*(1471), 1251-1263.

Ashrafian, H., & le Roux, C. W. (2009). Metabolic surgery and gut hormones—a review of bariatric entero-humoral modulation. *Physiol Behav, 97*(5), 620-631.

Attele, A. S., Shi, Z. Q., & Yuan, C. S. (2002). Leptin, gut, and food intake. *Biochem Pharmacol, 63*(9), 1579-1583.

Bado, A., Levasseur, S., Attoub, S., Kermorgant, S., Laigneau, J. P., Bortoluzzi, M. N., et al., (1998). The stomach is a source of leptin. *Nature, 394*(6695), 790-793.

Baicy, K., London, E. D., Monterosso, J., Wong, M. L., Delibasi, T., Sharma, A., et al., (2007). Leptin replacement alters brain response to food cues in genetically leptin-deficient adults. *Proc Natl Acad Sci U.S.A., 104*(46), 18276-18279.

Baile, C. A., McLaughlin, C. L., & Della-Fera, M. A. (1986). Role of cholecystokinin and opioid peptides in control of food intake. *Physiol Rev, 66*(1), 172-234.

Ballantyne, G. H., Farkas, D., Laker, S., & Wasielewski, A. (2006). Short-term changes in insulin resistance following weight loss surgery for morbid obesity: laparoscopic adjustable gastric banding versus laparoscopic Roux-en-Y gastric bypass. *Obes Surg, 16*(9), 1189-1197.

Balleine, B. W. (2005). Neural bases of food-seeking: affect, arousal and reward in corticostriatolimbic circuits. *Physiol Behav, 86*(5), 717-730.

Banks, W. A. (2008). The blood-brain barrier: connecting the gut and the brain. *Regul Pept, 149*(1-3), 11-14.

Banks, W. A., & Kastin, A. J. (1998). Differential permeability of the blood-brain barrier to two pancreatic peptides: insulin and amylin. *Peptides, 19*(5), 883-889.

Banks, W. A., Tschop, M., Robinson, S. M., & Heiman, M. L. (2002). Extent and direction of ghrelin transport across the blood-brain barrier is determined by its unique primary structure. *J Pharmacol Exp Ther, 302*(2), 822-827.

Barbas, H. (2000). Connections underlying the synthesis of cognition, memory, and emotion in primate prefrontal cortices. *Brain Res Bull, 52*(5), 319-330.

Baskin, D. G., Figlewicz Lattemann, D., Seeley, R. J., Woods, S. C., Porte, D., Jr., & Schwartz, M. W. (1999). Insulin and leptin: dual adiposity signals to the brain for the regulation of food intake and body weight. *Brain Res, 848*(1-2), 114-123.

Batterham, R. L., Cohen, M. A., Ellis, S. M., Le Roux, C. W., Withers, D. J., Frost, G. S., et al., (2003). Inhibition of food intake in obese subjects by peptide YY3-36. *N Engl J Med, 349*(10), 941-948.

Batterham, R. L., Cowley, M. A., Small, C. J., Herzog, H., Cohen, M. A., Dakin, C. L., et al., (2002). Gut hormone PYY(3-36) physiologically inhibits food intake. *Nature, 418*(6898), 650-654.

Batterham, R. L., ffytche, D. H., Rosenthal, J. M., Zelaya, F. O., Barker, G. J., Withers, D. J., et al., (2007). PYY modulation of cortical and hypothalamic brain areas predicts feeding behaviour in humans. *Nature, 450*(7166), 106-109.

Bellone, S., Rapa, A., Vivenza, D., Castellino, N., Petri, A., Bellone, J., et al., (2002). Circulating ghrelin levels as function of gender, pubertal status and adiposity in childhood. *J Endocrinol Invest, 25*(5), RC13-15.

Berthoud, H. R. (2004). Neural control of appetite: cross-talk between homeostatic and non-homeostatic systems. *Appetite, 43*(3), 315-317.

Berthoud, H. R. (2008a). Paying the price for eating ice cream: is excessive GLP-1 signaling in the brain the culprit? *Endocrinology, 149*(10), 4765-4767.

Berthoud, H. R. (2008b). Vagal and hormonal gut-brain communication: from satiation to satisfaction. *Neurogastroenterol Motil, 20 Suppl 1*, 64-72.

Berthoud, H. R., & Morrison, C. (2008). The brain, appetite, and obesity. *Annu Rev Psychol, 59*, 55-92.

Bjorntorp, P., & Rosmond, R. (2000). Neuroendocrine abnormalities in visceral obesity. *Int J Obes Relat Metab Disord, 24 Suppl 2*, S80-85.

Bloomgarden, Z. T. (2007). Gut hormones, obesity, polycystic ovarian syndrome, malignancy, and lipodystrophy syndromes. *Diabetes Care, 30*(7), 1934-1939.

Blum, K., Braverman, E. R., Wood, R. C., Gill, J., Li, C., Chen, T. J., et al., (1996). Increased prevalence of the Taq I A1 allele of the dopamine receptor gene (DRD2) in obesity with comorbid substance use disorder: a preliminary report. *Pharmacogenetics, 6*(4), 297-305.

Bose, M., Olivan, B., Teixeira, J., Pi-Sunyer, F. X., & Laferrere, B. (2009). Do Incretins play a role in the remission of type 2 diabetes after gastric bypass surgery: What are the evidence? *Obes Surg, 19*(2), 217-229.

Bragulat, V., Dzemidzic, M., Bruno, C., Cox, C. A., Talavage, T., Considine, R. V., et al., (2010). Food-Related Odor Probes of Brain Reward Circuits During Hunger: A Pilot fMRI Study. *Obesity (Silver Spring)*.

Bray, G. A. (1985). Autonomic and endocrine factors in the regulation of food intake. *Brain Res Bull, 14*(6), 505-510.

Bruce, A. S., Holsen, L. M., Chambers, R. J., Martin, L. E., Brooks, W. M., Zarcone, J. R., et al., (2010). Obese children show hyperactivation to food pictures in brain networks linked to motivation, reward and cognitive control. *Int J Obes (Lond)*.

Buffenstein, R., Poppitt, S. D., McDevitt, R. M., & Prentice, A. M. (1995). Food intake and the menstrual cycle: a retrospective analysis, with implications for appetite research. *Physiol Behav, 58*(6), 1067-1077.

Burnett, S., & Blakemore, S. J. (2009). Functional connectivity during a social emotion task in adolescents and in adults. *Eur J Neurosci, 29*(6), 1294-1301.

Butera, P. C. (2010). Estradiol and the control of food intake. *Physiol Behav, 99*(2), 175-180.

Butera, P. C., & Beikirch, R. J. (1989). Central implants of diluted estradiol: independent effects on ingestive and reproductive behaviors of ovariectomized rats. *Brain Res, 491*(2), 266-273.

Calandra, C., Musso, F., & Musso, R. (2003). The role of leptin in the etiopathogenesis of anorexia nervosa and bulimia. *Eat Weight Disord, 8*(2), 130-137.

Callahan, H. S., Cummings, D. E., Pepe, M. S., Breen, P. A., Matthys, C. C., & Weigle, D. S. (2004). Postprandial suppression of plasma ghrelin level is proportional to ingested caloric load but does not predict intermeal interval in humans. *J Clin Endocrinol Metab, 89*(3), 1319-1324.

Carlson, J. J., Turpin, A. A., Wiebke, G., Hunt, S. C., & Adams, T. D. (2009). Pre- and post-prandial appetite hormone levels in normal weight and severely obese women. *Nutr Metab (Lond), 6*, 32.

Carnell, S., Haworth, C. M., Plomin, R., & Wardle, J. (2008). Genetic influence on appetite in children. *Int J Obes (Lond), 32*(10), 1468-1473.

Carnell, S., & Wardle, J. (2008a). Appetite and adiposity in children: evidence for a behavioral susceptibility theory of obesity. *Am J Clin Nutr, 88*(1), 22-29.

Carnell, S., & Wardle, J. (2008b). Appetitive traits and child obesity: measurement, origins and implications for intervention. *Proc Nutr Soc, 67*(4), 343-355.

Carnell, S., & Wardle, J. (2009). Appetitive traits in children. New evidence for associations with weight and a common, obesity-associated genetic variant. *Appetite, 53*(2), 260-263.

Carroll, J. F., Kaiser, K. A., Franks, S. F., Deere, C., & Caffrey, J. L. (2007). Influence of BMI and gender on postprandial hormone responses. *Obesity (Silver Spring), 15*(12), 2974-2983.

Challis, B. G., Pinnock, S. B., Coll, A. P., Carter, R. N., Dickson, S. L., & O'Rahilly, S. (2003). Acute effects of PYY3-36 on food intake and hypothalamic neuropeptide expression in the mouse. *Biochem Biophys Res Commun, 311*(4), 915-919.

Chaudhri OB, S. V., Murphy KG, Bloom SR. (2008). Gastrointestinal Satiety Signals. *Annual Review of Physiology, 70*, 9.1—9.17.

Chelikani, P. K., Haver, A. C., Reeve, J. R., Jr., Keire, D. A., & Reidelberger, R. D. (2006). Daily, intermittent intravenous infusion of peptide YY(3-36) reduces daily food intake and adiposity in rats. *Am J Physiol Regul Integr Comp Physiol, 290*(2), R298-305.

Chen, H. Y., Trumbauer, M. E., Chen, A. S., Weingarth, D. T., Adams, J. R., Frazier, E. G., et al., (2004). Orexigenic action of peripheral ghrelin is mediated by neuropeptide Y and agouti-related protein. *Endocrinology, 145*(6), 2607-2612.

Chen, J., Scott, K. A., Zhao, Z., Moran, T. H., & Bi, S. (2008). Characterization of the feeding inhibition and neural activation produced by dorsomedial hypothalamic cholecystokinin administration. *Neuroscience, 152*(1), 178-188.

Chowdhury, U., & Lask, B. (2001). Clinical implications of brain imaging in eating disorders. *Psychiatr Clin North Am, 24*(2), 227-234.

Clegg, D. J., Brown, L. M., Woods, S. C., & Benoit, S. C. (2006). Gonadal hormones determine sensitivity to central leptin and insulin. *Diabetes, 55*(4), 978-987.

Clegg, D. J., Brown, L. M., Zigman, J. M., Kemp, C. J., Strader, A. D., Benoit, S. C., et al., (2007). Estradiol-dependent decrease in the orexigenic potency of ghrelin in female rats. *Diabetes, 56*(4), 1051-1058.

Coletta, M., Platek, S., Mohamed, F. B., van Steenburgh, J. J., Green, D., & Lowe, M. R. (2009). Brain activation in restrained and unrestrained eaters: an fMRI study. *J Abnorm Psychol, 118*(3), 598-609.

Comings, D. E., Gade, R., MacMurray, J. P., Muhleman, D., & Peters, W. R. (1996). Genetic variants of the human obesity (OB) gene: association with body mass index in young women, psychiatric symptoms, and interaction with the dopamine D2 receptor (DRD2) gene. *Mol Psychiatry, 1*(4), 325-335.

Cornier, M., Salzberg, A., Endly, D., Bessesen, D., Rojas, D., & Tregellas, J. (2009). The Effects of Overfeeding on the Neuronal Response to Visual Food Cues in Thin Reduced-Obese Individuals. *PLoS One, 4*(7), e6310.

Cornier, M., Von Kaenel, S., Bessesen, D., & Tregellas, J. (2007). Effects of overfeeding on the neuronal response to visual food cues. *Am J Clin Nutr, 86*(4), 965-971.

Corp, E. S., Melville, L. D., Greenberg, D., Gibbs, J., & Smith, G. P. (1990). Effect of fourth ventricular neuropeptide Y and peptide YY on ingestive and other behaviors. *Am J Physiol, 259*(2 Pt 2), R317-323.

Coutinho, W. F., Moreira, R. O., Spagnol, C., & Appolinario, J. C. (2007). Does binge eating disorder alter cortisol secretion in obese women? *Eat Behav, 8*(1), 59-64.

Crawley, J. N., & Beinfeld, M. C. (1983). Rapid development of tolerance to the behavioural actions of cholecystokinin. *Nature, 302*(5910), 703-706.

Cummings, D. E. (2009). Endocrine mechanisms mediating remission of diabetes after gastric bypass surgery. *Int J Obes (Lond), 33 Suppl 1*, S33-40.

Cummings, D. E., Overduin, J., & Foster-Schubert, K. E. (2004). Gastric bypass for obesity: mechanisms of weight loss and diabetes resolution. *J Clin Endocrinol Metab, 89*(6), 2608-2615.

Cummings, D. E., Overduin, J., Shannon, M. H., & Foster-Schubert, K. E. (2005). Hormonal mechanisms of weight loss and diabetes resolution after bariatric surgery. *Surg Obes Relat Dis, 1*(3), 358-368.

Cummings, D. E., Purnell, J. Q., Frayo, R. S., Schmidova, K., Wisse, B. E., & Weigle, D. S. (2001). A preprandial rise in plasma ghrelin levels suggests a role in meal initiation in humans. *Diabetes, 50*(8), 1714-1719.

Cummings, D. E., Weigle, D. S., Frayo, R. S., Breen, P. A., Ma, M. K., Dellinger, E. P., et al., (2002). Plasma ghrelin levels after diet-induced weight loss or gastric bypass surgery. *N Engl J Med, 346*(21), 1623-1630.

Dallman, M. F., Akana, S. F., Strack, A. M., Hanson, E. S., & Sebastian, R. J. (1995). The neural network that regulates energy balance is responsive to glucocorticoids and insulin and also regulates HPA axis responsivity at a site proximal to CRF neurons. *Ann N Y Acad Sci, 771*, 730-742.

Dallman, M. F., Pecoraro, N., Akana, S. F., La Fleur, S. E., Gomez, F., Houshyar, H., et al., (2003). Chronic stress and obesity: a new view of "comfort food." *Proc Natl Acad Sci U.S.A., 100*(20), 11696-11701.

Davidson, R. J. (2003). Affective neuroscience and psychophysiology: toward a synthesis. *Psychophysiology, 40*(5), 655-665.

Davis, C., Strachan, S., & Berkson, M. (2004). Sensitivity to reward: implications for overeating and overweight. *Appetite, 42*(2), 131-138.

de Araujo, I. E., Rolls, E. T., Kringelbach, M. L., McGlone, F., & Phillips, N. (2003). Taste-olfactory convergence, and the representation of the pleasantness of flavour, in the human brain. *Eur J Neurosci, 18*(7), 2059-2068.

De Vriese, C., & Delporte, C. (2008). Ghrelin: a new peptide regulating growth hormone release and food intake. *Int J Biochem Cell Biol, 40*(8), 1420-1424.

Del Parigi, A., Gautier, J. F., Chen, K., Salbe, A. D., Ravussin, E., Reiman, E., et al., (2002). Neuroimaging and obesity: mapping the brain responses to hunger and satiation in humans using positron emission tomography. *Ann N Y Acad Sci, 967*, 389-397.

Delgado, M. R., Gillis, M. M., & Phelps, E. A. (2008). Regulating the expectation of reward via cognitive strategies. *Nat Neurosci, 11*(8), 880-881.

DelParigi, A., Chen, K., Salbe, A. D., Hill, J. O., Wing, R. R., Reiman, E. M., et al., (2004). Persistence of abnormal neural responses to a meal in postobese individuals. *Int J Obes Relat Metab Disord, 28*(3), 370-377. doi: 10.1038/sj.ijo.0802558
0802558 [pii]

DelParigi, A., Chen, K., Salbe, A. D., Hill, J. O., Wing, R. R., Reiman, E. M., et al., (2007). Successful dieters have increased neural activity in cortical areas involved in the control of behavior. *Int J Obes (Lond), 31*(3), 440-448.

DelParigi, A., Chen, K., Salbe, A. D., Reiman, E. M., & Tataranni, P. A. (2005). Sensory experience of food and obesity: a positron emission tomography study of the brain regions affected by tasting a liquid meal after a prolonged fast. *Neuroimage, 24*(2), 436-443.

DePaula, A. L., Macedo, A. L., Schraibman, V., Mota, B. R., & Vencio, S. (2009). Hormonal evaluation following laparoscopic treatment of type 2 diabetes mellitus patients with BMI 20-34. *Surg Endosc, 23*(8), 1724-1732.

Di Chiara, G., Bassareo, V., Fenu, S., De Luca, M. A., Spina, L., Cadoni, C., et al., (2004). Dopamine and drug addiction: the nucleus accumbens shell connection. *Neuropharmacology, 47 Suppl 1*, 227-241.

Druce, M., & Bloom, S. R. (2006). The regulation of appetite. *Arch Dis Child, 91*(2), 183-187.

Dunn, J. P., Cowan, R. L., Volkow, N. D., Feurer, I. D., Li, R., Williams, D. B., et al., (2010) Decreased dopamine type 2 receptor availability after bariatric surgery: Preliminary findings. *Brain Res*, 2(1350), 123-30

Elimam, A., & Marcus, C. (2002). Meal timing, fasting and glucocorticoids interplay in serum leptin concentrations and diurnal profile. *Eur J Endocrinol, 147*(2), 181-188.

English, P. J., Ghatei, M. A., Malik, I. A., Bloom, S. R., & Wilding, J. P. (2002). Food fails to suppress ghrelin levels in obese humans. *J Clin Endocrinol Metab, 87*(6), 2984.

Epel, E., Lapidus, R., McEwen, B., & Brownell, K. (2001). Stress may add bite to appetite in women: a laboratory study of stress-induced cortisol and eating behavior. *Psychoneuroendocrinology, 26*(1), 37-49.

Essah, P. A., Levy, J. R., Sistrun, S. N., Kelly, S. M., & Nestler, J. E. (2007). Effect of macronutrient composition on postprandial peptide YY levels. *J Clin Endocrinol Metab, 92*(10), 4052-4055.

Eyzaguirre, F., & Mericq, V. (2009). Insulin resistance markers in children. *Horm Res, 71*(2), 65-74.

Farooqi, I. S., Bullmore, E., Keogh, J., Gillard, J., O'Rahilly, S., & Fletcher, P. C. (2007). Leptin regulates striatal regions and human eating behavior. *Science, 317*(5843), 1355.

Ferry, A. T., Ongur, D., An, X., & Price, J. L. (2000). Prefrontal cortical projections to the striatum in macaque monkeys: evidence for an organization related to prefrontal networks. *J Comp Neurol, 425*(3), 447-470.

Ford, A. L., Bergh, C., Sodersten, P., Sabin, M. A., Hollinghurst, S., Hunt, L. P., et al., (2010). Treatment of childhood obesity by retraining eating behaviour: randomised controlled trial. *BMJ, 340*, b5388.

Foschi, D., Corsi, F., Pisoni, L., Vago, T., Bevilacqua, M., Asti, E., et al., (2004). Plasma cholecystokinin levels after vertical banded gastroplasty: effects of an acidified meal. *Obes Surg, 14*(5), 644-647.

Fox, A. S., & Olster, D. H. (2000). Effects of intracerebroventricular leptin administration on feeding and sexual behaviors in lean and obese female Zucker rats. *Horm Behav, 37*(4), 377-387. Fried, S. K., Ricci, M. R., Russell, C. D., & Laferrere, B. (2000). Regulation of leptin production in humans. *J Nutr, 130*(12), 3127S-3131S.

Fruhbeck, G., Diez Caballero, A., & Gil, M. J. (2004). Fundus functionality and ghrelin concentrations after bariatric surgery. *N Engl J Med, 350*(3), 308-309.

Fuhrer, D., Zysset, S., & Stumvoll, M. (2008). Brain activity in hunger and satiety: an exploratory visually stimulated FMRI study. *Obesity (Silver Spring), 16*(5), 945-950.

Gainetdinov, R. R. (2007). Mesolimbic dopamine in obesity and diabetes. *Am J Physiol Regul Integr Comp Physiol, 293*(2), R601-602.

Garcia de la Torre, N., Rubio, M. A., Bordiu, E., Cabrerizo, L., Aparicio, E., Hernandez, C., et al., (2008). Effects of weight loss after bariatric surgery for morbid obesity on vascular endothelial growth factor-A, adipocytokines, and insulin. *J Clin Endocrinol Metab, 93*(11), 4276-4281.

Garcia-Fuentes, E., Garrido-Sanchez, L., Garcia-Almeida, J. M., Garcia-Arnes, J., Gallego-Perales, J. L., Rivas-Marin, J., et al., (2008). Different effect of laparoscopic Roux-en-Y gastric bypass and open biliopancreatic diversion of Scopinaro on serum PYY and ghrelin levels. *Obes Surg, 18*(11), 1424-1429.

Garcia-Mayor, R. V., Andrade, M. A., Rios, M., Lage, M., Dieguez, C., & Casanueva, F. F. (1997). Serum leptin levels in normal children: relationship to age, gender, body mass index, pituitary-gonadal hormones, and pubertal stage. *J Clin Endocrinol Metab, 82*(9), 2849-2855.

Garcia-Unzueta, M. T., Fernandez-Santiago, R., Dominguez-Diez, A., Vazquez-Salvi, L., Fernandez-Escalante, J. C., & Amado, J. A. (2005). Fasting plasma ghrelin levels increase progressively after biliopancreatic diversion: one-year follow-up. *Obes Surg, 15*(2), 187-190.

Gautier, J. F., Chen, K., Salbe, A. D., Bandy, D., Pratley, R. E., Heiman, M., et al., (2000). Differential brain responses to satiation in obese and lean men. *Diabetes, 49*(5), 838-846.

Geiger, B. M., Behr, G. G., Frank, L. E., Caldera-Siu, A. D., Beinfeld, M. C., Kokkotou, E. G., et al., (2008). Evidence for defective mesolimbic dopamine exocytosis in obesity-prone rats. *FASEB J, 22*(8), 2740-2746.

Geliebter, A., Gluck, M. E., & Hashim, S. A. (2005). Plasma ghrelin concentrations are lower in binge-eating disorder. *J Nutr, 135*(5), 1326-1330.

Geliebter, A., Ladell, T., Logan, M., Schneider, T., Sharafi, M., & Hirsch, J. (2006). Responsivity to food stimuli in obese and lean binge eaters using functional MRI. *Appetite, 46*(1), 31-35.

Geloneze, B., Tambascia, M. A., Pilla, V. F., Geloneze, S. R., Repetto, E. M., & Pareja, J. C. (2003). Ghrelin: a gut-brain hormone: effect of gastric bypass surgery. *Obes Surg, 13*(1), 17-22.

George, S. A., Khan, S., Briggs, H., & Abelson, J. L. (2010). CRH-stimulated cortisol release and food intake in healthy, non-obese adults. *Psychoneuroendocrinology, 35*(4), 607-612.

Gil-Campos, M., Aguilera, C. M., Ramirez-Tortosa, M. C., Canete, R., & Gil, A. (2010). Fasting and postprandial relationships among plasma leptin, ghrelin, and insulin in prepubertal obese children. *Clin Nutr,* 29(1), 54-9

Gluck, M. E., Geliebter, A., Hung, J., & Yahav, E. (2004). Cortisol, hunger, and desire to binge eat following a cold stress test in obese women with binge eating disorder. *Psychosom Med, 66*(6), 876-881.

Gluck, M. E., Geliebter, A., & Lorence, M. (2004). Cortisol stress response is positively correlated with central obesity in obese women with binge eating disorder (BED) before and after cognitive-behavioral treatment. *Ann N Y Acad Sci, 1032*, 202-207.

Grant, S., London, E. D., Newlin, D. B., Villemagne, V. L., Liu, X., Contoreggi, C., et al., (1996). Activation of memory circuits during cue-elicited cocaine craving. *Proc Natl Acad Sci U.S.A., 93*(21), 12040-12045.

Gutzwiller, J. P., Drewe, J., Goke, B., Schmidt, H., Rohrer, B., Lareida, J., et al., (1999). Glucagon-like peptide-1 promotes satiety and reduces food intake in patients with diabetes mellitus type 2. *Am J Physiol, 276*(5 Pt 2), R1541-1544.

Gutzwiller, J. P., Goke, B., Drewe, J., Hildebrand, P., Ketterer, S., Handschin, D., et al., (1999). Glucagon-like peptide-1: a potent regulator of food intake in humans. *Gut, 44*(1), 81-86.

Haase, L., Cerf-Ducastel, B., & Murphy, C. (2009). Cortical activation in response to pure taste stimuli during the physiological states of hunger and satiety. *Neuroimage, 44*(3), 1008-1021.

Hagan, M. M. (2002). Peptide YY: a key mediator of orexigenic behavior. *Peptides, 23*(2), 377-382.

Haltia, L. T., Rinne, J. O., Merisaari, H., Maguire, R. P., Savontaus, E., Helin, S., et al., (2007). Effects of intravenous glucose on dopaminergic function in the human brain in vivo. *Synapse, 61*(9), 748-756.

Haqq, A. M., Farooqi, I. S., O'Rahilly, S., Stadler, D. D., Rosenfeld, R. G., Pratt, K. L., et al., (2003). Serum ghrelin levels are inversely correlated with body mass index, age, and insulin concentrations in normal children and are markedly increased in Prader-Willi syndrome. *J Clin Endocrinol Metab, 88*(1), 174-178.

Hellstrom, P. M., Geliebter, A., Naslund, E., Schmidt, P. T., Yahav, E. K., Hashim, S. A., et al., (2004). Peripheral and central signals in the control of eating in normal, obese and binge-eating human subjects. *Br J Nutr, 92 Suppl 1*, S47-57.

Heyder, K., Suchan, B., & Daum, I. (2004). Cortico-subcortical contributions to executive control. *Acta Psychol (Amst), 115*(2-3), 271-289.

Heymsfield, S. B., Greenberg, A. S., Fujioka, K., Dixon, R. M., Kushner, R., Hunt, T., et al., (1999). Recombinant leptin for weight loss in obese and lean adults: a randomized, controlled, dose-escalation trial. *JAMA, 282*(16), 1568-1575.

Hirsch, J., Moreno, D. R., & Kim, K. H. (2001). Interconnected large-scale systems for three fundamental cognitive tasks revealed by functional MRI. *J Cogn Neurosci, 13*(3), 389-405.

Holsen, L. M., Zarcone, J. R., Brooks, W. M., Butler, M. G., Thompson, T. I., Ahluwalia, J. S., et al., (2006). Neural mechanisms underlying hyperphagia in Prader-Willi syndrome. *Obesity (Silver Spring), 14*(6), 1028-1037.

Holsen, L. M., Zarcone, J. R., Thompson, T. I., Brooks, W. M., Anderson, M. F., Ahluwalia, J. S., et al., Neural mechanisms underlying food motivation in children and adolescents 2005. *Neuroimage, 27*(3), 669-676.

Holsen, L. M., Zarcone, J. R., Thompson, T. I., Brooks, W. M., Anderson, M. F., Ahluwalia, J. S., et al., (2005). Neural mechanisms underlying food motivation in children and adolescents. *Neuroimage, 27*(3), 669-676.

Hukshorn, C. J., van Dielen, F. M., Buurman, W. A., Westerterp-Plantenga, M. S., Campfield, L. A., & Saris, W. H. (2002). The effect of pegylated recombinant human leptin (PEG-OB) on weight loss and inflammatory status in obese subjects. *Int J Obes Relat Metab Disord, 26*(4), 504-509.

James, R. J., Drewett, R. F., & Cheetham, T. D. (2004). Low cord ghrelin levels in term infants are associated with slow weight gain over the first 3 months of life. *J Clin Endocrinol Metab, 89*(8), 3847-3850.

James, R. J., James, A., Drewett, R. F., & Cheetham, T. D. (2007). Milk intake and feeding behavior in the first week of life and its relationship to cord blood ghrelin, leptin, and insulin concentrations. *Pediatr Res, 62*(6), 695-699.

Jankowiak, R., & Stern, J. J. (1974). Food intake and body weight modifications following medial hypothalamic hormone implants in female rats. *Physiol Behav, 12*(5), 875-879.

Jayo, J. M., Shively, C. A., Kaplan, J. R., & Manuck, S. B. (1993). Effects of exercise and stress on body fat distribution in male cynomolgus monkeys. *Int J Obes Relat Metab Disord, 17*(10), 597-604.

Jerlhag, E., Egecioglu, E., Dickson, S. L., Douhan, A., Svensson, L., & Engel, J. A. (2007). Ghrelin administration into tegmental areas stimulates locomotor activity and increases extracellular concentration of dopamine in the nucleus accumbens. *Addict Biol, 12*(1), 6-16.

Johnson, P. M., & Kenny, P. J. (2010). Dopamine D2 receptors in addiction-like reward dysfunction and compulsive eating in obese rats. *Nat Neurosci, 13*(5), 635-641.

Johnson, S. L. (2000). Improving Preschoolers' self-regulation of energy intake. *Pediatrics, 106*(6), 1429-1435.

Karamanakos, S. N., Vagenas, K., Kalfarentzos, F., & Alexandrides, T. K. (2008). Weight loss, appetite suppression, and changes in fasting and postprandial ghrelin and peptide-YY levels after Roux-en-Y gastric bypass and sleeve gastrectomy: a prospective, double blind study. *Ann Surg, 247*(3), 401-407.

Karhunen, L. J., Vanninen, E. J., Kuikka, J. T., Lappalainen, R. I., Tiihonen, J., & Uusitupa, M. I. (2000). Regional cerebral blood flow during exposure to food in obese binge eating women. *Psychiatry Res, 99*(1), 29-42.

Kastin, A. J., Akerstrom, V., & Pan, W. (2002). Interactions of glucagon-like peptide-1 (GLP-1) with the blood-brain barrier. *J Mol Neurosci, 18*(1-2), 7-14.

Kelley, A. E. (2004). Ventral striatal control of appetitive motivation: role in ingestive behavior and reward-related learning. *Neurosci Biobehav Rev, 27*(8), 765-776.

Kelley, A. E., Schiltz, C. A., & Landry, C. F. (2005). Neural systems recruited by drug- and food-related cues: studies of gene activation in corticolimbic regions. *Physiol Behav, 86*(1-2), 11-14.

Kellum, J. M., Kuemmerle, J. F., O'Dorisio, T. M., Rayford, P., Martin, D., Engle, K., et al., Gastrointestinal hormone responses to meals before and after gastric bypass and vertical banded gastroplasty 1990. *Ann Surg, 211*(6), 763-770.

Kersten, S. (2001). Mechanisms of nutritional and hormonal regulation of lipogenesis. *EMBO Rep, 2*(4), 282-286.

Killgore, W. D., Young, A. D., Femia, L. A., Bogorodzki, P., Rogowska, J., & Yurgelun-Todd, D. A. (2003). Cortical and limbic activation during viewing of high- versus low-calorie foods. *Neuroimage, 19*(4), 1381-1394.

Kim, K. H., Relkin, N. R., Lee, K. M., & Hirsch, J. (1997). Distinct cortical areas associated with native and second languages. *Nature, 388*(6638), 171-174.

Kissileff, H. R., Pi-Sunyer, F. X., Thornton, J., & Smith, G. P. (1981). C-terminal octapeptide of cholecystokinin decreases food intake in man. *Am J Clin Nutr, 34*(2), 154-160.

Koda, S., Date, Y., Murakami, N., Shimbara, T., Hanada, T., Toshinai, K., et al., (2005). The role of the vagal nerve in peripheral PYY3-36-induced feeding reduction in rats. *Endocrinology, 146*(5), 2369-2375.

Koo-Loeb, J. H., Costello, N., Light, K. C., & Girdler, S. S. (2000). Women with eating disorder tendencies display altered cardiovascular, neuroendocrine, and psychosocial profiles. *Psychosom Med, 62*(4), 539-548.

Korbonits, M., Goldstone, A. P., Gueorguiev, M., & Grossman, A. B. (2004). Ghrelin—a hormone with multiple functions. *Front Neuroendocrinol, 25*(1), 27-68.

Korner, J., Bessler, M., Cirilo, L. J., Conwell, I. M., Daud, A., Restuccia, N. L., et al., (2005). Effects of Roux-en-Y gastric bypass surgery on fasting and postprandial concentrations of plasma ghrelin, peptide YY, and insulin. *J Clin Endocrinol Metab, 90*(1), 359-365.

Korner, J., Inabnet, W., Febres, G., Conwell, I. M., McMahon, D. J., Salas, R., et al., (2009). Prospective study of gut hormone and metabolic changes after adjustable gastric banding and Roux-en-Y gastric bypass. *Int J Obes (Lond)*, 33(7), 786-95.

Kringelbach, M. L., O'Doherty, J., Rolls, E. T., & Andrews, C. (2003). Activation of the human orbitofrontal cortex to a liquid food stimulus is correlated with its subjective pleasantness. *Cereb Cortex, 13*(10), 1064-1071.

Le, D. S., Pannacciulli, N., Chen, K., Del Parigi, A., Salbe, A. D., Reiman, E. M., et al., (2006). Less activation of the left dorsolateral prefrontal cortex in response to a meal: a feature of obesity. *Am J Clin Nutr, 84*(4), 725-731.

Le, D. S., Pannacciulli, N., Chen, K., Salbe, A. D., Del Parigi, A., Hill, J. O., et al., (2007). Less activation in the left dorsolateral prefrontal cortex in the reanalysis of the response to a meal in obese than in lean women and its association with successful weight loss. *Am J Clin Nutr, 86*(3), 573-579.

le Roux, C. W., Aylwin, S. J., Batterham, R. L., Borg, C. M., Coyle, F., Prasad, V., et al., (2006). Gut hormone profiles following bariatric surgery favor an anorectic state, facilitate weight loss, and improve metabolic parameters. *Ann Surg, 243*(1), 108-114.

le Roux, C. W., Batterham, R. L., Aylwin, S. J., Patterson, M., Borg, C. M., Wynne, K. J., et al., (2006). Attenuated peptide YY release in obese subjects is associated with reduced satiety. *Endocrinology, 147*(1), 3-8.

le Roux, C. W., & Bloom, S. R. (2005). Peptide YY, appetite and food intake. *Proc Nutr Soc, 64*(2), 213-216.

Lenard, N. R., & Berthoud, H. R. (2008). Central and peripheral regulation of food intake and physical activity: pathways and genes. *Obesity (Silver Spring), 16 Suppl 3*, S11-22.

Levin, F., Edholm, T., Ehrstrom, M., Wallin, B., Schmidt, P. T., Kirchgessner, A. M., et al., (2005). Effect of peripherally administered ghrelin on gastric emptying and acid secretion in the rat. *Regul Pept, 131*(1-3), 59-65.

Levy, R., & Goldman-Rakic, P. S. (2000). Segregation of working memory functions within the dorsolateral prefrontal cortex. *Exp Brain Res, 133*(1), 23-32.

Liddle, R. A., Goldfine, I. D., Rosen, M. S., Taplitz, R. A., & Williams, J. A. (1985). Cholecystokinin bioactivity in human plasma. Molecular forms, responses to feeding, and relationship to gallbladder contraction. *J Clin Invest, 75*(4), 1144-1152.

Lim, G. E., Huang, G. J., Flora, N., LeRoith, D., Rhodes, C. J., & Brubaker, P. L. (2009). Insulin regulates glucagon-like peptide-1 secretion from the enteroendocrine L cell. *Endocrinology, 150*(2), 580-591.

Lin, E., Gletsu, N., Fugate, K., McClusky, D., Gu, L. H., Zhu, J. L., et al., (2004). The effects of gastric surgery on systemic ghrelin levels in the morbidly obese. *Arch Surg, 139*(7), 780-784.

Lin, H. C., & Chey, W. Y. (2003). Cholecystokinin and peptide YY are released by fat in either proximal or distal small intestine in dogs. *Regul Pept, 114*(2-3), 131-135.

Liu, Y., Gao, J. H., Liu, H. L., & Fox, P. T. (2000). The temporal response of the brain after eating revealed by functional MRI. *Nature, 405*(6790), 1058-1062.

Lomenick, J. P., Clasey, J. L., & Anderson, J. W. (2008). Meal-related changes in ghrelin, peptide YY, and appetite in normal weight and overweight children. *Obesity (Silver Spring), 16*(3), 547-552.

Lomenick, J. P., Melguizo, M. S., Mitchell, S. L., Summar, M. L., & Anderson, J. W. (2009). Effects of meals high in carbohydrate, protein, and fat on ghrelin and peptide YY secretion in prepubertal children. *J Clin Endocrinol Metab, 94*(11), 4463-4471.

Lovejoy, J. C. (1998). The influence of sex hormones on obesity across the female life span. *J Womens Health, 7*(10), 1247-1256.

Lovejoy, J. C. (2003). The menopause and obesity. *Prim Care, 30*(2), 317-325.

Maffeis, C., Manfredi, R., Trombetta, M., Sordelli, S., Storti, M., Benuzzi, T., et al., (2008). Insulin sensitivity is correlated with subcutaneous but not visceral body fat in overweight and obese prepubertal children. *J Clin Endocrinol Metab, 93*(6), 2122-2128.

Malik, S., McGlone, F., Bedrossian, D., & Dagher, A. (2008). Ghrelin modulates brain activity in areas that control appetitive behavior. *Cell Metab, 7*(5), 400-409.

Mantzoros, C. S., Rifas-Shiman, S. L., Williams, C. J., Fargnoli, J. L., Kelesidis, T., & Gillman, M. W. (2009). Cord blood leptin and adiponectin as predictors of adiposity in children at 3 years of age: a prospective cohort study. *Pediatrics, 123*(2), 682-689.

Matson, C. A., Reid, D. F., & Ritter, R. C. (2002). Daily CCK injection enhances reduction of body weight by chronic intracerebroventricular leptin infusion. *Am J Physiol Regul Integr Comp Physiol, 282*(5), R1368-1373.

Matsuda, M., Liu, Y., Mahankali, S., Pu, Y., Mahankali, A., Wang, J., et al., (1999). Altered hypothalamic function in response to glucose ingestion in obese humans. *Diabetes, 48*(9), 1801-1806.

McCabe, C., & Rolls, E. T. (2007). Umami: a delicious flavor formed by convergence of taste and olfactory pathways in the human brain. *Eur J Neurosci, 25*(6), 1855-1864.

Meeran, K., O'Shea, D., Edwards, C. M., Turton, M. D., Heath, M. M., Gunn, I., et al., (1999). Repeated intracerebroventricular administration of glucagon-like peptide-1-(7-

36) amide or exendin-(9-39) alters body weight in the rat. *Endocrinology, 140*(1), 244-250.

Moran, T. H. (2006). Gut peptide signaling in the controls of food intake. *Obesity (Silver Spring), 14 Suppl 5*, 250S-253S.

Morinigo, R., Casamitjana, R., Moize, V., Lacy, A. M., Delgado, S., Gomis, R., et al., (2004). Short-term effects of gastric bypass surgery on circulating ghrelin levels. *Obes Res, 12*(7), 1108-1116.

Morinigo, R., Moize, V., Musri, M., Lacy, A. M., Navarro, S., Marin, J. L., et al., (2006). Glucagon-like peptide-1, peptide YY, hunger, and satiety after gastric bypass surgery in morbidly obese subjects. *J Clin Endocrinol Metab, 91*(5), 1735-1740.

Murphy, K. G., & Bloom, S. R. (2006). Gut hormones and the regulation of energy homeostasis. *Nature, 444*(7121), 854-859.

Naslund, E., & Hellstrom, P. M. (2007). Appetite signaling: from gut peptides and enteric nerves to brain. *Physiol Behav, 92*(1-2), 256-262.

Neary, M. T., & Batterham, R. L. (2009). Gut hormones: implications for the treatment of obesity. *Pharmacol Ther, 124*(1), 44-56.

Nijhuis, J., van Dielen, F. M., Buurman, W. A., & Greve, J. W. (2004). Ghrelin, leptin and insulin levels after restrictive surgery: a 2-year follow-up study. *Obes Surg, 14*(6), 783-787.

Nonaka, N., Shioda, S., Niehoff, M. L., & Banks, W. A. (2003). Characterization of blood-brain barrier permeability to PYY3-36 in the mouse. *J Pharmacol Exp Ther, 306*(3), 948-953.

Ochner, C. N., Gibson, C., Carnell, S., Dambkowski, C., & Geliebter, A. (2010). The neurohormonal regulation of energy intake in relation to bariatric surgery for obesity. *Physiol Behav,* 100(5), 549-59.

Olszewski, P. K., Li, D., Grace, M. K., Billington, C. J., Kotz, C. M., & Levine, A. S. (2003). Neural basis of orexigenic effects of ghrelin acting within lateral hypothalamus. *Peptides, 24*(4), 597-602.

Ong, K. K., Ahmed, M. L., Sherriff, A., Woods, K. A., Watts, A., Golding, J., et al., (1999). Cord blood leptin is associated with size at birth and predicts infancy weight gain in humans. ALSPAC Study Team. Avon Longitudinal Study of Pregnancy and Childhood. *J Clin Endocrinol Metab, 84*(3), 1145-1148.

Ongur, D., & Price, J. L. (2000). The organization of networks within the orbital and medial prefrontal cortex of rats, monkeys and humans. *Cereb Cortex, 10*(3), 206-219.

Osmond, C., & Barker, D. J. (2000). Fetal, infant, and childhood growth are predictors of coronary heart disease, diabetes, and hypertension in adult men and women. *Environ Health Perspect, 108 Suppl 3*, 545-553.

Palmiter, R. D. (2008). Dopamine signaling in the dorsal striatum is essential for motivated behaviors: lessons from dopamine-deficient mice. *Ann N Y Acad Sci, 1129*, 35-46.

Pannacciulli, N., Le, D. S., Salbe, A. D., Chen, K., Reiman, E. M., Tataranni, P. A., et al., (2007). Postprandial glucagon-like peptide-1 (GLP-1) response is positively associated with changes in neuronal activity of brain areas implicated in satiety and food intake regulation in humans. *Neuroimage, 35*(2), 511-517.

Passamonti, L., Rowe, J. B., Schwarzbauer, C., Ewbank, M. P., von dem Hagen, E., & Calder, A. J. (2009). Personality predicts the brain's response to viewing appetizing foods: the neural basis of a risk factor for overeating. *J Neurosci, 29*(1), 43-51.

Pi-Sunyer, X., Kissileff, H. R., Thornton, J., & Smith, G. P. (1982). C-terminal octapeptide of cholecystokinin decreases food intake in obese men. *Physiol Behav, 29*(4), 627-630.

Pohjalainen, T., Rinne, J. O., Nagren, K., Lehikoinen, P., Anttila, K., Syvalahti, E. K., et al., (1998). The A1 allele of the human D2 dopamine receptor gene predicts low D2 receptor availability in healthy volunteers. *Mol Psychiatry, 3*(3), 256-260.

Porubska, K., Veit, R., Preissl, H., Fritsche, A., & Birbaumer, N. (2006). Subjective feeling of appetite modulates brain activity: an fMRI study. *Neuroimage, 32*(3), 1273-1280.

Pritchard, T. C., Schwartz, G. J., & Scott, T. R. (2007). Taste in the medial orbitofrontal cortex of the macaque. *Ann N Y Acad Sci, 1121*, 121-135.

Raspopow, K., Abizaid, A., Matheson, K., & Anisman, H. (2010). Psychosocial stressor effects on cortisol and ghrelin in emotional and non-emotional eaters: Influence of anger and shame. *Horm Behav,* 58(4), 677-84.

Ravussin, E., Smith, S. R., Mitchell, J. A., Shringarpure, R., Shan, K., Maier, H., et al., (2009). Enhanced weight loss with pramlintide/metreleptin: an integrated neurohormonal approach to obesity pharmacotherapy. *Obesity (Silver Spring), 17*(9), 1736-1743.

Reinehr, T., Enriori, P. J., Harz, K., Cowley, M. A., & Roth, C. L. (2006). Pancreatic polypeptide in obese children before and after weight loss. *Int J Obes (Lond), 30*(10), 1476-1481.

Richter-Levin, G., & Akirav, I. (2000). Amygdala-hippocampus dynamic interaction in relation to memory. *Mol Neurobiol, 22*(1-3), 11-20.

Rissanen, P., Makimattila, S., Vehmas, T., Taavitsainen, M., & Rissanen, A. (1999). Effect of weight loss and regional fat distribution on plasma leptin concentration in obese women. *Int J Obes Relat Metab Disord, 23*(6), 645-649.

Riedy, C. A., Chavez, M., Figlewicz, D. P., & Woods, S. C. (1995). Central insulin enhances sensitivity to cholecystokinin. *Physiol Behav, 58*(4), 755-760.

Roberts, C., Troop, N., Connan, F., Treasure, J., & Campbell, I. C. (2007). The effects of stress on body weight: biological and psychological predictors of change in BMI. *Obesity (Silver Spring), 15*(12), 3045-3055.

Rolls, E. T. (2000). The orbitofrontal cortex and reward. *Cereb Cortex, 10*(3), 284-294.

Rosenbaum, M., & Leibel, R. L. (1999). The role of leptin in human physiology. *N Engl J Med, 341*(12), 913-915.

Rosenbaum, M., Sy, M., Pavlovich, K., Leibel, R. L., & Hirsch, J. (2008). Leptin reverses weight loss-induced changes in regional neural activity responses to visual food stimuli. *J Clin Invest, 118*(7), 2583-2591.

Rosmond, R., Holm, G., & Bjorntorp, P. (2000). Food-induced cortisol secretion in relation to anthropometric, metabolic and haemodynamic variables in men. *Int J Obes Relat Metab Disord, 24*(4), 416-422.

Roth, C. L., Enriori, P. J., Harz, K., Woelfle, J., Cowley, M. A., & Reinehr, T. (2005). Peptide YY is a regulator of energy homeostasis in obese children before and after weight loss. *J Clin Endocrinol Metab, 90*(12), 6386-6391.

Roth, J. D., Roland, B. L., Cole, R. L., Trevaskis, J. L., Weyer, C., Koda, J. E., et al., (2008). Leptin responsiveness restored by amylin agonism in diet-induced obesity: evidence from nonclinical and clinical studies. *Proc Natl Acad Sci U.S.A., 105*(20), 7257-7262.

Rothemund, Y., Preuschhof, C., Bohner, G., Bauknecht, H. C., Klingebiel, R., Flor, H., et al., (2007). Differential activation of the dorsal striatum by high-calorie visual food stimuli in obese individuals. *Neuroimage, 37*(2), 410-421.

Ruter, J., Kobelt, P., Tebbe, J. J., Avsar, Y., Veh, R., Wang, L., et al., (2003). Intraperitoneal injection of ghrelin induces Fos expression in the paraventricular nucleus of the hypothalamus in rats. *Brain Res, 991*(1-2), 26-33.

Sahu, A. (1998). Leptin decreases food intake induced by melanin-concentrating hormone (MCH), galanin (GAL) and neuropeptide Y (NPY) in the rat. *Endocrinology, 139*(11), 4739-4742.

Sanderson, S. C., Persky, S., & Michie, S. (2009). Psychological and Behavioral Responses to Genetic Test Results Indicating Increased Risk of Obesity: Does the Causal Pathway from Gene to Obesity Matter? *Public Health Genomics* May 4. [Epub ahead of print]

Santollo, J., & Eckel, L. A. (2008). Estradiol decreases the orexigenic effect of neuropeptide Y, but not agouti-related protein, in ovariectomized rats. *Behav Brain Res, 191*(2), 173-177.

Savino, F., Liguori, S. A., Fissore, M. F., Oggero, R., Silvestro, L., & Miniero, R. (2005). Serum ghrelin concentration and weight gain in healthy term infants in the first year of life. *J Pediatr Gastroenterol Nutr, 41*(5), 653-659.

Schoppen, S., Riestra, P., Garcia-Anguita, A., Lopez-Simon, L., Cano, B., de Oya, I., et al., (2010). Leptin and adiponectin levels in pubertal children: relationship with anthropometric variables and body composition. *Clin Chem Lab Med, 48*(5), 707-711.

Schur, E. A., Kleinhans, N. M., Goldberg, J., Buchwald, D., Schwartz, M. W., & Maravilla, K. (2009). Activation in brain energy regulation and reward centers by food cues varies with choice of visual stimulus. *Int J Obes (Lond), 33*(6), 653-661.

Schwartz, M. W., Sipols, A. J., Marks, J. L., Sanacora, G., White, J. D., Scheurink, A., et al., (1992). Inhibition of hypothalamic neuropeptide Y gene expression by insulin. *Endocrinology, 130*(6), 3608-3616.

Schweinsburg, A. D., Nagel, B. J., & Tapert, S. F. (2005). fMRI reveals alteration of spatial working memory networks across adolescence. *J Int Neuropsychol Soc, 11*(5), 631-644.

Silha, J. V., Krsek, M., Skrha, J. V., Sucharda, P., Nyomba, B. L., & Murphy, L. J. (2003). Plasma resistin, adiponectin and leptin levels in lean and obese subjects: correlations with insulin resistance. *Eur J Endocrinol, 149*(4), 331-335.

Small, D. M., Jones-Gotman, M., & Dagher, A. (2003). Feeding-induced dopamine release in dorsal striatum correlates with meal pleasantness ratings in healthy human volunteers. *Neuroimage, 19*(4), 1709-1715.

Small, D. M., Zatorre, R. J., Dagher, A., Evans, A. C., & Jones-Gotman, M. (2001). Changes in brain activity related to eating chocolate: from pleasure to aversion. *Brain, 124*(Pt 9), 1720-1733.

Smeets, P. A., de Graaf, C., Stafleu, A., van Osch, M. J., & van der Grond, J. (2005). Functional MRI of human hypothalamic responses following glucose ingestion. *Neuroimage, 24*(2), 363-368.

Soares, J. B., & Leite-Moreira, A. F. (2008). Ghrelin, des-acyl ghrelin and obestatin: three pieces of the same puzzle. *Peptides, 29*(7), 1255-1270.

Sodowski, K., Zwirska-Korczala, K., Kuka, D., Kukla, M., Budziszewska, P., Czuba, B., et al., (2007). Basal and postprandial gut peptides affecting food intake in lean and obese pregnant women. *J Physiol Pharmacol, 58 Suppl 1*, 37-52.

Steele, K. E., Prokopowicz, G. P., Schweitzer, M. A., Magunsuon, T. H., Lidor, A. O., Kuwabawa, H., et al., Alterations of central dopamine receptors before and after gastric bypass surgery. *Obes Surg, 20*(3), 369-374.

Stice, E., Spoor, S., Bohon, C., & Small, D. M. (2008). Relation between obesity and blunted striatal response to food is moderated by TaqIA A1 allele. *Science, 322*(5900), 449-452.

Stice, E., Spoor, S., Bohon, C., Veldhuizen, M. G., & Small, D. M. (2008). Relation of reward from food intake and anticipated food intake to obesity: a functional magnetic resonance imaging study. *J Abnorm Psychol, 117*(4), 924-935.

Stice, E., Yokum, S., Bohon, C., Marti, N., & Smolen, A. Reward circuitry responsivity to food predicts future increases in body mass: moderating effects of DRD2 and DRD4. *Neuroimage, 50*(4), 1618-1625.

Stock, S., Leichner, P., Wong, A. C., Ghatei, M. A., Kieffer, T. J., Bloom, S. R., et al., (2005). Ghrelin, peptide YY, glucose-dependent insulinotropic polypeptide, and hunger responses to a mixed meal in anorexic, obese, and control female adolescents. *J Clin Endocrinol Metab, 90*(4), 2161-2168.

Stoeckel, L. E., Weller, R. E., Cook, E. W., 3rd, Twieg, D. B., Knowlton, R. C., & Cox, J. E. (2008). Widespread reward-system activation in obese women in response to pictures of high-calorie foods. *Neuroimage, 41*(2), 636-647.

Strader, A. D., & Woods, S. C. (2005). Gastrointestinal hormones and food intake. *Gastroenterology, 128*(1), 175-191.

Stunkard, A. J., & Messick, S. (1985). The three-factor eating questionnaire to measure dietary restraint, disinhibition and hunger. *J Psychosom Res, 29*(1), 71-83.

Sun, Y., Asnicar, M., & Smith, R. G. (2007). Central and peripheral roles of ghrelin on glucose homeostasis. *Neuroendocrinology, 86*(3), 215-228.

Suzuki, K., Simpson, K. A., Minnion, J. S., Shillito, J. C., & Bloom, S. R. (2010). The role of gut hormones and the hypothalamus in appetite regulation. *Endocr J, 57*(5), 359-372.

Suzuki, S., Ramos, E. J., Goncalves, C. G., Chen, C., & Meguid, M. M. (2005). Changes in GI hormones and their effect on gastric emptying and transit times after Roux-en-Y gastric bypass in rat model. *Surgery, 138*(2), 283-290.

Tang-Christensen, M., Larsen, P. J., Goke, R., Fink-Jensen, A., Jessop, D. S., Moller, M., et al., (1996). Central administration of GLP-1-(7-36) amide inhibits food and water intake in rats. *Am J Physiol, 271*(4 Pt 2), R848-856.

Tang-Christensen, M., Vrang, N., & Larsen, P. J. (2001). Glucagon-like peptide containing pathways in the regulation of feeding behaviour. *Int J Obes Relat Metab Disord, 25 Suppl 5*, S42-47.

Tataranni, P. A., Gautier, J. F., Chen, K., Uecker, A., Bandy, D., Salbe, A. D., et al., (1999). Neuroanatomical correlates of hunger and satiation in humans using positron emission tomography. *Proc Natl Acad Sci U.S.A., 96*(8), 4569-4574.

Tataranni, P. A., Larson, D. E., Snitker, S., Young, J. B., Flatt, J. P., & Ravussin, E. (1996). Effects of glucocorticoids on energy metabolism and food intake in humans. *Am J Physiol, 271*(2 Pt 1), E317-325.

Taylor, A. E., Hubbard, J., & Anderson, E. J. (1999). Impact of binge eating on metabolic and leptin dynamics in normal young women. *J Clin Endocrinol Metab, 84*(2), 428-434.

Thomas, G. N., Critchley, J. A., Tomlinson, B., Cockram, C. S., & Chan, J. C. (2001). Relationships between the taqI polymorphism of the dopamine D2 receptor and blood pressure in hyperglycaemic and normoglycaemic Chinese subjects. *Clin Endocrinol (Oxf), 55*(5), 605-611.

Tritos, N. A., Mun, E., Bertkau, A., Grayson, R., Maratos-Flier, E., & Goldfine, A. (2003). Serum ghrelin levels in response to glucose load in obese subjects post-gastric bypass surgery. *Obes Res, 11*(8), 919-924.

Tschop, M., Smiley, D. L., & Heiman, M. L. (2000). Ghrelin induces adiposity in rodents. *Nature, 407*(6806), 908-913.

Uher, R., Treasure, J., Heining, M., Brammer, M. J., & Campbell, I. C. (2006). Cerebral processing of food-related stimuli: effects of fasting and gender. *Behav Brain Res, 169*(1), 111-119.

Van Strien, T., Frijters, J. E., Bergers, G. P., Defares, P. B. (1986). The Dutch Eating Behavior Questionnaire (DEBQ) for assessment of restrained, emotional, and external eating behavior *International Journal of Eating Disorders, 5*, 295-315.

Verdich, C., Toubro, S., Buemann, B., Lysgard Madsen, J., Juul Holst, J., & Astrup, A. (2001). The role of postprandial releases of insulin and incretin hormones in meal-induced satiety—effect of obesity and weight reduction. *Int J Obes Relat Metab Disord, 25*(8), 1206-1214.

Vogt, B. A., Finch, D. M., & Olson, C. R. (1992). Functional heterogeneity in cingulate cortex: the anterior executive and posterior evaluative regions. *Cereb Cortex, 2*(6), 435-443.

Volkow, N. D., Fowler, J. S., & Wang, G. J. (2004). The addicted human brain viewed in the light of imaging studies: brain circuits and treatment strategies. *Neuropharmacology, 47 Suppl 1*, 3-13.

Volkow, N. D., Wang, G. J., Maynard, L., Jayne, M., Fowler, J. S., Zhu, W., et al., (2003). Brain dopamine is associated with eating behaviors in humans. *Int J Eat Disord, 33*(2), 136-142.

Volkow, N. D., Wang, G. J., Telang, F., Fowler, J. S., Thanos, P. K., Logan, J., et al., (2008). Low dopamine striatal D2 receptors are associated with prefrontal metabolism in obese subjects: possible contributing factors. *Neuroimage, 42*(4), 1537-1543.

Wadden, T. S. D., & Goldstein, D. (1996). Behavioral treatment of obesity *The Management of Eating Disorders*. Totowa, New Jersey: Humana Press.

Wang, G. J., Volkow, N. D., Logan, J., Pappas, N. R., Wong, C. T., Zhu, W., et al., (2001). Brain dopamine and obesity. *Lancet, 357*(9253), 354-357.

Wang, G. J., Volkow, N. D., Telang, F., Jayne, M., Ma, J., Rao, M., et al., (2004). Exposure to appetitive food stimuli markedly activates the human brain. *Neuroimage, 21*(4), 1790-1797.

Wang, L., Barachina, M. D., Martinez, V., Wei, J. Y., & Tache, Y. (2000). Synergistic interaction between CCK and leptin to regulate food intake. *Regul Pept, 92*(1-3), 79-85.

Weickert, M. O., Spranger, J., Holst, J. J., Otto, B., Koebnick, C., Mohlig, M., et al., (2006). Wheat-fibre-induced changes of postprandial peptide YY and ghrelin responses are not associated with acute alterations of satiety. *Br J Nutr, 96*(5), 795-798.

Weiss, R., & Caprio, S. (2006). Altered glucose metabolism in obese youth. *Pediatr Endocrinol Rev, 3*(3), 233-238.

West, D. B., Fey, D., Woods, S.C. (1984). Cholecystokinin persistently suppresses meal size but not food intake in free-feeding rats. *Am J Physiol Regul Integr Comp Physiol, 246*(5), 776-787.

Wolfe, B. E., Jimerson, D. C., Orlova, C., & Mantzoros, C. S. (2004). Effect of dieting on plasma leptin, soluble leptin receptor, adiponectin and resistin levels in healthy volunteers. *Clin Endocrinol (Oxf), 61*(3), 332-338.

Wolkowitz, O. M., Epel, E. S., & Reus, V. I. (2001). Stress hormone-related psychopathology: pathophysiological and treatment implications. *World J Biol Psychiatry, 2*(3), 115-143.

Woods, S. C., Lutz, T. A., Geary, N., & Langhans, W. (2006). Pancreatic signals controlling food intake; insulin, glucagon and amylin. *Philos Trans R Soc Lond B Biol Sci, 361*(1471), 1219-1235.

Wren, A. M., & Bloom, S. R. (2007). Gut hormones and appetite control. *Gastroenterology, 132*(6), 2116-2130.

Wren, A. M., Seal, L. J., Cohen, M. A., Brynes, A. E., Frost, G. S., Murphy, K. G., et al., (2001). Ghrelin enhances appetite and increases food intake in humans. *J Clin Endocrinol Metab, 86*(12), 5992.

Wynne, K., & Bloom, S. R. (2006). The role of oxyntomodulin and peptide tyrosine-tyrosine (PYY) in appetite control. *Nat Clin Pract Endocrinol Metab, 2*(11), 612-620.

Yada, T., Dezaki, K., Sone, H., Koizumi, M., Damdindorj, B., Nakata, M., et al., (2008). Ghrelin regulates insulin release and glycemia: physiological role and therapeutic potential. *Curr Diabetes Rev, 4*(1), 18-23.

Yanovski, S. Z. (2003). Binge eating disorder and obesity in 2003: could treating an eating disorder have a positive effect on the obesity epidemic? *Int J Eat Disord, 34 Suppl*, S117-120.

Zwirska-Korczala, K., Konturek, S. J., Sodowski, M., Wylezol, M., Kuka, D., Sowa, P., et al., (2007). Basal and postprandial plasma levels of PYY, ghrelin, cholecystokinin, gastrin and insulin in women with moderate and morbid obesity and metabolic syndrome. *J Physiol Pharmacol, 58 Suppl 1*, 13-35.

In: Pathways to Obesity and Main Roads to Recovery
Editor: Piergiuseppe Vinai
ISBN: 978-1-61122-740-6

Chapter IV

Psychiatric, Psychological, and Familial Parameters in Childhood Obesity

Daniel Stein*[1], *Yael Latzer*[2], *Laurel Edmunds*[3], *Silvana Fennig*[4], *Moria Golan*[5], *Eitan Gur*[6], *Ze'ev Hochberg*[7], *Diane Levin-Zamir*[8], *Eynat Zubery*[9] and *Phyllis Speiser*[10]

[1]Pediatric Psychosomatic Department, the Edmond and Lily Safra Children's Hospital, The Chaim Sheba Medical Center, Tel Hashomer, affiliated with The Sackler Faculty of Medicine, Tel Aviv University, Tel Aviv, Israel

[2]Eating Disorders Clinic, Psychiatric Division, Rambam Medical Center, Haifa, Israel, affiliated with The Faculty of Social Welfare & Health Sciences, Haifa University, Haifa, Israel

[3]Bristol Royal Hospital for Children, Bristol, UK

[4]Inpatient Psychiatric Unit, Schneider Children's Medical Center, Feinberg Child Study Center, affiliated with The Sackler Faculty of Medicine, Tel Aviv University, Tel Aviv, Israel

[5]School of Nutritional Sciences, Faculty of Agricultural, Food and Environmental Quality Sciences, The Hebrew University of Jerusalem, and Shahaf Community Services for Eating Disorders, Naan and Tel Aviv, Israel

[6]Department of Eating and Weight Disorders, The Chaim Sheba Medical Center, Tel Hashomer, and The Hebrew University, Faculty of Medicine, Jerusalem, Israel

[7]Meyer Children's Hospital, Rambam Medical Center, and Technion—Israel Institute of Technology, Haifa, Israel

[8]Department of Health Education and Promotion, Clalit Health Services, Israel

[9]Eating Disorders Unit, Davidson Clinic, Shalvata Mental Health Center, Clalit Health Services, affiliated with The Sackler Faculty of Medicine, Tel Aviv University, Israel

[10]Schneider Children's Hospital, New Hyde Park, NY, and New York University School of Medicine, New York, NY, USA

Abstract

The current review focuses on an updated critical analysis of the most relevant psychiatric and psychosocial issues in childhood overweight issues. It is rooted on a comprehensive systematic literature search from PUBMED, PSYCHLIT, PSYCHINFO, and ERIC from 1991-2010.

A rise in the prevalence of childhood overweight issues has occurred in Western and non-Western countries around the globe during the last three decades. Overweight issues in children and adolescents may be associated with psychological and social problems such as reduced school and social performance, less favorable quality of life, societal victimization and peer teasing, lower self-and body-esteem, and neuropsychological dysfynctioning. Whereas community samples of obese youngsters do not show elevated psychopathology, clinically referred overweight children have elevated depression, anxiety, behavior problems and disordered eating. Parents' perceptions of their children being overweight highly influence how a child perceives himself. Obese youngsters often share the overall negative perception of their normal-weight peers about being overweight.

Introduction

The investigation of the psychosocial aspects of childhood obesity has been the focus of long-standing theoretical and empirical endeavors (Renman et al., 1999; Strauss, 2000). Obesity is a well-defined term in adults; but in children and adolescents, its definition is less consistent. The U.S. Center for Disease Control (CDC) growth charts include gender-specific body mass index (BMI) growth charts for ages 2 to 19 years (CDC, 2004). Obesity among individuals 2 to 19 years old is defined as the 95th percentile or greater of BMI for age, and being overweight is defined as the 85th percentile or greater, but less than the 95th percentile of BMI for age (CDC, 2004). Because of the likelihood of stigmatization associated with the term "obesity," several leading authorities in the field have suggested to define a "risk for overweight" as BMI between 85 to 95%, and overweight as a BMI>95% (see for example, Ogden et al., 2006; Puhl & Latner, 2007). An international forum of consensus development, the International Obesity Task Force (IOTF) (Bellizzi & Dietz, 1999), has recently recommended adopting the risk-related cut-off concept of Cole et al., (2000), who developed age- and sex-specific cut-off points using the BMI. These charts extrapolate risk from the adult experience to children. The IOTF defines childhood overweight as a BMI of approximately 91% or greater and obesity as a BMI of approximately 99% or greater (Bellizzi & Dietz, 1999). In this review, we will relate to the classical definitions of obesity and being overweight. We will relate to the following psychosocial dimensions: the influence of parents on the consequences of being overweight in their children, psychosocial functioning, self- and body esteem and psychopathology of overweight youngsters, and the influence of children's perception of themselves as being overweight on their well-being. The review is based on a comprehensive systematic literature search of the PUBMED, PSYCHLIT, PSYCHINFO, and ERIC between 1991 and 2010.

Epidemiology

Childhood obesity is epidemic around the globe and on the rise in both industrialized and developing countries. Thus, whereas the prevalence of child and adolescent obesity has been relatively stable during the 1960s and early 1970s, it has begun to accelerate since the late 1970s (McGinnis et al., 2006; Sweeting et al., 2008). Accordingly, in the U.S., the prevalence of overweight has doubled among youngsters 6 to 11 years of age and tripled among those 12 to 17 years of age between 1976 and 1980 and 1999 and 2002, respectively (McGinnis et al., 2006). The prevalence of overweight people in the United States around the end of the 1990s has been estimated around 10.4%, 15.3% and 15.5% for children 5 to 10, 6 to 11, and 12 to 19 years old, respectively (Ogden et al., 2002). From 2007 to 2008, 9.5% of American infants and toddlers were at or above the 95th percentile of the weight-for-recumbent-length growth charts. Among American children and adolescents aged 2 through 19 years, 11.9% were at or above the 97th percentile of the BMI-for-age growth charts; 16.9% were at or above the 95th percentile; and 31.7% at or above the 85th percentile of BMI for age (Ogden et al., 2010).

In the UK, the rate of people who are overweight, including obesity, has risen from 17 to 22% and from 20 to 25% in two- to five-year-old boys and girls, respectively, between the early 1990s and early 2000s (Hawkins et al., 2008). Similarly, high rates of childhood obesity have been found recently in other Western countries. For example, the prevalence of overweight and obesity among children in Argentina in 2004, has been estimated as 19 and 18.4%, respectively (Hirschler et al., 2006). Comparison of cross-sectional data from school-based surveys conducted in 1997 and 1998, in 13 European countries, Israel, and the United States, have shown that the United States, Greece, Israel, and Portugal have the highest prevalence of overweight in children (Lissau et al., 2004). Furthermore, it is estimated that by 2010, 50% of the children in North America and almost 40% of children in the European Union will be overweight (Wang & Lobstein, 2006). Some even predict that by the year 2025, childhood obesity will be the world's number one health problem (Vaidya, 2006).

High rates of pediatric obesity have been observed also in non-Western countries in recent years. For example, in China, the overall prevalence of obesity overwieght among children ages two to six years was 10.7% and 4.2%, respectively, in the first years of the 21st century (Jiang et al., 2006). Interestingly, studies in some countries have found a stabilization in the rate of pediatric overweight and obesity in recent years. This has been noted, for example, in the USA from 2000 to 2008 (Ogden et al., 2010), and in France from 2000 to 2007 (Salanave et al., 2009).

Genetic factors account for around 50% of the risk for being overweight and obesity among children (Hebebrand & Hinney, 2009), whereas specific genetic or endocrine diseases account for less than 10% of all cases, and hypothalamic injuries and drug-induced obesity are even less common. As the gene pool has likely not changed during the past two to three decades, environmental, social and psychological factors are largely thought to account for the high prevalence of being overweight and obesity in recent years. It is important to note that while the individual effect sizes of most environmental factors are likely to be small and the validation of their causality is not straight-forward (Hebebrand & Hinney, 2009), the simultaneous change in many socio-environmental risk factors from the second half of the 20th century may explain the parallel changes in the prevalence of childhood obesity (Ogden et al., 2002, Speiser et al., 2005).

Parental Influence on the Consequences of Being Overweight in their Children

Parents of overweight/obese children may be either not worried (Campbell et al., 2006b; Crawford et al., 2006; Genovesi et al., 2005; Jain et al., 2001; Lampard et al., 2008; Stern 2000) about their children's weight, or, alternatively, over-concerned with and critical about it (Baughcum et al., 2000; 33; Burdette et al., 2006). Not surprisingly, ignoring weight may be more considerable in parents of overweight children (above 80%), than in parents of obese children (less than 20%) (Crawford et al., 2006; Lampard et al., 2008; West et al., 2008). Furthermore, parents are more concerned about their young children being underweight than overweight (Pagnini et al., 2007a). Accordingly, one study has shown that more than 50% of mothers who perceive their children to be overweight or obese are not concerned about it (Genovesi et al., 2005).

One explanation for the inconsistencies in parental perceptions of their children weight problems likely relates to the tendency of parents to be unaware (Crawford et al., 2006), misperceive (Dubois & Girad, 2007; Watkins et al., 2007), or disconnect between the perceived and actual weight of their children (Doolen et al., 2009; West et al., 2008). For example, over 70% of mothers of overweight children see them as being of similar weight to their peers, as being equally or more active than other children, and as having a diet at least as healthy as their peers (Campbell et al., 2006a). Parents mostly underestimate their children's weight, with more than 50% of parents of obese and overweight children being unable to recognize when their child is overweight (Adams et al., 2005; Crawford et al., 2006; Hackie & Bowles, 2007; Hirscler et al., 2006; Parry et al., 2008; West et al., 2008). Still, in some studies, parents have been found to overestimate their overweight children's weights (Dubois & Girad, 2007).

The inclination for misperception is greater for boys than for girls (Dubois & Girad, 2007). In addition, parents of young overweight children misperceive their children's weight to a greater extent than parents of overweight adolescents (65% vs. 51% respectively, West et al., 2008). Interestingly, parents tend to perceive their children's weight significantly less accurately than their own (Genovesi et al., 2005; Nazario Rodriguez et al., 2008). There is some debate whether the inaccuracy in the perception of the child's weight is related to parents being overweight. Whereas some studies have found no association between parental perceptional inaccuracy and overweight parents (Hackie & Bowles, 2007; West et al., 2008), others have shown a significant difference in the proportion of distorted perception of shape between mothers of normal-weight children vs. those of overweight and obese children (17 vs. 87.5%, respectively, see Hirschler et al., 2006). This inaccuracy in perception is not related to socio-economic status or education level in some studies (Hackie & Bowles, 2007; West et al., 2008), whereas others (Genovesi et al., 2005) have shown greater misperception in families with lower education levels. In addition, African-American parents have been found twice as likely to underestimate as Caucasians (West et al., 2008). BMI screening and feedback may improve parental perception to some extent (West et al., 2008).

In addition to parental misperception about overweight, mothers may exhibit poor overall ability to estimate the way their overweight and obese children eat (Campbell et al., 2006a; Genovesi et al., 2005). A significant difference may, thus, be found in the proportion of distorted perception of eating habits between mothers of normal-weight children vs. those of overweight and obese children (36.3 vs. 90.8%, see Hirschler et al., 2006). Eighty-four and

96% of mothers of obese and overweight children, respectively, in that study, have actually thought that their children ate right or too little (Hirschler et al., 2006). Most importantly, mothers' distorted perceptions of shape and eating habits of their overweight children (Hirschler et al., 2006), found already during infancy (Kroke et al., 2006), may become significant independent risk factors for the prediction of frank obesity in later life.

Parental attitudes toward obesity in their children may be associated with the child's gender and age, as well as with their own ethnic background and/or level of education. For example, parents of boys (Campbell et al., 2006a), or of African-American descent, or with less education (Nsiah-Kumi et al., 2009), have been shown to associate lower risk with their children being overweight. Parents with less education are also less inclined to take action to prevent unhealthy weight gain in their children (Crawford et al., 2006). Parents of overweight children tend not to include weight in their distinction of health and have been found to be more concerned with their child's health than with his/her weight (Goodell et al., 2009).

Unfortunately, not only parental lack of concern (Hirschler et al., 2006), but also their over concern (Brudette et al., 2006), may be associated with elevated BMI and adiposity in their children. Factors increasing parental weight concern include higher child BMI, less parental underestimation of child body size, and lower child health-related quality of life (Lampard et al., 2008). In other studies, parents have been found to be concerned about being overweight among children and adolescents in general, but are reluctant to address it with their own children (Booth et al., 2009). Conversely, some researchers reported no difference in the manner in which parents of normal and overweight children estimate their weights, with both groups likely inclining towards underestimation (Kersey et al., 2010).

One of the most important factors affecting parental attitude toward their children being overweight is the manner in which parents perceive and are preoccupied with their own weight. Accordingly, parents are more likely to worry about their children's potential for future weight if they or the other parent are, or have been, overweight (Campbell et al., 2006a). In addition, parents may become over concerned with their children being overweight as the result of problematic consultations they have had with health care professionals (Edmunds, 2005). Lastly, although parents appreciate the role of diet and inactivity in the causation of being overweight, they tend to underestimate the difficulties involved in their children's attempts to change maladaptive eating behaviors (Cullen et al., 2000; Jain et al., 2001; Rainey et al., 1998).

Parents may endorse and transmit weight-based stereotypes to their children (Puhl & Latner, 2007). Moreover, children's perceptions about their own being overweight have been found to be influenced to a greater extent by the manner in which their parents relate to their being overweight than by their actual BMI For example, for overweight girls, their mothers' weight-related over-reacting, likely leading to restriction of food, and their fathers' overt criticism about their weights, are among the factors that have the most detrimental influence on their self-perceptions (Davison & Birch, 2001; Birch et al., 2003), and well-being (Rumpel & Harris, 1994). By contrast, lack of parental criticism with respect to the child's being overweight may be a protective factor for the child's self-esteem (Zametkin et al., 2004). The latter youngsters tend to use adaptive compensatory methods for the regulation of self-esteem, such as reducing the importance of areas in which they are less competent and increasing the importance of domains in which they perform well (Israel & Ivanova, 2002; Manus & Killeen, 1995).

Another important factor in the well-being of obese children relates to the influence of parental psychopathology and distress on the emotional condition of the overweight child. For example, maternal anxiety may predict the overweight child's severity of depression and anxiety (Roth et al., 2008). Nevertheless, the presence of adequate coping strategies in the child may considerably reduce the impact of the mother's mental state on his/her well-being (Roth et al., 2008).

The Psychosocial Functioning of Overweight Youngsters

Being overweight in children and adolescents may be associated with a host of psychological and social problems, which can have a considerable deleterious impact on the psychological development and the quality of life of the overweight youngster. In addition, the school and social performance of obese children is often (Krukowski et al., 2009; Pinhas-Hamiel et al., 2006), although not always (Li et al., 2008; Wang & Veugelers, 2008) less favorable in comparison to normal-weight youngsters. One explanation for this finding is that overweight children are absent from school significantly more than normal-weight children. Thus, the obese category remains a significant contributor to the number of days absent from school even after adjusting for age, race/ethnicity, and gender (Geier et al., 2007). Obese children are, in addition, at increased risk of psychosocial distress relative to their non-obese peers (Janicke et al., 2008), and their overall quality of life (Pinhas-Hamiel et al., 2006; Wallander et al., 2009; Yackobovitch-Gavan et al., 2009) and emotional well-being (Cornette, 2008; Wille et al., 2008) are often less favorable. Lastly, lower school performance during childhood and adolescence is an important predictor for the development of obesity in later life (Alatupa et al., 2010). Psychosocial factors such as global self-concept, body dissatisfaction (Wallander et al., 2009), and weight-based teasing (Kestilä et al., 2009; Krukowski et al., 2009) may mediate in the influence of overweight/obesity on the performance of children and adolescents in their required age-specific developmental tasks and their well-being.

Interestingly, lower childhood IQ scores may be associated with an increased prevalence of adult obesity, this relation largely mediated via educational attainment and the adoption of healthy diets in later life (Chandola et al., 2006). From a different perspective, children and adolescents whose diets are nutritious and whose participation in physical activity is high have been found to perform better on various measures of cognitive performance and academic achievement (Sigfúsdóttir et al., 2007). Thus, in one cross- sectional study of school children in Iceland, BMI, diet and physical activity have explained up to 27% of the variance in academic achievement when controlling for gender, parental education, family structure, absenteeism, depressed mood, and self-esteem (Sigfúsdóttir et al., 2007). Moreover, an association has been recently found between overweight/obesity and decreased visuo-spatial organization in 8 to 16 years old (Li et al., 2008), and reduced motor, verbal, cognitive and social skills in four- to nine-year old (Mond et al., 2007), and even in two- to three-year old (Cawley & Speiss, 2008) children, particularly, although not exclusively, in boys. The finding of less than normal visuo-spatial functioning in obese youngsters retains its significance after adjusting for confounding variables such as parental/familial characteristics, sports participation, physical activity, hours spent watching TV, psychosocial development, blood pressure, and serum lipid profile (Li et al., 2008). Although these studies do not provide causal explanations for their findings, the implications of the reduced skill attainment during infancy and childhood on the likelihood of less favorable academic performance in overweight adolescents and adults are crucial (Cawley & Speiss, 2008; Mond et al., 2007).

Self- and Body-Esteem in Overweight Youngsters

The association between being overweight and global self-esteem in youngsters is not straight forward. Thus, some studies have indicated that overweight youngsters have lower self-esteem than non-obese teens (Cole et al., 2000; French et al., 1995; Harris et al., 2009; Li et al., 2007; Manus & Killeen, 1995; Shin & Shin, 2008; Wang & Veugelers, 2008; Wang et al., 2009), whereas other studies have shown no difference in the self-esteem of overweight and normal-weight youngsters (Gortmaker et al., 1993; Marsh et al., 2007; Renman et al., 1999). Still other studies have found that self-esteem is no longer lower in overweight children when controlling for the influence of body image and body dissatisfaction (Pesa et al., 2000). The lack of association between being overweight and self-esteem in some studies may reflect the inclination of most obese youngsters assessed in the community (as opposed to clinical samples) to be mostly unconcerned with their weight (although obese adolescents are more concerned with their weight than normal-weight teens; see Sweeting et al., 2008).

Self esteem in overweight children and adolescents varies with gender, with females being at a greater risk of developing low self-esteem than males (Nowicka et al., 2009; Zametkin et al., 2004). The influence of age on self-esteem is not clear cut. Thus, some studies have shown that young overweight children are at particular risk for lower self-esteem (Coronette, 2008), whereas in others, adolescents are more vulnerable than younger children (Nowicka et al., 2009; Pesa et al., 2000). Additional factors that may potentially influence self-esteem include the severity of being overweight and socio-cultural status. For example, being overweight may influence self-esteem in Caucasian and Latin American but not in African-American girls (Maynard et al., 2009; Strauss, 2000), or in Australian as opposed to Hong Kong youngsters (Marsh et al., 2007). Still other studies have shown no association in obese youngsters between BMI levels and self-esteem (Nowicka et al., 2009). Fourthly, low self-esteem in overweight youngsters may be also related to the presence of dieting behavior and preoccupation with weight and shape (Pesa et al., 2000; Wang & Veugelers, 2008), and to an overall inactive lifestyle (Wang & Veugelers, 2008), particularly among overweight females, these being in some cases even more influential than the actual weight problem.

The findings concerning the association of body image with being overweight are more consistent in comparison to self-esteem. Favorable body image and perception have been found to be inversely correlated with the actual weight, and overweight youngsters usually show more body image disturbances and more body-related negative attitudes than their normal-weight counterparts (Israel & Ivanova, 2002; Marsh et al., 2007; Philips RG, Hill, 1998; Renman et al., 1999; Shin & Shin, 2008; Stradmeijer et al., 2000; Strauss, 2000). In some studies (Li et al., 2007; Pesa et al., 2000; Shin & Shin, 2008), body dissatisfaction has been found to mediate the association between obesity and self-esteem, with obese children with greater body dissatisfaction having significantly lower self-esteem. Still other studies have shown no mediating effect of body image on self-esteem (Marsh et al., 2007).

Influence of Children's Perceptions of Being Overweight on Overall Well-Being and Self-Esteem

Adiposity is very visible to youngsters, and even young children tend to rate disease and minor deformities as less detrimental than obesity and to ascribe more negative attitudes to being overweight than to normal-weight youngsters (Puhl & Latner, 2007). Studies assessing attributes that are primarily related by children to obesity emphasize those of laziness, selfishness, lower intelligence, social isolation, poor social functioning and low academic success (Israel & Ivanova, 2002). Overweight children are also perceived by their normal-weight peers as being less healthy, eating less well, and exercising significantly less (Israel & Ivanova, 2002). This stigmatization stems from children's beliefs that weight is under one's own personal control (Puhl & Latner, 2007).

In addition, children as young as five years old are very aware of their own weight, which has a considerable influence on the more derogatory manner in which they perceive their own appearance, athletic ability, physical competence, social competence, self-worth, and general health (Birch & Davidson, 2001; Epstein et al., 2001; McCullough et al., 2009; Puhl & Latner, 2007; Wille et al., 2008). These findings support the notion that on the whole, children share the overall negative parental and societal perceptions towards those who are overweight or obese, independent of their own weight status or gender.

Considering the issue of popularity, overweight preadolescent girls are significantly less likely to be considered pretty, although they may not differ in popularity (Neumark-Sztainer et al., 2002). A considerable decrease in popularity occurs during adolescence, as weight teasing in these age groups is highly correlated with actual weight. Weight-related teasing is greater in girls than in boys and in adolescents than in younger children (Krukowski et al., 2008). Moreover, overweight girls may report more victimization compared with their average-weight peers and are less likely to date than their peers (Pearce et al., 2002; Puhl & Latner, 2007). Similarly, overweight children and adolescents are often liked less, chosen less as friends, and more rejected, isolated and peripheral to social networks than their normal-weight peers (Puhl & Latner, 2007; Strauss RS, Pollack, 2003). Indeed, large-scale community-based studies have shown a greater prevalence of overweight and obesity among preschool children showing problematic relations with their peers in comparison to children with adaptive peer relationships (Boneberger, et al., 2009).

There is currently a growing amount of literature showing that overweight and obese children and adolescents are targets of societal stigmatization and teasing by peers, educators, and even parents (Falkner et al., 2001; Kestilä et al., 2009; Krukowski et al., 2008, 2009; Levine & Smolak, 2008; Neumark-Sztainer et al., 2002; Puhl & Latner, 2007; Vaidya, 2006; Young-Hyman et al., 2006). Puhl and Latner (2007) have recently critically analyzed the findings about the association between obesity, teasing, and health among youth. According to these authors and others (Young-Hyman et al., 2006), higher BMI is associated with more frequent and intense stigmatization in children and adolescents of both sexes. Internalization of this weight stigma in overweight and obese youth has been found to be associated with lower self-esteem, decreased physical activity, and elevated depression, anxiety, suicide, and body dissatisfaction. Among the socio-cultural affecting children's weight-related attitudes, greater media use, in particular magazine and videogame use, have been significantly correlated with more negative reactions to obese girls and boys among ten- to thirteen-year-old youngsters (Latner et al., 2007).

Childhood Overweight/Obesity and Psychopathology

Childhood obesity per se is not considered a behavioral or psychiatric disturbance, but rather a general medical condition (Epstein et al., 2001; WHO, 1992). Although being overweight may sometimes accompany depression, anxiety, and other psychiatric disorders, most overweight young individuals do not show significant psychiatric morbidity (Whitaker, 1997). Accordingly, in most studies of non-clinical overweight populations, the psychological condition of the youngster is found to be within normal ranges of healthy behavior (Ackard et al., 2003; Epstein et al., 1994; Vaidya, 2006; Wadden et al., 1991), and being overweight is usually not associated with elevated depression and anxiety (Philips & Hill, 1998; Shin & Shin, 2008). Nevertheless, in several community-based studies (Falkner et al., 2001; Mellin et al., 2002), overweight boys and girls have been more likely to report the presence of emotional problems as compared with normal-weight adolescents. Similarly, another recent study has found that 23% of non-referred obese youngsters (mean age around 14 years) meet criteria for at least one mental disorder (in comparison to 37.5% of youngsters referred for overweight treatment; Van Vlierberghe et al., 2009).

In contrast to community populations, elevated rates of psychopathological disturbances, primarily depression, anxiety, somatoform disorders and eating disorders, are usually reported in clinical populations of overweight youngsters (Vaidya, 2006; Janicke et al., 2008). It is not surprising thus to find that in many studies (Flodmark, 2005), although not all (Pinhas-Hamiel et al., 2006), clinical samples of obese children have a less favorable quality of life and self-esteem than community samples. One explanation for the difference between referred and non-referred obese youngsters is that the former group demonstrates significantly greater severity of being overweight (Van Vlierberghe et al., 2009). Alternatively, the neuroendocrine changes associated with stress, depression, and anxiety may cause metabolic changes that predispose and perpetuate obesity in clinically referred children (Vaidya, 2006). Research has shown that between 30 to 60% of overweight children aged five to 18 years referred for treatment show at least one internalizing or externalizing mental disorder (Van Vlierberghe et al., 2009; Vaidya, 2006; Janicke et al., 2008). This rate is higher in comparison with children with many other chronic physical disorders (Janicke et al., 2008).

Specifically, between 30 to 50% of clinical samples of obese children and adolescents show moderate to severe depression, and around a third have high levels of anxiety (Isnard et al., 2003; Wallace et al., 1993). Conversely, latency children and adolescents suffering from depression and anxiety are at greater risk to develop elevated BMI (Anderson et al., 2006), including obesity (Rofey et al., 2009) in later life in comparison to healthy controls, although some studies have not found such an association (Tanofsky-Kraft et al., 2006). In addition, overweight boys and girls have been found to engage in significantly more unhealthy risk-taking behaviors and to experience psychosocial distress to a greater extent than their non-overweight peers (Young-Hyman et al., 2006). In particular, overweight girls have attempted suicide to a greater extent than normal-weight girls.

Psychopathology in overweight children is correlated with gender (girls reporting more problems than boys), ethnicity (African-American youngsters reporting more problems than Caucasians), peer teasing, obesity-induced distress, body dissatisfaction and parental overweight and overall psychopathology (Janicke et al., 2008; Park et al., 2009; Young-Hyman et al., 2006; Zametkin et al., 2004). Interestingly, actual BMI is found less influential than these parameters in inducing psychological disturbances in obese and overweight youngsters. Reduction of physical activity may also mediate in the association of depression with childhood obesity (Gray et al., 2008).

Behavioral problems are also found to a greater extent in overweight youngsters compared to their normal-weight peers, particularly in pre-pubertal children (Stradmeijer et al., 2000). Moreover, youngsters with disruptive disorders are found to have a higher BMI than subjects without disruptive disorders (Anderson et al., 2006), and behavioral problems during childhood and early adolescence may be associated with a greater risk to develop overweight issues and obesity in early adulthood (Duarte et al., 2010; Mamun et al., 2009). These associations remain consistent also after adjusting for a variety of paternal characteristics (i.e., demographics and lifestyle), child dietary patterns, family meals, television watching, and participation in sports and exercise during childhood (Mamun et al., 2009). For the most part, the behavioral problems of overweight children do not reach the intensity of full-blown behavioral disorders. Nevertheless, over a half of obese school-age children may be diagnosed with full-blown attention deficit hyperactivity disorder (ADHD; Agranat-Meged et al., 2005), and overweight children show a greater preponderance of ADHD symptoms of both inattention, for example, deficits in set shifting and attention abilities, and impulsivity in comparison to normal-weight youngsters (Braet et al., 2007; Cserjési et al., 2007).

Eating Disorders and Obesity in Children and Adolescents

The rate of eating disorders (EDs), including anorexia nervosa (AN), bulimia nervosa (BN), binge eating disorder (BED), and/or ED not otherwise specified (ED-NOS), is found to be significantly greater in clinically referred overweight youngsters compared to population-based overweight groups (Britz et al., 2000; Schuetzmann et al., 2008; Van Vlierberghe et al., 2009). Moreover, clinically referred patients with childhood-onset obesity have a significantly higher lifetime prevalence of EDs in general, and of BN in particular, than adult-onset obesity patients (Guerdjikova et al., 2007). Still, although psychological traits associated with disordered eating, for example, pursuit of thinness and body dissatisfaction, appear among community samples of obese patients, being close in the respect to young ED patients, these obese youngsters do not usually show clinically full-blown EDs (Lundstedt et al., 2006). Furthermore, if an overweight youngster has an ED, its course and outcome are less favorable if the ED develops in the context of pre-morbid normal weight, in comparison to pre-morbid overweight (Bean et al., 2004).

Although obesity per se is not classified as an ED, it shares important psychosocial antecedents with EDs. Accordingly, peer teasing, disturbed self- and body-esteem, and self-directed and naturalistic dieting may be all precursors for the development of both disturbances (Field et al., 2003; Puhl & Latner, 2007; Tanofsky-Kraft et al., 2006). Furthermore, elevated weight may increase the risk for the development of an ED (Levine and Smolak, 2008), and, conversely, disturbed eating, in particular binge eating, may predict an increase in body fat in children at risk to develop later obesity (Tanofsky-Kraft et al., 2006). It is, thus, not surprising that the prevention programs targeted for both problems are similar in many cardinal aspects (Levine and Smolak, 2008), and programs aimed toward reducing the risk of one may often improve also the condition of the other (Neumark-Sztainer et al., 2007).

Binge Eating Disorder (BED) in Childhood Obesity

BED is defined as a subcategory of the ED-NOS diagnosis in which uncontrolled binge eating episodes occur at least twice a week for a period of no less than three consecutive months, with no evidence of weight-reduction compensatory behaviors (APA, 1994). Two patterns of BED have been identified in both adults and adolescents, in that the onset of binge eating may occur either before or after the onset of dieting. Whereas in the dieting-associated BED subtype, binge eating usually appears in late adolescence, in non-dieting BED, it may appear as early as 11 to 13 years of age (Latner et al., 2007; Marcus & Kalcharian, 2003; Tzischinsky & Latzer, 2006 a,b).

BED is currently considered a major clinical problem in overweight individuals (Philips & Hill, 1998; Spitzer et al., 1993) in that 20 to 40% of severely obese adults (Marcus et al., 1992; Yanovski et al., 1993) and adolescents (Ackard et al., 2003; Berkowitz et al., 1993; Britz et al., 2000; Decaluwe et al., 2003; Philips & Hill, 1998; Severi et al., 1993) seeking treatment report significant binge eating symptomatology (Glasofer et al., 2007; Goossens et al., 2009a; Lock, 2007; Tanofsky-Kraff et al., 2005).

The prevalence of BED among adult overweight individuals in the general community is much lower (five to eight percent) (Marcus, 1995). Although the findings for children and adolescents are still inconclusive (Marcus & Kalcharian, 2003), some studies have shown that up to 5.3% of overweight children six to ten years of age may be diagnosed with BED (Morgan et al., 2002).

Studies that have associated binge eating only with eating a large amount of food have shown that boys report more binges and recurrent bingeing behaviors, but girls are more embarrassed and self-critical about their binges (Whitaker, 1989). By contrast, studies that define binge eating as including loss of control over eating as well have found a greater extent of bingeing behaviors among girls, in keeping with findings in adults (Croll et al., 2002; Goldschmidt et al., 2008; Goossens et al., 2007; Tanofsky-Kraff et al., 2008; Tanofsky-Kraff et al., 2009). With respect to age, binge eating has been found to increase with age for Caucasian youngsters and decrease with age for African-American youngsters, independent of gender (Johnson et al., 2002). Compensatory weight reduction purging and non-purging restricting behaviors occur only infrequently in overweight youngsters.

For both children and adolescents, a personal and family history of obesity likely increases the risk for the development of binge eating problems when adverse childhood experiences, problematic family relationships and/or maladaptive parental eating-related attitudes, weak social support, and risk factors for psychiatric morbidity (particularly depression, but also emotional disinhibition) are also present (Fisher & Birch, 2002; Johnson et al., 2002). It is not yet clear whether binge eating or BED in childhood and adolescence continuous to BED in adulthood (Marcus & Kalcharian, 2003).

The implications of binge-eating behavior have been repeatedly investigated in overweight adults, but only a few studies have evaluated this behavior in overweight children and adolescents. The presence of binge eating behavior in overweight individuals signifies overall greater eating-related and non-eating related lifetime morbidity in comparison to non-binge eating overweight, although an inclination towards more severe overweight has been found only in adult (French et al., 1999) but not in adolescent binge eaters. Non-bingeing severely overweight adults (Renman et al., 1999) and adolescents (Philips & Hill, 1998) report relatively few psychological difficulties, although they do score low on self-esteem and may show considerable social difficulties. By contrast, overweight children and adolescents with binge eating behavior and BED, characterized by a loss of control over eating above and beyond overeating, show problematic eating behaviors (particularly eating in the absence of hunger and eating in secrecy) (Eddy et al., 2007; Fisher & Birch, 2002; Tanofsky-Kraff et al., 2004). These youngsters eat significantly more, have greater weight and shape concerns, as well as significantly elevated levels of depressive and anxiety symptoms and significantly lower self-esteem when compared to non-bingeing overweight youngsters (Goossens et al., 2009b; Morgan et al., 2002; Philips & Hill, 1998; Tanofsky-Kraff et al., 2004). In addition, the greater the severity of bingeing behavior among overweight youngsters, the more these youngsters are at risk to develop depression, anxiety, and self- and body-esteem problems (Philips & Hill, 1998; Goossens et al., 2009b).

Both adult and adolescent overweight binge eaters do not usually compensate for bingeing episodes by restricting food intake between episodes (Epstein et al., 1994), and loss of control over eating in pediatric binge eating is usually not associated with dieting (Morgan et al., 2002). Dieting behavior is usually not a necessary factor for the development of binge eating in overweight children (Marcus & Kalcharian, 2003), whereas adult binge-eating individuals do diet more frequently than overweight non-binge eaters. From a different perspective, studies among adults have shown that BED and BN represent different syndromes on a continuum of disturbed eating that are likely associated with different etiological factors (Marcus & Kalcharian, 2003). Accordingly BN patients show an overall greater eating-related and non-eating related psychopathology (Salvemini et al., 2000). This phenomenon has not been investigated yet in adolescents, but apparently BED in youngsters does not develop into BN in later life (Marcus & Kalcharian, 2003).

Binge eating behavior can be identified early in childhood (Morgan et al., 2002; Tanofsky-Kraff et al., 2007), is relatively frequent among young overweight individuals, and can lead to considerable emotional distress and psychiatric morbidity (Goossens et al., 2009b; Marcus & Kalcharian, 2003; Tanofsky-Kraff et al., 2004). Nevertheless, although binge eating is defined identically in children, adolescents and adults, converging evidence indicates that it is difficult to systematically diagnose BED in young children with accepted adult criteria (APA, 1994; Goldschmidt et al., 2007). Factors considered of particular relevance for this diagnostic ambiguity are the inclination of children either not to understand the meaning of loss of control when it comes to binge-eating or to frankly deny such behaviors when asked about their eating habits, out of shame and embarrassment (Eddy et al., 2007; Spitzer et al., 1993; Tanofsky-Kraff et al., 2004). Additionally, parents also tend to deny such behaviors in their children for similar reasons. Large-scale community studies that apply broad, less stringent and developmentally appropriate criteria for the characterization of BED (for example, inclusion of food seeking in the absence of hunger, and sneaking or hiding food), and that use age appropriate interview techniques for both children and parents are required for a better characterization of BED in younger age groups (Goldschmidt et al., 2007; Marcus & Kalcharian, 2003; Tanofsky-Kraff et al., 2007).

Conclusion

Several important findings are highlighted in the present review. Parents may often not worry about their children being overweight, as they tend to underestimate the severity and to misperceive what their children actually eat. Nevertheless, overweight children are negatively influenced to a greater extent by their parents' criticism than by their actual BMI. In contrast, lack of parental criticism about the child being overweight may be a protective factor for the child's self-esteem and overall coping and well-being.

The school and social performance of obese children and their overall quality of life are often less favorable compared to their normal-weight peers. This is related to greater school absenteeism and overall social stress, less nutritious diet and physical activity, and less favorable neuropsychological functioning.

Not all obese youngsters show low self esteem, and the association between the extent of being overweight and global self-esteem is not straightforward. By contrast, negative body esteem is usually correlated with the severity of being overweight. Normal-weight children tend to show negative attitudes towards their overweight peers. Obese adolescents are usually considered less popular than normal-weight teens, and being overweight during childhood and adolescence may be associated with considerable societal victimization and peer teasing. Moreover, obese children themselves perceive negatively many of their own characteristics and attach them to their being overweight.

Overweight children in community-based samples do not usually show a greater extent of psychiatric morbidity in comparison to normal-weight populations. By contrast, clinically referred youngsters show elevated rates of depression, anxiety, behavioral disturbances, attention deficit hyperactivity disorder, and eating disorders. BED in youngsters does not usually follow a course of dieting. Its presence in overweight children increases the likelihood of overall psychopathology. BED may be difficult to diagnose during childhood, and adult criteria are often not suitable for children.

In line with the main findings of our review, we recommend that the psychological assessment of overweight/obese young individuals should be performed with age- and developmentally appropriate criteria and tools. Any psychological assessment should relate to the parents' and children's attitudes with respect to being overweight and should assess the children's overall psychological functioning and psychiatric condition, their strengths as well as their weaknesses.

The limitations of the present status of the research in pediatric and adolescent overweight issues, reflected also in the present review, should be outlined. There is a paucity of well-designed studies that would encourage primary health care professionals to integrate the relevant psychosocial issues described in this review and others in their evaluation procedures and intervention strategies. In particular, the use of adult psychosocial assessment tools, adult psychiatric diagnoses, and adult intervention strategies has not been validated in younger populations. Future research requires the design of prospective and longitudinal studies with appropriate sample sizes, age-appropriate assessment techniques, inclusion of the families and social organizations in the interventions, and adequate long-term follow-up.

References

Ackard, D., Neumark-Sztainer, D., Story, M. & Perry, C. (2003). Overeating among adolescents: Prevalence and associations with weight-related characteristics and psychological health. *Pediatrics, 111,* 67-74.

Adams, A.K., Quinn, R.A. & Prince, R.J. (2005). Low recognition of childhood overweight and disease risk among Native- American caregivers. *Obesity Research, 13*, 146–152.

Agranat-Meged, D. C., Goldzweig, G., Leibenson, L., Stein, M. & Galili-Weisstub, E. (2005). Childhood obesity and attention deficit/hyperactivity disorder: a newly described comorbidity in obese hospitalized children. *International Journal of Eating Disorders, 37*, 357-359.

Alatupa, S., Pulkki-Råback, L., Hintsanen, M., Ravaja, N., Raitakari, O.T., Telama, R., Viikari, J.S. & Keltikangas-Järvinen, L. (2010). School performance as a predictor of adulthood obesity: a 21-year follow-up study. *European Journal of Epidemiology*, Feb 4. [Epub ahead of print]

American Psychiatric Association. (1994). *Diagnostic and Statistical Manual of Mental Disorders,* (4th Edition). Washington, DC: American Psychiatric Association. pp. 549-550.

Anderson, S.E., Cohen, P., Naumova, E.N. & Must, A. (2006). Relationship of childhood behavior disorders to weight gain from childhood into adulthood. *Ambulatory Pediatrics, 6*, 297-301.

Baughcum, A.E., Chamberlin, L.A., Deeks, C.M., Powers, S.W. & Whitaker, R.C. (2000). Maternal perceptions of overweight preschool children. *Pediatrics, 106,* 1380-1386.

Bellizzi, M.C. & Dietz, W.H. (1999). Workshop on childhood obesity: summary of the discussion. *American Journal of Clinical Nutrition*, *70*, 173S-175S.

Berkowitz, R., Stunkard, A.J. & Stallings, V.A. (1993). Binge-eating disorder in obese adolescent girls. *Annals of the New York Academy of Sciences, 699,* 200-206.

Birch, L.L., Fisher, J.O. & Davison, K.K. (2003). Learning to overeat: Maternal use of restrictive feeding practices promotes girls eating in the absence of hunger. *American Journal of Clinical Nutrition, 78,* 215-220.

Boneberger, A., von Kries, R., Milde-Busch, A., Bolte, G., Rochat, M.K. & Rückinger, S. (2009). GME Study Group. Association between peer relationship problems and childhood overweight/obesity. *Acta Paediatrica, 98*, 1950-1955.

Booth, M.L., King, L.A., Pagnini, D.L., Wilkenfeld, R.L. & Booth, S.L. (2009). Parents of school students on childhood overweight: the Weight of Opinion Study. *Journal of Paediatrics and Child Health, 45*, 194-198.

Braet, C., Claus, L., Verbeken, S. & Van Vlierberghe, L. (2007). Impulsivity in overweight children. *European Child and Adolescent Psychiatry, 16*, 473-483.

Britz, B., Siegfried, W. & Ziegler, A. (2000). Rates of psychiatric disorders in a clinical study group of adolescents with extreme obesity and in obese adolescents ascertained via population based study. *International Journal of Obesity*, *24,* 1707-1714.

Burdette, H.L., Whitaker, R.C., Hall, W.C. & Daniels, S.R. (2006). Maternal infant-feeding style and children's adiposity at 5 years of age. *Archives of Pediatrics and Adolescent Medicine, 160*, 513-520.

Campbell, M.W., Williams, J., Hampton, A. & Wake, M. (2006a). Maternal concern and perceptions of overweight in Australian preschool-aged children. *Medical Journal of Australia, 184*, 274-277.

Campbell, K.J., Crawford, D.A. & Ball, K. (2006b). Family environment and dietary behaviors likely to promote fatness in 5–6-year-old children. *International Journal of Obesity, 30*, 1272–1280.

Cawley, J. & Spiess, C.K. (2008). Obesity and skill attainment in early childhood. *Economics and Human Biology, 6*, 388-397.

Center for Disease Control and Prevention. (2004). *Overweight among* U.S. *Children and adolescents. National Health and Nutrition Examination Survey*. January 2004.

Chandola, T., Deary, I.J., Blane, D. & Batty, G.D. (2006). Childhood IQ in relation to obesity and weight gain in adult life: the National Child Development (1958) Study. *International Journal of Obesity, 30*, 1422-1432.

Cole, T.J., Bellizzi, M.C., Flegal, K.M. & *Dietz,* W.H. (2000). Establishing a standard definition for child overweight and obesity worldwide: international survey. *British Medical Journal, 320*, 1240-1243.

Cornette, R. (2008). The emotional impact of obesity on children. *Worldviews Evidence Based Nursing, 5*, 136-141.

Cullen, K.W., Baranowski, T., Rittenberry, L. & Olvera, N. (2000). Social-environmental influences on children's diets: Results from focus groups with African-, Euro- and Mexican-American children and their parents. *Health Education Research*, *15*, 581-590.

Crawford, D., Timperio, A., Telford, A. & Salmon, J. (2006). Parental concerns about childhood obesity and the strategies employed to prevent unhealthy weight gain in children. *Public Health Nutrition, 9*, 889-895.

Croll, J., Neumark-Sztainer, D., Story, M. & Ireland, M. (2002). Prevalence and risk and protective factors related to disordered eating behaviors among adolescents. Relationship to gender and ethnicity. *Journal of Adolescent Health, 31*, 166-175.

Cserjési, R., Molnár, D., Luminet, O. & Lénárd, L. (2007). Is there any relationship between obesity and mental flexibility in children? *Appetite, 49,* 675-678.

Davison, K.K. & Birch, L.L. (2001). Weight status, parent reaction, and self-concept in 5-year-old girls. *Pediatrics*, *107*, 46-53.

Decaluwe, V., Braet, C. & Fairburn, C.G. (2003) Binge eating in obese children and adolescents. *International Journal of Eating Disorders, 33*, 78-84

Doolen, J., Alpert, P.T. & Miller, S.K. (2009). Parental disconnect between perceived and actual weight status of children: a metasynthesis of the current research. *Journal of American Academy of Nurse Practitioner, 2*, 160-166.

Duarte, C.S., Sourander, A., Nikolakaros, G., Pihlajamaki, H., Helenius, H., Piha, J., Kumpulainen, K., Moilanen, I., Tamminen, T., Almqvist, F. & Must, A. (2010). Child mental health problems and obesity in early adulthood. *Journal of Pediatrics, 156*, 93-97.

Dubois, L. & Girad, M. (2007). Accuracy of maternal reports of pre-schoolers' weights and heights as estimates of BMI values. *International Journal of Epidemiology, 36*, 132-138.

Eddy, K., Tanofsky-Kraff, M., Thompson-Brenner, H., Herzog, D., Brown, T. & Ludwig, D. (2007). Eating disorder pathology among overweight treatment-seeking youth: Clinical correlates and cross-sectional risk modeling. *Behavior Research and Therapy, 45*, 2360-2371.

Edmunds, L.D. (2005). Parents' perceptions of health professionals' responses when seeking help for their overweight children. *Family Practice, 22*, 287-292.

Epstein, L.H., Klein, K.R. & Wisniewski, L. (1994). Child and parent factors that influence psychological problems in obese children. *International Journal of Eating Disorders*, *15*, 151-157.

Epstein, L.H., Valoski, A., Wing, R.R. & McCurley, J. (1994). Ten years follow-up of behavioral, family-based treatment for obese children. *Health Psychology*, *13*, 373-383.

Epstein, L.H., Roemmich, J.N. & Raymor, H.A. (2001). Behavioral therapy in the treatment of pediatric obesity. *Pediatric Clinics of North America*, *48,* 981-993.

Falkner, N.H., Neumark-Sztainer, D. & Story, M. (2001). Social, educational, and psychological correlates of weight status in adolescents. *Obesity Research*, *9,* 32-42.

Field, A., Austin, S.B., Taylor, C.B., Malspeis, S., Rosner, B., Rockett, H., Gillman, M. & Colditz, G. (2003). Relation between dieting and weight change among preadolescents and adolescents. *Pediatrics, 112*, 900-906.

Fisher, J.O. & Birch, L.L. (2002). Eating in the absence of hunger and overweight in girls from 5-7 years of age. *American Journal of Clinical Nutrition*, *76,* 226-231.

Flodmark, C.E. (2005). The happy obese child. International Journal of Obesity, 29, S31-S33.

French, S.A., Story, M. & Perry, C.L. (1995). Self-esteem and obesity in children and adolescents: a literature review. *Obesity Research, 3*, 479-490.

French, S.A., Jeffery, R.W. & Sherwood, N.E. (1999). Prevalence and correlates of binge eating in a nonclinical sample of women enrolled in a weight gain prevention program. *International Journal of Obesity, 23,* 576-585.

Geier, A.B., Foster, G.D., Womble, L.G., McLaughlin, J., Borradaile, K.E., Nachmani, J., Sherman, S., Kumanyika, S. & Shults, J. (2007). The relationship between relative weight and school attendance among elementary schoolchildren. *Obesity, 15*, 2157-2161.

Genovesi, S., Giussani, M., Faini, A., Vigorita, F., Pieruzzi, F., Strepparava, M.G., Stella, A. & Valsecchi, M.G. (2005). Maternal perception of excess weight in children: a survey conducted by pediatricians in the province of Milan. *Acta Paediatrica, 94*, 747-752.

Glasofer, D., Tanofsky-Kraff, M., Eddy, K., Yanovski, S., Theim, K., Mirch, M., Ghorbani, S., Ranzenhofer, L.M., Haaga, D. & Yanovski, J.A. (2007). Binge eating in overweight treatment-seeking adolescents. *Journal of Pediatric Psychology, 32*, 95-105.

Goldschmidt, A., Doyle, A. & Wilfley, D. (2007). Assessment of binge eating on overweight youth using a questionnaire version of the child eating disorder examination with instructions. *International Journal of Eating Disorders, 40*, 460-467.

Goldschmidt, A., Jones, M., Manwaring, J., Luce, K., Osborne, M., Cunning, D., Taylor, K.L., Doyle, A.C., Wilfley, D.E. & Taylor, C.B. (2008). The clinical significance of loss of control over eating in overweight adolescents. *International Journal of Eating Disorders, 41*, 153-158.

Goodell, S.L., Pierce, M.B., Bravo, C.M. & Ferris, A.M. (2008). Parental perceptions of overweight during early childhood. *Qualitative Health Research, 18*, 1548-1555.

Goossens, L., Braet, C. & Decaluwe, V. (2007). Loss of control over eating in obese youngsters. *Behavior Research and Therapy, 45(1)*, 1-9.

Goossens, L., Soenens, B. & Braet, C. (2009a). Prevalence and Characteristics of Binge Eating in an Adolescent Community Sample. *Journal of Clinical Child and Adolescents Psychology, 38(3)*, 342-353.

Goossens, L., Braet, C., Van Vlierberghe, L. & Mels, S. (2009b). Loss of Control Over Eating in Overweight Youngsters: The Role of Anxiety, Depression and Emotional Eating. *European Eating Disorders Review, 17(1)*, 68-78.

Gortmaker, S.L., Must, A., Perrin, J.M., Sobol, A.M. & Dietz, W.H. (1993). Social and economic consequences of overweight in adolescence and young adulthood. *New England Journal of Medicine, 329,* 1008-1012.

Gray, W.N., Janicke, D.M., Ingerski, L.M., Silverstein, J.H. (2008). The impact of peer victimization, parent distress and child depression on barrier formation and physical activity in overweight youth. *Journal of Developmental and Behavioral Pediatrics, 29,* 26-33.

Guerdjikova, A.I., McElroy, S.L., Kotwal, R., Stanford, K. & Keck, P.E. Jr. (2007). Psychiatric and metabolic characteristics of childhood versus adult-onset obesity in patients seeking weight management. *Eating Behaviors, 8*, 266-276.

Hackie, M. & Bowles, C.L. (2007). Maternal perception of their overweight children. *Public Health Nursing, 24*, 538-546.

Harris, J.L., Pomeranz, J.L., Lobstein, T. & Brownell, K.D. (2009). A crisis in the marketplace: how food marketing contributes to childhood obesity and what can be done. A crisis in the marketplace: how food marketing contributes to childhood obesity and what can be done. *Annual Review of Public Health, 30,* 211-225.

Hawkins, S.S., Cole, T.J. & Law, C. (2008). Maternal employment and early childhood overweight: findings from the UK Millennium Cohort Study. *International Journal of Obesity, 32*, 30-38.

Hebebrand, J. & Hinney, A. (2009). Environmental and genetic risk factors in obesity. *Child and Adolescent Psychiatric Clinics of North America, 18*, 83-94.

Hirschler, V., Gonzalez, C., Talgham, S. & Jadzinsky, M. (2006). Do mothers of overweight Argentinean preschool children perceive them as such? *Pediatric Diabetes, 7*, 201-204.

Israel, A.C. & Ivanova, M.Y. (2002). Global and dimensional self-esteem in preadolescent and early adolescent children who are overweight: age and gender differences. *International Journal of Eating Disorders, 3,* 424-429.

Jain, A., Sherman, S.N., Chamberlin, D.L., Carter, Y., Powers. S.W. & Whitaker, R.C. (2001). Why don't low-income mothers worry about their preschoolers being overweight? *Pediatrics, 107*, 1138-1146.

Janicke, D.M., Harman, J.S., Kelleher, K.J. & Zhang, J. (2008). Psychiatric diagnosis in children and adolescents with obesity-related health conditions. *Journal of Developmental and Behavioral Pediatrics, 29*, 276-284.

Jiang, J., Rosenqvist, U., Wang, H., Greiner, T., Ma, Y. & Toschke, A.M. (2006). Risk factors for overweight in 2- to 6-year-old children in Beijing, China. *International Journal of Pediatric Obesity, 1*, 103-108.

Johnson, W.G., Rohan, K.J. & Kirk, K.K. (2002). Prevalence and correlates of binge eating in white and African American adolescents. *Eating Behaviors, 3,* 179-189.

Johnson, J.G., Cohen, P., Kotler, L., Kasen, S. & Brooks, J.S. (2002). Psychiatric disorders associated with the risk for the development of eating disorders during adolescence and early adulthood. *Journal of Consulting and Clinical Psychology, 70,* 1119-1128.

Kersey, M., Lipton, R., Quinn, M.T. & Lantos, J.D. (2010). Overweight in Latino preschoolers: do parental health beliefs matter? *American Journal of Health Behavior, 34*, 340-348.

Kestilä, L., Rahkonen, O., Martelin, T., Lahti-Koski, M. & Koskinen, S. (2009). Do childhood social circumstances affect overweight and obesity in early adulthood? *Scandinavian Journal of Public Health, 37*, 206-219

Kroke, A., Strathmann, S. & Günther, A.L. (2006). Maternal perceptions of her child's body weight in infancy and early childhood and their relation to body weight status at age 7. *European Journal of Pediatrics, 165*, 875-883.

Krukowski, R.A., West, D.S., Siddiqui, N.J., Bursac, Z., Phillips, M.M. & Raczynski, J.M. (2008). No change in weight-based teasing when school-based obesity policies are implemented. *Archives of Pediatrics and Adolescent Medicine, 162*, 936-942.

Krukowski, R.A., West, D. S., Perez, A. P., Bursac, Z., Phillips, M.M. & Raczynski, J.M. (2009). Overweight children, weight-based teasing and academic performance. *International Journal of Pediatric Obesity, 4*, 274-280.

Lampard, A.M., Byrne, S.M., Zubrick, S.R. & Davis, E.A. (2008). Parents' concern about their children's weight. *International Journal of Pediatric Obesity, 3*, 84-92.

Latner, J.D., Rosewall, J.K. & Simmonds, M.B. (2007). Childhood obesity stigma: association with television, videogame, and magazine exposure. *Body Image, 4*, 147-155.

Latner, J., Hildebrandt, T., Rosewall, J., Chisholm, A. & Hayashi, K. (2007). Loss of control over eating reflects eating disturbances and general psychopathology. *Behavior Research and Therapy, 45(9)*, 2203-2211.

Levine, M.P. & Smolak, L. (2008). "What exactly are we waiting for?" The case for universal-selective eating disorders prevention programs. *International Journal of Child and Adolescent Health, 1*, 295-304.

Li, Y.P., Ma, G.S., Schouten, E.G., Hu, X.Q., Cui, Z.H., Wang, D. & Kok, F.J. (2007). Report on childhood obesity in China (5): body weight, body dissatisfaction, and depression symptoms of Chinese children aged 9-10 years. *Biomedical and Environmental Sciences, 20*, 11-18.

Li, Y., Dai, Q., Jackson, J.C. & Zhang, J. (2008). Overweight is associated with decreased cognitive functioning among school-age children and adolescents. *Obesity, 16*, 1809-1815.

Lissau, I., Overpeck, M.D., Ruan, W.J., Due, P., Holstein, B.E. & Hediger, M.L. (2004). Body mass index and overweight in adolescents in 13 European countries, Israel, and the United States. *Archives of Pediatric and Adolescent Medicine, 158*, 27-33.

Lock, J. (2007). Classification of child and adolescent eating disturbances—Workgroup for classification of eating disorders in children and adolescents (WCEDCA). *International Journal of Eating Disorders, 40*, S117-S122.

Lundstedt, G., Edlund, B., Engström, I., Thurfjell, B. & Marcus, C. (2006). Eating disorder traits in obese children and adolescents. *Eating and Weight Disorders, 11*, 45-50.

Mamun, A.A., O'Callaghan, M.J., Cramb, S.M., Najman, J.M., Williams, G.M. & Bor, W. (2009). Childhood behavioral problems predict young adults' BMI and obesity: evidence from a birth cohort study. *Obesity, 17*, 761-766.

Manus, H.E. & Killeen, M.R. (1995). Maintenance of self-esteem by obese children. *Journal of Child and Adolescence Psychiatric Nursing, 8,* 17-27.

Marcus, M.D., Smith, D. & Santelli, R. (1992). Characterization of eating disordered behavior in obese binge eaters. *International Journal of Eating Disorders, 12,* 249-255.

Marcus, M. (1995). Binge Eating and Obesity. In: Brownell KD, Fairburn CG, eds. *Eating disorders and obesity, a comprehensive book.* 1st Ed. New York: The Guilford Press. pp 441-444.

Marcus, M.D. & Kalcharian, M.A. (2003). Binge eating in children and adolescents. *International Journal of Eating Disorders, 34*(Suppl.), S47-S57.

Marsh, H.W., Hau, K.T., Sung, R.Y. & Yu, C.W. (2007). Childhood obesity, gender, actual-ideal body image discrepancies, and physical self-concept in Hong Kong children: cultural differences in the value of moderation. *Developmental Psychology, 43*, 647-662.

Maynard, M.J., Baker, G., Rawlins, E., Anderson, A. & Harding, S. (2009). Developing obesity prevention interventions among minority ethnic children in schools and places of worship: The DEAL (DiEt and Active Living) study. *BMC Public Health, 9*, 480-490.

McCullough, N., Muldoon, O. & Dempster, M. (2009). Self-perception in overweight and obese children: a cross-sectional study. *Child Care Health and Development, 35*, 357-364.

McGinnis, J.M., Gootman, J.A. & Kraak, V.I. (Eds.) (2006). *Food Marketing to Children and Youth: Threat or Opportunity?* Washington, D.C.: National Academies Press.

Mond, J.M., Stich, H., Hay, P.J., Kraemer, A. & Baune, B.T. (2007). Associations between obesity and developmental functioning in pre-school children: a population-based study. *International Journal of Obesity, 31*, 1068-1073.

Morgan, C.M., Yanoveski, S.Z. & Nguyan, T.T. (2002). Loss of control over eating adiposity and psychopathology in overweight children. *International Journal of Eating Disorders, 31*, 430-431.

Nazario Rodriguez, I.J., Figueroa, W.I., Rosado, J. & Parrilla Idel C. (2008). Perception of parents regarding their children's weight. *Boletin- Asociacion Medica de Puerto Rico, 100*, 33-38.

Neumark-Sztainer, D., Falkner, N., Story, M., Perry, C., Hannan, P. & Mulert, S. (2002). Weight-teasing among adolescents: Correlations with weight status and disordered eating behaviors. *International Journal of Obesity and Related Metabolic Disorders, 26,* 123-131.

Nsiah-Kumi, P.A., Ariza, A.J., Mikhail, L.M., Feinglass, J. & Binns, H.J. (2009). Pediatric Practice Research Group. Family history and parents' beliefs about consequences of childhood overweight and their influence on children's health behaviors. *Academic Pediatric, 9*, 53-59.

Nowicka, P., Höglund, P., Birgerstam, P., Lissau, I., Pietrobelli, A. & Flodmark, C.E. (2009). Self-esteem in a clinical sample of morbidly obese children and adolescents. *Acta Paediatrica, 98*, 153-158.

Ogden, C.L., Flegal, K.M., Carroll, M.D. & Johnson, C.L. (2002). Prevalence and trends in overweight among U.S. children and adolescents, 1999-2000. *JAMA, 288*, 1728-1732.

Ogden, C.L., Carroll, M.D., Curtin, L.R., McDowell, M.A., Tabak, C.J. & Flegal, K.M. (2006). Prevalence of overweight and obesity in the United States, 1999–2004. *JAMA, 295*, 1549–1555.

Ogden, C.L., Carroll, M.D., Curtin, L.R., Lamb, M.M. & Flegal, K.M. (2010). Prevalence of high body mass index in U.S. children and adolescents, 2007-2008. *JAMA, 303*, 242-249.

Pagnini, D.L., Wilkenfeld, R.L., King, L.A., Booth, M.L. & Booth, S.L. (2007a). Mothers of pre-school children talk about childhood overweight and obesity: The Weight Of Opinion Study. *Journal of Paediatrics and Child Health, 43*, 806-810.

Park, C.M., Kim, M.D., Hong, S.C., Kim, Y., Hyun, M.Y., Kwak, Y.S., Lee, C.I., Park, M.J., Jang, Y.H., Moon, J.H., Seok, E.M., Song, Y.J. & Ju, K. H. (2009). Effects of obesity and obesity-induced stress on depressive symptoms in Korean elementary school children. *International Journal of Social Psychiatry, 55*, 322-335.

Parry, L.L., Netuveli, G., Parry, J. & Saxena, S. (2008). A systematic review of parental perception of overweight status in children. *Journal of Ambulatory Care Management, 31*, 253-268.

Pearce, M.J., Boergers, J. & Prinstein, M.J. (2002). Adolescent obesity, overt and relational peer victimization, and romantic relationships. *Obesity Research, 10,* 386-393.

Pesa, J.A., Syre, T.R. & Jones, E. (2000). Psychosocial differences associated with body weight among female adolescents: The Importance of Body Image. *Journal of Adolescence Health*, *26,* 330-337.

Philips, R.G. & Hill, A.J. (1998). Fat, plain, but not friendless: self esteem and peer acceptance of obese pre-adolescent girls. *International Journal of Obesity and Related Metabolic Disorders*, *22,* 287-293.

Pinhas-Hamiel, O., Singer, S., Pilpel, N., Fradkin, A., Modan, D. & Reichman, B. (2006). Health-related quality of life among children and adolescents: associations with obesity. *International Journal of Obesity, 30*, 267-272.

Puhl, R.M. & Latner, J.D. (2007). Stigma, obesity, and the health of the nation's children. *Psychological Bulletin, 133*, 557-580.

Rainey, C.J., Kemper, K.A., Poling, R. & Tucker, S. (1998). Parents' perceptions of influences on child eating behaviors: An attitudinal approach. *Journal of Health Education*, *29*, 223-229.

Renman, C., Engstrom, I., Silverdal, S.A. & Aman, J. (1999). Mental health and psychosocial characteristics in adolescent obesity: a population based case-control study. *Acta Paediatrica*, *88*, 998-1003.

Rofey, D.L., Kolko, R.P., Iosif, A.M., Silk, J.S., Bost, J.E., Feng, W., Szigethy, E.M., Noll, R.B., Ryan, N.D. & Dahl, R.E. (2009). A longitudinal study of childhood depression and anxiety in relation to weight gain. *Child Psychiatry and Human Development, 40*, 517-526.

Roth, B., Munsch, S., Meyer, A., Isler, E. & Schneider, S. (2008). The association between mothers' psychopathology, children's competences and psychological well-being in obese children. *Eating and Weight Disorders, 13*, 129-136

Rumpel, C. & Harris, T. (1994). The influence of weight on adolescent self-esteem. *Journal of Psychosomatic Research*, *38,* 547-556.

Salanave, B., Peneau, S., Rolland-Cachera, M.F., Hercberg, S. & Castetbon, K. (2009). Stabilization of overweight prevalence in French children between 2000 and 2007. *International Journal of Pediatric Obesity, 4*, 66-72.

Salvemini, V., Berna, G., Foca, F., Indrimi, M., Sammartino, F., Spinosa, L. & Tulli, F. (2000). Differences and similarities in the personality structure of 327 women with eating disorders. *Eating and Weight Disorders, 5,* 108-115.

Schuetzmann, M., Richter-Appelt, H., Schulte-Markwort, M. & Schimmelmann, B.G. (2008). Associations among the perceived parent-child relationship, eating behavior, and body weight in preadolescents: results from a community-based sample. *Journal of Pediatric Psychology, 33*, 772-782.

Severi, F., Verri, A. & Livieri, C. (1993). Eating behavior and psychological profile in childhood obesity. *Advances in Bioscience*, *90,* 329-336.

Shin, N.Y. & Shin, M.S. (2008). Body dissatisfaction, self-esteem, and depression in obese Korean children. *Journal of Pediatrics, 152*, 502-506.

Sigfúsdóttir, I.D., Kristjánsson, A.L. & Allegrante, J.P. (2007). Health behavior and academic achievement in Icelandic school children. *Health Education Research, 22*, 70-80.

Speiser, P.W., Rudolf, M.C.J., Anhalt, H., Camacho-Hubner, C., Chiarelli, F., Eliakim, A., Freemark, M., Gruters, A., Hershkovitz, E., Iughetti, L., Krude, H., Latzer, Y., Lustig, R.H., Hirsch Pescovitz, O., Pinhas-Hamiel, O., Rogol, A.D., Shalitin, S., Sultan, C., Stein, D., Vardi, P., Werther, G.A., Zadik, Z., Zuckerman-Levin, N. & Hochberg, Z. (2005). CONSENSUS STATEMENT: Childhood Obesity. *The Journal of Clinical Endocrinology & Metabolism*, *90,* 1871–1887.

Spitzer, R.L., Yanovski, S.Z. & Wadden, T. (1993). Binge eating disorder: Its further validation in a multisite study. *International Journal of Eating Disorders*, *13,* 137-153.

Stern, J.S. (2000). Survey of parental attitudes on their children's weight. Bethesda USA. 2. Conference Proceeding.

Stradmeijer, M., Bosch, J., Koops, W. & Seidell, J. (2000). Family functioning and psychosocial adjustment in overweight youngsters. *International Journal of Eating Disorders*, *27,* 110-114.

Strauss, R.S. (2000). Childhood obesity and self-esteem. *Pediatrics*, *105*, 1-5.

Strauss, R.S. & Pollack, H.A. (2003). Social marginalization of overweight children. *Archives of Pediatric and Adolescents Medicine, 157,* 746-752.

Sweeting, H., West, P. & Young, R. (2008). Obesity among Scottish 15 year olds 1987-2006: prevalence and associations with socio-economic status, well-being and worries about weight. *BMC Public Health, 8*, 404-410.

Tanofsky-Kraff, M., Yanovski, S., Wilfley, D., Marmarosh, C., Morgan, C. & Yanovski, J. (2004). Eating-disordered behaviors, body fat, and psychopathology in overweight and normal-weight children. *Journal of Consulting and Clinical Psychology, 72(1)*, 53-38.

Tanofsky-Kraff, M., Faden, D., Yanovski, S., Wilfley, D. & Yanovski, J. (2005). The perceived onset of dieting and loss of control eating behaviors in overweight children. *International Journal of Eating Disorders, 38(2)*, 112-122.

Tanofsky-Kraff, M., Goossens, L., Eddy, K., Ringham, R., Goldschmidt, A. &, Yanovski, S. (2007). A multisite investigation of binge eating behaviors in children and adolescents. *Journal of Consulting and Clinical Psychology, 75(6)*, 901-913.

Tanofsky—Kraff, M., Marcus, M., Yanovski, S. & Yanovski, J. (2008). Loss of control eating disorder in children age 12 years and younger: Proposed research criteria. *Eating Behaviors. 9*, 360-365.

Tanofsky-Kraff, M., Yanovski, S.Z., Schvey, N.A., Olsen, C.H., Gustafson, J. & Yanovski, J.A. (2009). A Prospective Study of Loss of Control Eating for Body Weight Gain in Children at High Risk for Adult Obesity. *International Journal of Eating Disorders, 42(1)*, 26-30.

Tanofsky-Kraff, M., Yanovski, S.Z., Schvey, N.A., Olsen, C.H., Gustafson, J. & Yanovski, J.A. (2009). A prospective study of loss of control eating for body weight gain in children at high risk for adult obesity. *International Journal of Eating Disorders, 42*, 26-30.

Tzischinsky, O. & Latzer, Y. (2006). Sleep-wake cycles in obese adolescents with and without binge eating episodes. *European Eating Disorders Review*, *14(2)*, 111-117.

Tzischinsky, O. & Latzer, Y. (2006). Sleep-wake cycles in obese children with and without binge-eating episodes. *Journal of Paediatrics and Child Health, 42(11)*, 688-693.

Vaidya, V. (2006). Psychosocial aspects of obesity. *Advances in Psychosomatic Medicine, 27*, 73-85.

Van Vlierberghe, L., Braet, C., Goossens, L. & Mels, S. (2009). Psychiatric disorders and symptom severity in referred versus non-referred overweight children and adolescents. *European Child and Adolescent Psychiatry, 18*, 164-173.

Wadden, T.A., Brown, G., Foster, G.D. & Linowitz, J.R. (1991). Salience of weight-related worries in adolescent males and females. *International Journal of Eating Disorders, 10*, 407-414.

Wallander, J.L., Taylor, W.C., Grunbaum, J.A., Franklin, F.A., Harrison, G.G., Kelder, S.H. & Schuster, M.A. (2009). Weight status, quality of life, and self-concept in African American, Hispanic, and white fifth-grade children. *Obesity, 17*, 1363-1368.

Wang, Y. & Lobstein, T. (2006). Worldwide trends in childhood overweight and obesity. *International Journal of Pediatric Obesity, 1*, 11–25.

Wang, F. & Veugelers, P.J. (2008). Self-esteem and cognitive development in the era of the childhood obesity epidemic. *Obesity Reviews, 9*, 615-623.

Wang, F., Wild, T.C., Kipp, W., Kuhle, S. & Veugelers, P.J. (2009). The influence of childhood obesity on the development of self-esteem. *Health Reports, 20*, 21-27.

Watkins, M.G., Clark, K.M., Foster, C.M., Welch, K.B. & Kasa-Vubu, J.Z. (2007). Relationships among body mass index, parental perceptions, birth weight and parental weight after referral to a weight clinic. *Journal of the National Medical Association, 99*, 908-913.

West, D.S., Raczynski, J.M., Phillips, M.M., Bursac, Z., Heath Gauss, C. & Montgomery, B.E. (2008). Parental recognition of overweight in school-age children. *Obesity, 16*, 630-636.

Whitaker, R.C., Wright, J.A., Pepe, M.S., Seidel, K.D. & Dietz, W.H. (1997). Predicting obesity in young adulthood from childhood and parental obesity. *New England Journal of Medicine, 37*, 869-873.

Whitaker, A., Davies, M., Shaffer, D., Johnson, J., Abrams, S., Walsh, B.T. & Kalikow, K. (1989). The struggle to be thin: A survey of anorexic and bulimic symptoms in non-referred adolescent populations. *Psychological Medicine, 19*, 143-163.

Willc, N., Erhart, M., Petersen, C. & Ravens-Sieberer, U. (2008). The impact of overweight and obesity on health-related quality of life in childhood—results from an intervention study. *BMC Public Health, 8*, 421-428,

World Health Organization (1992). *The ICD-10 Classification of Mental and Behavioral Disorders*. Geneva, Switzerland.

Yackobovitch-Gavan M., Nagelberg N., Phillip M., Ashkenazi-Hoffnung L., Hershkovitz E., Shalitin S. (2009)The influence of diet and/or exercise and parental compliance on health-related quality of life in obese children. *Nutr Res., 29*, 397-404.

Yanovski S.Z., Nelson J.E., Dubbert B.K. (1993). Association of binge eating disorder and psychiatric comorbidity in obese subjects. *American Journal of Psychiatry, 150*, 1472-1479.

Young-Hyman D., Tanofsky-Kraff M., Yanovski S.Z., Keil M., Cohen M.L., Peyrot M., Yanovski J.A. (2006). Psychological status and weight-related distress in overweight or at-risk-for-overweight children. *Obesity, 14*, 2249-58.

Zametkin A.J., Zoon C.K., Klein H.W., Munson S. (2004). Psychiatric aspects of child and adolescent obesity: A review of the past 10 years. *Journal of the American Academy of Child Adolescent Pychiatry, 43*, 134-150.

In: Pathways to Obesity and Main Roads to Recovery
Editor: Piergiuseppe Vinai
ISBN: 978-1-61122-740-6

Chapter V

Emotions Becoming Food: The Binge Eating Disorder

Piergiuseppe Vinai and Patrizia Todisco
No Profit Research Group Cuneo, Studi Cognitivi Post Graduate Psychotherapy School Research Group. Milan, Italy
Villa Margherita Eating Disorders Unit Vicenza, Italy

Abstract

Binge Eating Disorder (BED) is a quite common syndrome among obese individuals; clinical studies have shown a prevalence of BED up to 30% among obese persons seeking bariatric surgery. It is characterized by recurrent episodes of binge eating with a sensation of loss of control. Currently it is included in the Appendix B of the DSM IV TR as a disorder requiring further study, but the majority of researchers agree with clinicians in recognizing BED as a distinct eating disorder with specific clinical and psychopathological characteristics: impulsivity, low self-esteem and difficulties in regulating emotions. High levels of perceived stress and negative mood can trigger the binge episodes. The influence of the diagnosis of BED on the outcome of behavioral and surgical treatments for obesity is still an open question

Introduction

Frequently, obese patients seeking help to lose weight complain about their difficulty to control food intake. They often refer episodes in which they eat large amounts of food with a sensation of loss of control; this behavior makes vain any attempt to lose weight. In these cases, it is worth investigating the possible presence of Binge Eating Disorder (BED): a syndrome characterized by recurrent episodes of binge eating associated with other clinical characteristics and specific psychopathological features. It has been included in the Appendix

B of the DSM IV TR (APA 2000) as a disorder with research criteria requiring further study. This collocation is due to the intense debate that is going on in the scientific community regarding the opportunity to consider BED a specific pathology among eating disorders. Several researchers sustained that the differences between Bulimia Nervosa (BN) without compensatory behaviors and BED are more quantitative than qualitative, so they consider it a variant of this pathology. They hypothesize that bingeing is the common symptom of the Binge Spectrum Disorders including purging BN, non-purging BN and BED. According to this model, BED represents the less severe and unstable form of Bulimia Nervosa (Hay & Fairburn 1998). Other authors (Stunkard & Allison 2003) thought that BED emerges when obesity and depressive diathesis co-occur and consider binge episodes a marker of psychopathology among obese individuals. In the last years, the majority of clinicians, including ourselves, agree that BED is a diagnostic construct identifying a peculiar and stable pathology associated with elevated psychiatric co-morbidity, psychosocial impairment, medical problems, and it needs a specific treatment.

Diagnostic Criteria

Binge eating is common among obese individuals (Grissett, Fitzgibbon 1996), but Binge Eating Disorder affects not all the subjects who binge. This syndrome is characterized by recurrent episodes of binge eating i.e., to eat a larger amount of food than normal during a short period of time (within any two-hour period) experiencing a lack of control over eating during the episode: "*I cannot stop eating.*" Although the amount of food required is not quantified, several studies found that there is a concordance between BED patients and control subjects in defining the minimal quantity of eaten food necessary to have a binge.

The core characteristic of this symptom is the sensation of loss of control; it is not considered a bulimic episode to have second helpings during a meal or to exaggerate with food during a party with friends. A binge is associated with at least three of the following behavioral indicators of loss of control:

1. Eating until feeling uncomfortably full;
2. Eating large amounts of food when not feeling physically hungry;
3. Eating much more rapidly than usual;
4. Eating alone because of being embarrassed by how much one is eating;
5. Feeling disgusted, depressed, or guilty after overeating. Moreover a marked distress regarding binge eating is present, and this eating behavior is not associated with the regular use of inappropriate compensatory conducts (i.e., purging, excessive exercise, etc.) and doesn't occur during the course of bulimia or anorexia nervosa. The DSM IV definition states that symptoms take place at least two days a week for six months, but this criterion is currently under discussion. Probably in the next edition of the DSM, the frequency of binge eating and the time period necessary to diagnose the BED will be reduced respectively to once a week and three months for analogy with the diagnostic criteria of bulimia nervosa and because this option has the most empirical support (Wilson & Sysko, 2009). We highlight that in current apa criteria for BED is not mentioned neither patients'

weight nor over-concern about weight and shape unduly influencing self-esteem, while more recent research has tended to emphasize the relationship of BED to obesity (Wonderlich et al., 2009).

Epidemiology

Given the relatively recent definition of BED diagnostic criteria, epidemiologic research is limited. For instance, patients considered binge eaters in previous studies didn't meet current diagnostic criteria. Moreover, assessment strategies (self-reports versus interview-based assessments) influence prevalence results (Hoek, 2003). The overlap between epidemiologic studies regarding obesity and BED and the variability of BMI cut off to define obesity may also condition findings (Striegel-Moore, Franko, 2003). The literature has been focused on the association between obesity and Binge Eating Disorder (Yanovski, 2003; Reas DL, Grilo, 2007) but, despite the strong connection between obesity and eating disorders, the increase in obesity rates has not been followed by an increase in eating disorders rates.

Clinical studies have shown a prevalence of BED up to 30% among obese persons seeking bariatric surgery, (Dymek-Valentine et al., 2004; de Zwaan et al., 2003) and of 10% among persons seeking nonsurgical weight reduction. (de Man LJ, Ghaderi, 2006) Population-based studies of correlates to eating disorders have found obesity to be one of the few specific risk factors for BED (Fairburn et al., 1998) A review by Hoek and van Hoeken (2003) found that the estimated prevalence of BED was at least 1%, that is slightly higher than in subsequent studies. However, a similar rate of 1.2% was found by Ghaderi and Scott when examining the female Swedish population. Favaro et al., suggested lifetime EDNOS and BED figures of 4.7% and 0.6%, respectively. (Zachrisson et al., 2008). The Sesto Fiorentino Study (Faravelli et al., 2006), a community-based survey, found a lifetime prevalence of 0.32% for binge eating disorder.

Studies in the United States found prevalence of 1% to 3% in the general population (Striegel-Moore RH, Franko)., but not all applied population-based sampling strategies. Available evidence suggests that BED may be the most common eating disorder, had a later age of onset and a longer duration compared to AN or BN (Hudson et al., 2007). Furthermore, it is frequently associated with obesity, even though the precise contribution of BED to obesity remains an open question. Binge eating disorder is accompanied by substantial distress, impairment, and co-morbidity (Pike et al., 2001; Striegle-Moore et al., 2003; Hudson et al., 2007). Striegle-Moore and colleagues (2007) found that is well represented in Black women even though White women are more likely to have any of ED. In another study (Pike et al., 2001) regarding BED and non-BED women, the former showed higher BMI and prevalence of obesity. Additionally, there were some racial differences among BEDs: Black subjects were more likely to be obese, while White subjects had lower levels of psychiatric co-morbidity and eating-disordered psychopathology (Pike et al., 2001). As far as we know, BED is well represented in racial minorities and in older people (adults 30 to 40 y.o.) with a story of previous disordered eating around their twenties (usually binge-eating preceding food restriction: Binge First 81% vs. Diet First 19%) (Santonastaso et al., 1999). Moreover, all social classes are affected by this pathology, with lower classes slightly preeminent (Striegel-Moore 2000).

According to literature, almost 40% of BED subjects are male (age between 25 and 35 years), and the difference in the prevalence between the two sexes is not so in favor of females like in other EDs, the proportion being 3:2. There are few studies about the distribution of BED in the male population. One of them was conducted in Austria (Kinzl et al., 1999) and involved 1,000 males (age 18 to 88 years), interviewed by dietitians. The total prevalence of ED was 14.9% and 0.8% of the sample satisfied BED diagnostic criteria, while 4.2% had a sub-threshold binge eating syndrome, 9.4% an eating disorder not otherwise specified and 0.5% BN. These data support that, in non-clinical samples, BED is rarely found among men, while partial or atypical ED are more common (Kinzl et al., 1999).

These studies further reinforce the view that BED may affect a demographically more diverse group than AN or BN and may be more frequently found in obese than non-obese groups (Striegel-Moore RH, Franko DL. 2003; Wonderlich 2009). Besides, the results, relying on large community-based samples, imply that BED differs from other ED in a host of epidemiologic variables including age of onset, racial composition, association with obesity, and psychiatric co-morbidity.

Genetic

There are two approaches to the study of genetic influence on BED: family/twin studies and molecular genetics. As far as the first is concerned, family studies are unable to distinguish between genetic and environmental factors; twin studies, in contrast, are able to decompose liability to a trait into genetic and environmental influences. In a twin study regarding subjects who binged (although not BED patients), Bulik, Sullivan & Kendler (1998) evidenced a genetic influence on the vulnerability to binge-eating.

The disorder appears to aggregate in families (Hudson et al., 2006), but the contribution of genetic factors to this aggregation is unclear. In two smaller family studies of BED, Fowler and Bulik (1997) found significant evidence for familial aggregation (60%) and Lee et al., (1999) showed an effect size (odds ratio of 1.9), although the value was not statistically significant. A population-based study of Norwegian twins between 18 and 31 years old demonstrated a heritability estimate of 41% for BED, with the remaining variance attributable to environment both in female and male subjects. (Reichborn-Kjennerud T et al., 2004) In a recent case-control family study (Javaras et al.2008), findings were similar: BED aggregates in families, and its heritability, is estimated as 57% (CI: 30–77%). It is likely that the genetic factors for this disorder are only partially shared with those for obesity. The Boston family study (Javaras et al., 2008), for instance, demonstrated that there is a partial overlap between the familial factors for BED and obesity. A previous twin study (Bulik et al., 2003) showed separate, as well as shared, genetic factors for bingeing and obesity. Additional studies will be needed to determine the specific genes involved in BED, including those in common with obesity.

Only few molecular genetic studies on BED have been published. One of them (Branson et al., 2003) found an association of melanocortin-4 receptor mutations with BED in obese individuals, but two subsequent studies (Hebebrand et al., 2004, Lubrano-Berthelier et al., 2006) failed to replicate these findings. Other research has reported an association of BED with the Leu72Met polymorphism of the ghrelin gene (Monteleone et al., 2006, 2007), and with a polymorphism of the promoter of the serotonin transporter gene. Summarizing, BED appears to aggregate in families and have a significant genetic component, but further evidence is needed given the exiguity of data at the moment.

Clinical Features

The majority of researchers agree with clinicians in recognizing BED as a distinct eating disorder with specific clinical and psychopathological characteristics. BED shares with BN a common symptom, but it is evident the difference between binge episodes of these two types of patients: the second ones are not related to any dietary restriction but are closely linked to emotional distress (Masheb & Grilo, 2006). Since the first sessions, we can recognize a BED patient. He/she is focused on weight gain due to excessive food intake, not only during binge episodes (Sysko et al., 2007), and feels a fatalistic sense of lack of control on eating behavior. This is a quite different attitude from that of bulimic patients, always complaining of their loss of control over eating and completely absorbed in their anguished thoughts about food, weight and shape. Even though BED patients often feel ashamed of their weight and shape, the influence of body image on their self-esteem is lower than in other ED. They wanted to be thinner than they are, but this desire is justified by their real aspect; often they are objectively overweight or obese. Anywhere they don't have a drive for thinness as bulimic patients have (Masheb, Grilo, 2003; Stein, Corte, 2003).

The emotion that most frequently precedes binge episode is anxiety followed by sadness, loneliness, fatigue and hunger, rarely happiness (Masheb, Grilo, 2006). Compared to bulimic patients, BEDs experience less an antecedent negative mood before bingeing episodes and also a concomitant negative cognitions about food/eating and stress (Hilbert, Tuschen-Caffier, 2007). Binges start with a feeling of distress that is followed by a temporary wellness due to the hedonic effect of food and fullness; but soon, the sense of guilt for the excessive food intake worsens mood. Several patients choose foods according to their emotions: when they feel anxiety, they usually prefer salty and fat foods, with higher consistency, while when they are depressed, they choose sweets and chocolate. These clinical observations have a bio-chemical and neuro-endocrine correlate as demonstrated by some studies (Monteleone, 2003, 2008) and confirmed by functional magnetic resonance imaging evidences. (Killgore, Yurgelun-Todd, 2006).

A core feature of BED is the absence of compensatory behaviors. Actually, bingers occasionally purge, but they don't have the immediate need to eliminate food after binge; they only are distressed by the amount of food eaten when they became conscious of their weight increasing day after day. For this reason, these subjects have periods in which they put on a diet trying to lose weight with rigid attitude, but shortly they leave up their intentions.

Psychopathological Features

The most part of BED patients share several psychological characteristics that can contribute to the development of the pathology: negative self-evaluation, low self-esteem, inefficacy and inadequacy (Mussell et al., 2000), emotional vulnerability, impulsivity (Galanti et al., 2007) and difficulties regulating emotions (Whiteside et al., 2007)). Moreover, BED patients worrying about weight and shape have higher levels of eating psychopathology and social impairment (Mond et al., 2006)

Subjects affected by personality disorders are more likely to develop binge eating and obesity. Fassino et al., (2002) found that the strongest predictor for the development of the Binge Eating Disorder was a low score on the self-directedness scale of the Temperamental Character Inventory (Cloninger, 1994).

Trigger and Maintenance Factors

High levels of perceived stress seem to precede the onset of BED (Striegel-Moore, Dohm, Kramer et al., 2007) and patients refer negative moods in bingeing days (Wegner et al., 2002). In BED, patients' negative emotions may trigger off a binge; among them there are those induced by food deprivation and the difficulties of losing weight (Todisco, Vinai, 2008). Emotions more frequently experienced by these subjects are sadness, anxiety, loneliness, tiredness, anger and boredom (Masheb, Grilo, 2006). However, it is a clinical impression that different BED patients are sensible to different emotions, but every emotion is likely to trigger a binge if it exceeds the subject's level of tolerance. It is arguable this may be partially explained by the presence of a difficulty in differentiating emotions from sensations and a low emotion tolerance in these subjects.

Explicative Models of Bed

Two categories of models have been hypothesized to explain the onset and maintenance of binge eating in patients suffering from BED: the *restraint theory* (Howard and Porzelius, 1999) and the *affect driven models* (Stein et al., 2007). Nowadays, the first appears to be insufficient to explain binge eating both in bulimia nervosa and BED. According to this model, the bulimic episodes are induced by the extreme dietary restriction due to a pathologic preoccupation for weight and shape. A lot of studies have demonstrated that the emotional aspects play a preeminent role, particularly negative emotions. The *trade off theory* (Stice et al., 2001) affirms that in the face of negative mood, binge eating is a way to substitute a less aversive affective condition, such as guilt for bingeing, for the more aversive emotional state that precedes the binge episode. The *escape from self awareness* model (Heatherton, Baumeister, 1991) proposes that the bulimic behavior narrows the focus of the patient's attention toward an immediate gratification (food) in order to block out the perception of negative emotions. The *masking theory* suggests that (Polivy, Herman, 1999) binge eating serves to mask the real cause inducing negative emotions, attributing them to the alimentary excess.

The *blocking model* (Root, Fallon, 1989) was developed to explain the maintenance of the bulimic behavior; the subject learns to binge in order to block emotions when they become too hard to afford and then tends to behave the same when similar situations occur.

None of these models seems to be sufficient to completely explain the onset and the maintenance of BED, and some authors suggested that the combination of two or more of these mechanisms could be more exhaustive.

In our opinion (Vinai Todisco, 2007; Todisco Vinai, 2008), in BED patients, the blocking model has peculiar characteristics because they have difficulties to control impulses, alexithymic traits and (Sassaroli, Ruggiero, 2005) a low level of tolerance of emotions. They have a sort of *narrow emotional window* (Vinai Todisco, 2007), (Table 5.1); i.e., they don't perceive the emotions until they are very intense, while as soon as they start feeling them, they cannot bear anymore. So they continuously balance between the unpleasant sensation of boredom due to the absence of emotions and the anxiety for the emotional arousal. Besides, if they are used to employ food as a multifunctional solution to whatever problem and have impulsive traits, it is likely that they will front either negative or perceived absence of emotions bingeing. Then the binge episode leads to an intolerable sense of guilt and shame opening the road to further binges.

Overeating represents a defective solution to front the emotional distress; nevertheless, patients go on with this behavior following the dysfunctional belief that it is easier to deal with binges then with external cues inducing intolerable emotions.

Psychiatric Co-morbidity

The available literature (Grilo, White and Masheb, 2009) shows high rates of co-occurring psychiatric disorders among BED patients; however, studies regarding the relationship between co-morbidity and eating-disordered psychopathology reached controversial results. Wilfley et al., in a study of 162 patients found that 77% of them met criteria for at least another lifetime psychiatric disorder (mood, substance-use, and anxiety disorders were the most common); but co-morbidity was related neither to BMI, nor to eating disorder psychopathology or binge eating frequency Another study including 84 women with BED found opposite results: co-occurrence of psychiatric diseases was significantly associated with elevated levels of eating-disorder psychopathology (Peterson et al., 2005) Recently Grilo, White and Masheb (2009) reported a frequent lifetime (74%) and current (43%) additional psychiatric disorder in 404 BED patients seeking treatment and assessed using semi-structured interviews.

Table 5.1. The narrow emotional window of patients affected by BED

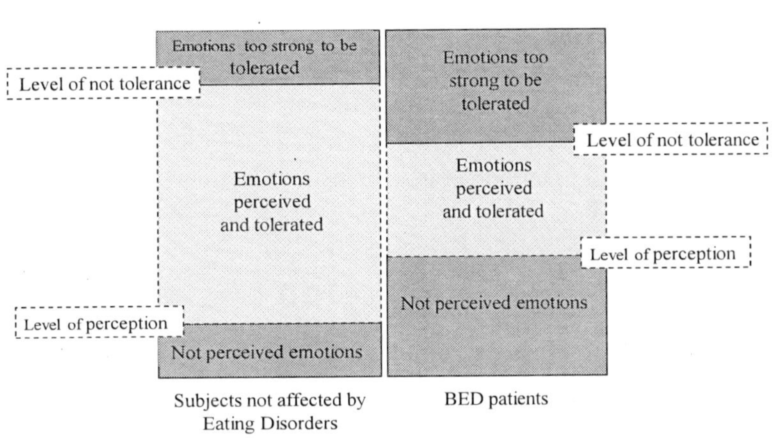

The most common co-morbidities were mood (lifetime 54.2% versus current 26.0%), anxiety (37.1% vs. 24.5%), and substance use disorders (24.8% vs. 2.7%). The authors found that current, but not lifetime, history of psychiatric disorders is associated with elevated levels of eating disorder psychopathology, higher depression scores, lower self-esteem and more severe clinical picture of BED. Hudson et al., (2007) compared individuals with AN, BN, and BED in terms of co-morbid mental disorders. They found that, of the participants with eating disorders, individuals with BN were at the highest risk for co-morbid disorders [94.5%; odds ratio: 4.7 (4.3–7.5)], followed by individuals with BED [(78.9%; odds ratio: 2.3 (2.6–3.7)], and that individuals with AN were at the lowest risk (relatively) for co-morbid disorders [56.2%; 2.1 (1.2– 2.9)]. These controversial findings support the necessity to assess BED patients for psychiatric co-morbidity to clear up its prognostic significance and implications for treatment outcome.

Clinical Implications for Obesity Treatment

It is an open question whether the diagnosis of BED influences the outcome of behavioral and surgical treatments for obesity. Gorin et al., (2008) found among diabetic obese BED patients that baseline BED diagnosis did not influence the outcome of diets, but individuals who retained their BED diagnosis at the end of treatment lost less weight than subjects who failed to meet diagnostic criteria at the end of treatment. In their review on validity and clinical utility of BED, Wonderlich et al., (2009) evaluated the moderating effect of a BED diagnosis on behavioral and surgical treatments for obesity reporting that the influence of BED on weight loss treatments is unclear and limited by the paucity of relevant studies. The authors suggest that specificity treatments are superior to behavioral weight loss for reducing binge eating and associated psychopathology in BED.

The influence of BED on outcome of bariatric surgery is mixed. Busetto et al., (2005) didn't find any difference in weight loss between BED and non BED patients at five-year follow-up after bariatric surgery, but BED patients had a greater likelihood of surgical complications. Burgmer and colleagues (2005) failed to find evidence that preoperative binge eating predicted weight loss at 12-month follow-up, but in this study, the number of DSM-IV BED patients was insufficient for an optimal test of the diagnostic construct. (Wonderlich et al., 2009) On the other hand, Sallet et al., (2007) found that two years after Roux-en-y surgery, patients affected by BED lost less weight than other obese subjects. In conclusion, according to Wonderlich et al., (2009), the hypothesis that BED will moderate the effectiveness of behavioral weight loss programs or bariatric surgery is inconsistently supported by the literature. The authors suggest that behavioral weight loss specialists and bariatric surgeons should not modify their treatments for individuals with BED.

Conclusion

There is evidence that individuals with BED display rates of eating disorder psychopathology, subjective distress, impairments in quality of life, and psychiatric co-morbidity at a level that is similar to other eating disorder diagnoses, but with some peculiar clinical and biological characteristics. Thus, in relationship to other eating disorders, the diagnosis of BED seems to represent a diagnostically distinct entity that carries clinically useful information. Nevertheless, data supporting that BED predicts a clinical course associated with negative medical and psychiatric outcomes are limited.

References

Bulik, C.M., Sullivan, P.F., Kendler, K.S. (2003) Genetic and environmental contributions to obesity and binge eating. *International Journal of Eating Disorders,* 33, 293–298.

Bulik, C.M., Sullivan, P.F., Kendler, K.S. (1998) Heritability of binge-eating and broadly defined bulimia nervosa. *Biol Psychiatry*, 44, 1210–1218

Burgmer, R., Grigutsch, K., Zipfel S, Wolf, A.M., de Zwaan, M., Husemann, B., et al., (2005) The influence of eating behavior and eating pathology on weight loss after gastric restriction operations. *Obes Surg*,15, 684–691.

Busetto, L., Gegato, G., De Luca, M., De Marchi, F., Foletto, M., Vianello, M. et al., (2005) Weight loss and postoperative complications in morbidly obese patients with binge eating disorder treated by laparoscopic adjustable gastric banding. *Obes Surg,*15:195–201

Cloninger, C.R (1994). *The temperament and character inventory (TCI): A guide to its development and use.* St. Louis, MO: Washington University.

de Man, L.J., Ghaderi, A., Norring, C. (2006) Eating disorders and disordered eating among patients seeking non-surgical weight-loss treatment in Sweden. *Eat Behav*,7,15–26.

de Zwaan, M., Mitchell, J.E., Howell. L.M., Monson, N., Swan-Kremeier, L., Crosby, R.D., et al., (2003) Characteristics of morbidly obese patients before gastric bypass surgery. *Compr Psychiatry,* 44, 428– 434.

Dymek-Valentine, M., Rienecke-Hoste, R., Alverdy, J. (2004) Assessment of binge eating disorder in morbidly obese patients evaluated for gastric bypass: SCID versus QEWP-R. *Eat Weight Disord,* 9, 211–216. 7.

Fairburn, C.G., Doll, H.A., Welch, S.L., Hay, P.J., Davies, B.A., O'Connor ME. (1998) Risk factors for binge eating disorder. A community based, case-control study. *Arch Gen Psychiatry,* 55, 425– 432.

Faravelli, C., Ravaldi, C., Truglia, E., Zucchi, T., Cosci F, Ricca, V. (2006) Clinical epidemiology of eating disorders: results from the Sesto Fiorentino study. *Psychother Psychosom.,* 75, 376-83

Fassino, S., Leombruni, P., Pierò, A. et al., (2002). Temperament and character in obese women with and without Binge Eating Disorder. *Comprehensive Psychiatry*, 6, 431-437

Favaro, A., Ferrara, S., Santonastaso, P. (2003) The spectrum of eating disorders in young women: A prevalence study in a general population sample. *Psychosom Med*, 65, 701–708.

Fowler, S.J., Bulik, C.M. (1997) Family environment and psychiatric history in women with binge-eating disorder and obese controls. *Behav Change*, 14, 106–112.

Galanti, K., Gluck, M.E., Geliebter, A. (2007). Test meal intake in obese binge eaters in relation to impulsivity and compulsivity. *International Journal of Eating Disorders*, 40, 727-732.

Ghaderi, A., Scott, B. (1999) Prevalence and psychological correlates of eating disorders among females aged 18–30 years in the general population. *Acta Psychiatr Scand*, 99, 261–266.

Gorin, A.A., Hogan, P., Di Lillo, V.G., Wadden, T.A., Williamson, D., Niemeier, HM., et al., (2008) Binge eating and weight loss outcomes in overweight and obese individuals with type 2 diabetes: Results from the LOOK AHEAD trial. *Arch Gen Psych*, 65, 1447–1455.

Grissett N.I., Fitzgibbon M.L. (1996). The clinical significance of binge eating in an obese population: support for BED and questions regarding its criteria. *Addictive Behaviors, 21,* 57-66.

Hay, P., Fairburn, C. (1998) The validity of the DSM-IV scheme for classifying bulimic eating disorders. *International Journal of Eating Disorders, 23*, 7-15

Heatherton, T.F., Baumeister, R.F. (1991). Binge eating as escape from self-awareness. *Psychological Bulletin,* 110, 86-108.

Hilbert, A., Tuschen-Caffier, B. (2007) Maintenance of binge eating through negative mood: a naturalistic comparison of binge eating disorder and bulimia nervosa. *International Journal of Eating Disorders,* 40, 521-30.

Hoek, H.W., van Hoeken, D. (2003) Review of the prevalence and incidence of eating disorders. *International Journal of Eating Disorders,* 34, 383–396.

Howard, C.E., Porzelius, L.K. (1999) The role of dieting in binge eating disorder: etiology and treatment implications. *Clin Psychol Rev.*, 19, 25-44.

Hudson, J.I., Hiripi, E., Pope, H.G. Jr, Kessler, R.C. (2007) The prevalence and correlates of eating disorders in the National Comorbidity Survey Replication. *Biol Psychiatry*, 61, 348-58.

Hudson, J.I., Lalonde, J.K., Berry, J.M., Pindyck, L.J., Bulik, C.M., Crow, S.J., et al., (2006) Binge eating disorder as a distinct familial phenotype in obese individuals. *Arch Gen Psychiatry*, 63, 313–319.

Javaras, K.N., Laird, N.M., Reichborn-Kjennerud, T., Bulik, C.M., Pope, H.G., Hudson, J.I. (2008) Familiarity and Heritability of Binge Eating Disorder: Results of a Case-Control Family Study and a Twin Study. *International Journal of Eating Disorders,* 41, 174–179.

Killgore, W.D., Yurgelun-Todd, D.A. (2006) Affect modulates appetite-related brain activity to images of food. *International Journal of Eating Disorders,* 39, 357-63.

Kinzl, J.F., Traweger, C., Trefalt, E. et al., (1999). Binge eating disorder in males: A population- based investigation. *Eating and Weight Disorders*, 4, 169-174.

Lee, Y.H., Abbott, D.W., Seim, H., Crosby, R.D., Monson, N., Burgard, M., et al., (1999) Eating disorders and psychiatric disorders in the first degree relatives of obese probands with binge eating disorder and obese non-binge eating disorder controls. *International Journal of Eating Disorders,* 26, 322–332.

Lewinsohn, P.M., Striegel-Moore, R.H., Seeley, J.R. (2000) Epidemiology and natural course of eating disorders in young women from adolescence to young adulthood. *J Am Acad Child Adolesc Psychiatry,* 39, 1284-92.

Masheb, R.M., Grilo, C.M. (2003) The nature of body image disturbance in patients with binge eating disorder. *International Journal of Eating Disorders,* 33, 333-41.

Masheb, R.M., Grilo, C.M. (2006). Emotional overeating and its associations with eating disorder psychopathology among overweight patients with Binge Eating Disorder. *International Journal of Eating Disorders, 39*, 141-146.

Mond, J.M., Hay, P.J., Rodgers, B. et al., (2006). Recurrent binge eating with and without the "undue influence of weight or shape on self-evaluation": implications for the diagnosis of binge eating disorder. *Behavior Research and Therapy*, 45, 929-938.

Monteleone, P., Bencivenga, R., Longobardi, N., Serritella, C., Maj, M. (2003) Differential responses of circulating ghrelin to high-fat or high-carbohydrate meal in healthy women. *J Clin Endocrinol Metab.*, 88, 5510-4.

Mussell, M.P., Bindford, R.B., Fulkerson, J.A. (2000). Eating Disorders: summary of risk factors, prevention programming, and prevention research. *The Counseling Psychologist*, 28, 764-796.

Peterson, C.B., Miller, K.B., Crow, S.J., Thuras, P. Mitchell, J.E. (2005) Subtypes of binge eating disorder based on psychiatric history. *International Journal of Eating Disorders*, 38, 273–276.

Pike, K.M., Dohm, F.A, Striegel-Moore, R.H., Wilfley, D.E., Fairburn, C.G. (2001) A comparison of black and white women with binge eating disorder. *Am J Psychiatry*, 158, 1455-60.

Polivy, J., Herman, C.P. (1999). Distress and eating: why do dieters overeat?. *International Journal of Eating Disorders*, 26, 153-164.

Reas, D.L., Grilo, C.M. (2007) Timing and sequence of the onset of overweight, dieting, and binge eating in overweight patients with binge eating disorder. *International Journal of Eating Disorders,* 40, 165–170

Reichborn-Kjennerud, T., Bulik, C.M., Tambs, K., Harris, J.R. (2004) Genetic and environmental influences on binge eating in the absence of compensatory behaviors: A population-based twin study. *International Journal of Eating Disorders,* 36, 307–314.

Root, M.P.P., Fallon, P. (1989). Treating the victimized bulimic. *Journal of Interpersonal Violence*, 4, 90-100

Sallet, P.C., Sallet, J.A., Dixon, J.B., Collis, E., Pisani, C.E., Levy, A., et al., (2007) Eating behavior as a prognostic factor for weight loss after gastric bypass. *Obes Surg*, 17, 445–451.

Santonastaso, P., Ferrara, S., Favaro, A. (1999) Differences between binge eating disorder and nonpurging bulimia nervosa. *International Journal of Eating Disorders,* Mar, 25, 215-8.

Sassaroli, S., Ruggiero, G.M. (2005). The role of stress in the association between low self-esteem, perfectionism, and worry, and eating disorders. *International Journal of Eating Disorders,* 37, 135-141.

Stein, K.F., Corte,. CM. (2003) Ecologic momentary assessment of eating-disordered behaviors. *International Journal of Eating Disorders,* 34, 349-60.

Stein, R.I., Kenardy, J., Wiseman, C.V., Dounchis, J.Z., Arnow, B.A., Wilfley, D.E. (2007) What's driving the binge in binge eating disorder?: A prospective examination of precursors and consequences. *International Journal of Eating Disorders,* 40, 195-203.

Stice, E., Agras, W.S., Telch, C.F., Halmi, K.A., Mitchell, J.E., Wilson, T. (2001). Subtyping binge eating-disordered women along dieting and negative affect dimensions. *International Journal of Eating Disorders,* 30, 11-27

Striegel-Moore, R.H., Dohm, F.A., Kraemer, H.C., Schreiber, G.B., Taylor, C.B., Daniels, S.R. (2007) Risk factors for binge-eating disorders: an exploratory study. *International Journal of Eating Disorders*, 40, 481-7.

Striegel-Moore, R.H., Franko, D.L. (2003) Epidemiology of binge eating disorder. *International Journal of Eating Disorders,* 34, 19-S29.

Stunkard, A.J., Allison, K.C. (2003) Binge eating disorder: disorder or marker? *International Journal of Eating Disorders, 34,* 107-16.

Sysko, R., Devlin M.J., Walsh, B.T., Zimmerli, E., Kissileff, H.R. (2007) Satiety and test meal intake among women with binge eating disorder. *International Journal of Eating Disorders, 40*, 554-61.

Todisco, P., Vinai, P. (2008) *La fame infinita*. Torino: Centro Scientifico Editore.

Vinai, P., Todisco, P. (2007) *Quando le emozioni diventano cibo*. Milano: Libreria Cortina.

Wegner, K.E., Smyth, J.M., Crosby, R.D. et al., (2002). An evaluation of the relationship between mood and binge eating in the natural environment using ecological momentary assessment. *International Journal of Eating Disorders*, 32, 352-361

Whiteside, U., Chen, E., Neighbors, C. et al., (2007). Difficulties regulating emotions: do binge eaters have fewer strategies to modulate and tolerate negative affect?. *Eating Behaviors,* 8, 162-169.

Wilfley, D.E., Friedman, M.A., Dounchis, J.Z., Stein, R.I., Welch, R.R., Ball, S.A. (2000) Comorbid psychopathology in binge eating disorder: Relation to eating disorder severity at baseline and following treatment. *J Consult Clin Psychol,* 68, 641–649.

Wilson GT, Sysko R. (2009). Frequency of Binge Eating Episodes in Bulimia Nervosa and Binge Eating Disorder: Diagnostic Considerations. *International Journal of Eating Disorders, 42,* 603–610.

Wonderlich, S.A., Gordon, K.H., Mitchell, J.E., Crosby, R.D., Engel, S.G. (2009) The validity and clinical utility of binge eating disorder. *International Journal of Eating Disorders,* 42, 687-705.

Wonderlich, S.A., Gordon, K.H., Mitchell, J.E., Crosby, R.D., Engel, S.G. (2009)The Validity and Clinical Utility of Binge Eating Disorder. *International Journal of Eating Disorders,* 42, 687–705.

Yanovski SZ. (2003) Binge eating disorder and obesity in 2003: Could treating an eating disorder have a positive effect on the obesity epidemic? *International Journal of Eating Disorders,* 34, 117–120.

Zachrisson, H.D., Vedul-Kjelsås, E., Götestam, K.G., Mykletun, A. (2008) Time trends in obesity and eating disorders. *International Journal of Eating Disorders,* 41, 673-80.

In: Pathways to Obesity and Main Roads to Recovery
Editor: Piergiuseppe Vinai
ISBN: 978-1-61122-740-6

Chapter VI

The Night Eating Syndrome

Piergiuseppe Vinai, Gabriella Carpegna, Paola Vallauri, Silvia Cardetti and Noemi Ferrato
GNOSIS: No Profit Research Group. Cuneo; Studi Cognitivi Post Graduate Psychotherapy Cognitive School Research Group, Milan, Italy

Abstract

More than fifty years after the first description of the night eating syndrome (NES), the research on this pathology is growing. The diagnostic criteria of the syndrome have been changed many times during the year, and only in 2008, a consensus among the researchers has been reached. Despite the blossom of studies and the high prevalence of NES among obese subjects, healthcare providers are often unaware of NES and its treatment. In this chapter are summarized the current diagnostic criteria and recent findings on pathogenetic mechanisms of the syndrome.

Introduction

NES was firstly described in 1955, by Stunkard, Grace et Wolff in a group of obese subjects. The first diagnostic criteria included morning anorexia, evening hyperphagia, insomnia, lower mood in the evening and emotional distress. Many peculiar characteristics of these patients have been described in the subsequent 50 years of descriptions, and diagnostic criteria have been modified many times. In 1986, Kuldau and Rand reported that NES patients feel tense, upset or anxious as bedtime nears. In 1996, Stunkard and colleagues suggested to modify the criteria, considering necessary to eat the 50% of daily calories after 7 pm to be diagnosed as affected by NES. The emotional distress, a core characteristic of Stunkard's original definition in 1955, reappeared among diagnostic criteria only in 1997, when Rand, Macgregor and Stunkard recommended again to consider it as a core characteristic of the syndrome. Experts from European countries (Adami et al., 1999) noted that the hour of evening meal differs cross-culturally and suggested to consider as nocturnal ingestion as eating something after the evening meal before going to sleep. This suggestion has been accepted by the majority of the researchers. The presence of insomnia has been cited since 1955, but the relation of NES with sleep disorders has not been further investigated and the nocturnal awakenings with food ingestion were included by Birketvedt in 1999, among the criteria to diagnose the NES.

To further confound the matter, in 1990, the sleep disorder experts community included a new syndrome in the International Classification of Sleep Disorder (ICSD-1 1990): the Night Eating and Drinking Syndrome (NEDS), characterized by nocturnal ingestions of food with full awareness; the diagnostic criteria didn't indicate any amount of food necessary to be diagnosed as NEDS. Luckily, this syndrome was no more included into the second edition of the ICSD (2005).

Since today, 20 different sets of diagnostic criteria have been suggested (Striegel Moore et al., 2006). Only nine papers on NES were published between 1955 and 1991, seven of which were case reports, but in the last ten years 75, research articles about this topic have been published. Nevertheless, this syndrome has not been included in the Diagnostic and Statistical Manual of Mental Disorders. This was mainly due to the lack of an agreement on an unambiguous definition of the syndrome. Vinai and colleagues (Allison et al., 2008) identify the presence of NES in sample of 202 obese persons seeking bariatric surgery according to four sets of different diagnostic criteria: the number of subjects diagnosed as affected by the syndrome varied from 32 to 23, but remarkably, only one subject met the diagnostic criteria of all the four classifications. This ambiguity makes it difficult to clinically recognize the syndrome with accuracy, compare the results of the different researches and to define the most effective treatment.

For these reasons, in 2008, during the First International Night Eating Symposium in Minneapolis, expert investigators in this area reached a consensus on a set of provisional diagnostic criteria for NES that have been recently published (Allison et al., 2010).

Clinical Features and Diagnostic Criteria

Core Criteria

1. An abnormally increased food intake in the evening and at night-time, manifested by the consumption of at least 25% of intake after the evening meal and/or nocturnal awakenings with ingestions at least twice a week.
2. Awareness of the eating episodes.
3. Significant distress or impairment in functioning.

Today, NES is widely believed to entail a defect in the circadian cycle of food ingestion, inducing an evening hyperphagia, with the ingestion, after dinner, of at least 25% of the daily caloric intake. The majority of patients have nocturnal awakenings with food ingestion. They are aware of their nocturnal ingestions even if sometimes affirm to eat in an automatic way; but, if solicited, they have memory of this behavior and remember what they eat. Moreover, frequently, their awareness increases during the therapy. Patients never ingest inedible objects. This is a main difference with those affected by Sleep-Related Eating Disorder (SRED). (See chapter VI).

The eating behavior is accompanied by significant distress, manifested by guilt-related feelings: for example, for eating snacks that are normally intended for children or for being incapable of keeping below the caloric intake prescribed by a dietician. Sometimes, a strong evening anxiety is present, related to the thought that a weight increase will follow their evening ingestion, or to the idea that the following day they will feel tired or sleepy because of nocturnal awakenings.

The symptoms must have a minimum duration of three months, and the nocturnal eating must not be due to other psychiatric or medical disorders or a side effect of medications.

Besides these core symptoms, to diagnose a NES, at least three factors between those indicated as "descriptors" have to be present.

Descriptors

Three of the following five symptoms are requested:

1. Morning anorexia.
2. Strong desire or urge to eat between dinner and sleep initiation and/or upon awakening at night from sleep.
3. Sleep onset and insomnia.
4. The belief that one must eat in order to get to sleep.
5. Depressed mood.

Morning anorexia can be described both as a lack of desire to eat in the morning and as the habit to skip breakfast almost every day (Gluck, Geliebter A, Satov, 2001) It has been comprised between the necessarily present symptoms since the first description of the syndrome (Stunkard, Grace, Wolff, 1955), but subsequent researches pointed out that it is a quite common behavior among obese subjects; for this reason, it has been included among the descriptors, instead of considering it a core diagnostic criterion for the syndrome.

A *strong desire or urge to* eat between dinner and sleep initiation and/or upon awakening at night from sleep was yet present between the requirements for the assessment in the diagnostic questionnaire prepared by Allison and colleagues (2008), and it is confirmed as core criterion. To satisfy this urge, the patients don't need a large amount of food. Craving for specific foods is sometimes present.

No differences have been found between night eaters and control subjects in sleep onset and offset was found by actigraphy among out-patients (O'Reardon et al., 2004) and by polysomnography among in-patients (Rogers et al., 2006). But night eaters manifested significantly greater sleep disturbance than control subjects with more frequent awakenings (Birketvedt et al., 1999). Rogers et al., found that sleep efficiency of night eaters was lower than that of control subjects (Rogers et al., 2006). *Onset and maintenance insomnia* are described in the symptomatology of NES by many researchers (Allison, Engel, Crosby, de Zwaan et al., 2008). Reported rates of insomnia range from 57% to 66%.

The *belief that one must eat in order to get to sleep* was used by Vinai and colleagues (Allison et al., 2008) as an important distinguishing feature between night eaters and patients affected by binge eating disorder (BED) or obesity. Among NES patients, they found a correlation between anxiety and the presence of the belief that one can't get to sleep without ingesting food. This was not present among BED or obese people not affected by any eating disorders. They hypothesize that the belief that to ingest some food will enable them to sleep supports the evening hyperphagia and the ingestion of food during the nocturnal awakenings. When waking up, NES patients immediately eat something; this reinforces the conviction that food works as a sleeping-tablet, so every time the patient wakes up he ingests "a pill of food." This also explains why about 25% of the patients don't consider their symptoms as a problem: for them, eating at night is the solution to their problems with anxiety and insomnia. In fact, their main problem is the fear of not sleeping enough; furthermore, their convictions regarding sleep are "all or nothing", a single nocturnal awakening is, for them, enough to be sure that nothing will work the next day if they do not go back to sleep immediately. This conviction is not so different from that of other insomniac patients: the more they are fearing of not being efficient and fit the next day, the less easily they are able to go back to sleep. However, different from other insomniac patients, those affected by NES believe they cannot go back to sleep unless they eat.

A depressed mood is frequently present; sometimes it is worsening in the evening and is connected to the idea of losing control on food, followed by sense of guilt and shame for the incapability of keeping the body weight and following a diet.

Prevalence

There are differences in the reported prevalence of community samples of NES; this is due to the differences between diagnostic criteria used to diagnose the syndrome. They range from 1.1% (Lamerz et al., 2005), to 1.6% (Striegel-Moore et al., 2006). Higher prevalence has been found among diabetic subjects: 3.8% (Allison et al., 2007), patients seeking weight loss, (rates from 4.3% (Colles et al., 2007), to 6%) (Adami, Meneghelli, Scopinaro, 1999), or candidates to bariatric surgery: 8% (Allison et al., 2006). An increase in the prevalence of NES with increasing BMI was reported by Colles et al., (2007) in both a weight loss group and among patients seeking for bariatric surgery. The highest prevalence, 12%, has been found by Lundgren et al., (2006) in psychiatric clinics; in this study, patients with substance-use disorders showed an increased risk of NES. A population-based study of the prevalence of NES utilizing the Swedish Twin Registry found a prevalence of night eating among 4.6% of men and 3.4% of women (Tholin et al., 2009). It also showed that the nocturnal eating was respectively 2.5 and 2.8 times more common among obese men and women than among normal-weight men and women.

Stunkard and colleague (2009) report that there are only two (Andersen et al., 2004; Gluck et al., 2008) prospective studies of NES as a risk factor for weight gain: the Danish MONICA study and a prospective study involving 117 Pima Indian and 43 Caucasian men and women (Gluck et al., 2008).

In the first research, obese women night eaters averaged a six-year weight gain of 5.2 kg, whereas non-night eating gained only 0.9 kg. There was no association between night eating and weight change in men or non-obese women. In the second study, night-time over-eaters gained significantly more weight (6.2 kg) than did non-night eaters (1.7 kg; $P = 0.03$) (Gluck et al., 2008) Despite the high prevalence of NES in multiple studies, healthcare providers are often unaware of NES and its treatment. Goncalves et al., (2009) contacted 154 persons with NES from our files regarding their experience with their physicians. Only 27% (42/159) of their doctors had definitely heard of NES, and 41% had "definitely" or "probably" dismissed their symptoms of NES.

Diagnostic Controversial

Some ambiguity still remains about Night Eating Syndrome. The hypothesis that NES is a form of disordered eating present only among obese persons seems to be disconfirmed by psychological differences found between NES and other obese patients. Comparing 20 patients affected by NES and 50 obese subjects not affected by any eating disorder, Vinai et al. (2006) found that Night Eaters differed significantly from obese subjects on subscales of the Eating Disorders Inventory: bulimia, ineffectiveness, perfectionism and interceptive awareness. Moreover the dysfunctional belief "I cannot sleep without eating" was significantly more frequent among obese night eaters than it is among other obese insomniac subjects who don't eat at night. They found a significant difference between patients affected by NES, obese subjects not affected by any eating disorder and subjects affected by BED.

It is an open question if NES represents a risk factor for obesity or if obesity is a risk factor for NES. The first hypothesis is supported by the research of Napolitano and coll. (2001), who found that NES patients appeared to have an earlier age of onset of obesity compared with non-eating-disordered individuals. However, no differences were found among NES patients, binge eaters, patients with dual diagnosis of NES and BED, and obese subjects on current weight and BMI. A research of De Zwaan et al (2006) supports the second hypothesis: the 60% of the obese participants in their study reported that they were already overweight before their night eating began, and there was no significant difference in the age of onset between normal and overweight participants. Lundgren et al., (2006) found that obese and overweight psychiatric patients were respectively 5.2 and 2.5 times more likely to meet criteria for night eating syndrome than normal-weight psychiatric patients. Finally, Striegel- Moore et al., did not find any relationship between obesity and nocturnal eating in a large epidemiological trial (2005). In conclusion, we need further studies in order to better understand the relationship between NES and obesity.

NES and BED

Several clinicians consider NES as a subtype of BED; but the relationship between the two pathologies needs further studies. Many BED patients are affected by evening hyperphagia, such as BED and BN share bingeing episodes; to have common symptoms doesn't mean necessarily share a common pathogenesis. Among NES patients, nocturnal eating has been correlated with nocturnal anxiety, but among BED patients, even if they binge at night, there is no correlation between their nocturnal eating behavior and their nocturnal anxiety (Sassaroli et al., 2009). Further, usually the size of nocturnal ingestions is not so large (about 300 kcals) among NES patients, as it is in those affected by BED. It has been reported that from 7 to 25% of patients affected by NES also meet criteria for BED (Stunkard et al., 1996; Tzischinsky et al., 2004; Goel et al., 2009) and that the prevalence of NES among individuals with BED can reach 24%, but other studies didn't find any overlap between the two diagnoses. (Spaggiari et al., 1994; Tzischinsky et al., 2004; Grilo & Masheb 2004). Examining whether NES is simply a subtype of BED , Cerú-Björk, Andersson and Rössner (2001) found that night eaters had binge eating problems, according to Binge Eating Scale, to the same extent as other obese subjects, differing from patients affected by BED. De Zwaan et al., (2006) found that there was a modest overlap between the two pathologies in a sample of 106 obese patients. Only nine met diagnostic criteria for current BED (8.5%) and fifteen (14.2%) for lifetime BED. These rates are similar to those found in previous studies. Only 5% of the patients studied by Striegel Moore et al., (2005) met criteria for both NES and BED. Napolitano et al., (2001) in a sample of 83 patients, found a rate of 15.7% of overlap between BED and NES. Among patients affected by NES, 37.1% met criteria for BED, a percentage similar to that (44%) found by Stunkard et al., in 1996. Additionally, in a study of 207 BED patients (Grilo & Masheb 2004), 28% of them reported nocturnal eating behavior during the previous 28 days. The double diagnosis has been associated with higher BMI, higher emotional distress, a greater likelihood of personality disorders and increased eating-related psychopathology.

NES and Bulimia Nervosa

Only two studies have assessed the symptoms of NES in individuals diagnosed with BN. Both of the NES groups had low sleep efficiency, as measured by actigraphy, compared to the control groups. The mean number of nocturnal ingestions was 3.9 ± 2.2 per night for the BED group and 3.0 ± 2.2 for the BN group. The Mini Sleep Questionnaire revealed severe subjective sleep disorders, and clinical data revealed high rates of traumatic life events (sexual and physical abuse) and high levels of psychiatric co-morbidity among the NES groups. Additionally, timing of sexual abuse coincided temporarily with NES onset (Tzischinsky, 2004). Approximately 5% of the outpatients presenting annually in the clinic were self-identified as having problems with night eating. The results may indicate that NES in BED and BN are gathered as a discriminate subgroup of eating disorders.

The second study included 31 adult women enrolled in an outpatient cognitive-behavioral treatment study for BN who were assessed with the NEQ. Nighttime eating behavior was common: 35.4% percent reported the consumption of 25% or more of total daily food intake after dinner. Similarly, 38.7% reported nocturnal ingestions of food sometimes or more frequently upon awakening at night during the month previous to the assessment. More research is needed on the antecedents and correlates of nocturnal ingestions of food among the bulimic population to determine if both disorders can occur independently, or if BN patients are simply engaging in bulimic behaviors primarily in the evening.

Psychopathology

We reviewed the international literature to find out if night eaters have peculiar psychopathological or personality traits. There are few studies on psychopathologic characteristics of NES and those regarding personality disorders among these patients are scarce and anecdotal.

Mood

A peculiar characteristic of the syndrome is the variation of mood during the day; frequently, it is lower in the evening than in the morning, differing from that of patients affected by major depressive disorder, in which mood is classically lower in the morning.

Stunkard (1955) reported that NES patients had depressive symptoms when trying to follow a diet. Depressed mood has also been associated with NES in many studies (Tzischinsky et al., 2000; 2004, de Zwaan et al., 2006); it is typically related to the lack of control and sense of helplessness related to nocturnal eating and feelings of guilt and shame. A high prevalence of current and lifetime depression has been confirmed by many researchers, (Birketvedt et al., 1999; Gluck et al., 2001; Striegel-Moore et al., 2005). Given that NES is frequent among overweight and obese persons, depression could be more due to obesity-related distress than to NES. To find out if there is a relationship between BMI and mood among Night Eaters, Marshall et al.(2004) studied 80 subjects recruited on a website and 21 outpatients. Participants were grouped by BMI status: a) less than 25 kg/m^2, and b) greater than 30 kg/m^2. No significant differences were found between the groups. The results suggest that low mood is related to the diagnosis of NES, but there are no studies investigating if it is either one of the causes or an effect of the eating disorder.

Few studies found no significant difference (Powers and al., 1999) between NE and control subjects for mood. Lundgren J.D. (2010) and Friedman (2004), assessing NES among patients affected by psychiatric disorders, did not find a relationship between mood disorders and NES.

Anxiety and Stress

Globally considering all of the studies, only 225 NES patients were tested for anxiety. The exiguity of the studies requires further research about anxiety and NES, particularly nocturnal anxiety.

Stunkard (1955) reported that persons with NE experienced severe anxiety during diets and Rand, Macgregor and Stunkard included evening tension and/or feeling upset before bedtime among diagnostic criteria of the syndrome in 1997. Subsequently the presence of elevated stress and anxiety among these patients was confirmed by Pawlow, O'Neil and Malcom (2003). Both State and Trait Anxiety levels were above the normal range and consistent with elevated stress; baseline salivary cortisol levels were above the normal range during the early morning hours. This supports the findings of Birketvedt et al., (2002) reporting that NES patients had significantly higher levels of plasma cortisol levels than control subjects throughout the most part of the day. The role of anxiety in NES has been confirmed by Striegel-Moore et al., in 2006.

Stress seems to play a primary role in the onset of the pathology. Stunkard, Allison, and O'Reardon (2005) found that the seventy-four percent of their patients started to eat at night during a period of life stress. However, Napolitano et al., (2001) found that patients exclusively diagnosed with NES scored significantly lower on anxiety than BED patients and patients with dual diagnoses (BED & NES). Individuals who met criteria both for NES and BED reported the highest levels of state and trait anxiety. The authors suggested that the combination of night eating and bingeing rather than night eating alone is related to greater levels of state anxiety. These findings suggest that individuals with dual diagnoses of NES and BED could experience an higher psychological distress and may be using the food a way of coping with these problems.

We found (Sassaroli et al., 2009) that nocturnal anxiety amongst obese night eaters was significantly higher than among other obese patients. There is a correlation between the Sleep Disturbance Questionnaire's mental anxiety subscale scores of NES patients and two of the Night Eating Questionnaire subscales: Evening Hyperphagia and Mood and Sleep Disturbance. This fact could play a primary role in the onset of nocturnal eating. Waking up during the night confused and agitated, they think that only a little food will calm them down and help them to go back to sleep. This way a vicious circle is maintained: the eating behavior is followed by negative emotions linked to the idea of not being able to control themselves, having a negative impact on sleep quality and so on. The day after, they feel guilty for the food consumed during the night and try to remedy to the excessive caloric intake by skipping breakfast, a common behavior of many obese patients, who try to begin a new diet every day.

Pathogenesis

Following Stunkard et al., (2009), genetic, neuroendocrine and psychological factors (stress) play a role in pathogenesis of NES.

The preliminary results of a large study using the Swedish twin register support the influence of genetic factors (Rasmussen, 2007) on NES that may increase the vulnerability to stress. (Stunkard et al., 2009). Birketvedt et al., (2002) found cortisol levels to be significantly higher among night eaters than among control subjects and Geliebter et al., (2002) reported that a cold pressor test produced significantly higher cortisol levels among night eaters than among control subjects. A central aspect of NES is its delayed circadian rhythm of meal times (Stunkard et al., 2009). Compared to control subjects (Goel et al., 2009), circadian rhythms of night eaters' caloric, carbohydrate and fat intake were significantly delayed by about 1.5 h and that of protein non-significantly delayed by about the same amount. The night eaters' delay in meal timing was accompanied by a significant delay in the circadian rhythm of two food regulatory hormones: insulin and leptin, while ghrelin had a phase advance of 5.2 hours (Goel et al., 2009). The authors (Stunkard 2009) hypothesize that three neuroendocrine systems can be involved in the NES: the glucocorticoid, the melanocortin and the serotonergic—for the last one there is the most evidence. The glucocorticoid system is a candidate for the mechanism of NES because glucocorticoids (Zakrzewska et al., 1999; Jeanrenaud and Rohner-Jeanrenaud, 2000; Dallman et al., 2007) have an appetite-promoting action, stress is involved in the secretion of glucocorticoids (Akana et al., 1999) and the Hypothalamic-Pituitary–Adrenal axis response to stress plays an important part in NES (Birketvedt, Sundsfjord, Florholmen, 2002). Research on the effects of glucocorticoids in NES patients had controversial results. Some studies have found elevated levels of serum cortisol among night eaters, across the 24 h (Birketvedt et al., 1999) and following a cold presser test (Geliebter, Gluck, and Yahav, 2002), but other studies didn't confirm these results (Allison et al., 2005; Birketvedt, Sundsfjord and Florholmen, 2002).

Leptin is an appetite-suppressing hormone, playing an important role in the glucocorticoid system. Chronic stress decreases leptin levels, disinhibiting the glucocorticoid system (Lu et al., 2006). Among night eaters (Birketvedt et al., 1999), there is a failure of leptin to rise at night presumably due to the effects of stress. This failure of leptin-induced inhibition of food intake may contribute to the characteristic night eating of NES. The melanocortin system is involved in the temporal organization of food intake. MC-3receptor regulates circadian rhythm in response to food cues (Sutton et al., 2008), and AgRP levels rise during the dark period in mice when feeding is active (Huszar et al., 1997); but currently no relevant findings in humans are available.

Serotonin regulates the release of stress hormones in response to stress (Birketvedt et al., 2002) and serotonin receptors modulate food intake (Clifton, Kennett, 2006) and circadian rhythms (Frazer, 1997). A decreased serotonin transmission impairs the circadian rhythms of food intake, so a disruption of serotonin function may be responsible of the evening hyperphagia of NES patients. An increased reuptake of serotonin by the elevated serotonin transporter (SERT) binding impairs postsynaptic serotonin transmission (Frazer, 1997), which may contribute to NES. Single photon emission computed tomography (SPECT) among night eaters showed greater levels of midbrain SERT binding than among control subjects, suggesting decreased synaptic serotonin (Lundgren et al., 2008). Administration of SSRIs (see chapter XVIII) increases postsynaptic serotonin restoring circadian rhythm and satiety. Stunkard et al., developed a bio-behavioral model of NES suggesting that the interaction of stress and genetic vulnerability elevates SERT levels in the midbrain, leading to increased reuptake of serotonin. The consequent decrease in serotonin at the synapse leads to circadian delay and decreased satiety. The various studies noted above have been assembled into a bio-behavioral model of NES (Stunkard, 2009). It suggests that the interaction of stress and genetic vulnerability elevates SERT levels in the midbrain, leading to increased reuptake of serotonin. The consequent decrease in serotonin at the synapse leads to circadian delay and decreased satiety.

References

Adami, G.H., Meneghelli, A., Scopinaro, N. (1999) Night eating and binge eating disorder in obese patients. *Int J Eat Disord, 25,* 335–338.

Akana, S.F., Strack, A.M., Hanson, E.S., Horsley, C.J., Milligan, E.D., Bhatnagar, S., Dallman, M.F. (1999) Interactions among chronic cold, corticosterone and puberty on energy intake and deposition. *Stress, 3,* 131–146.

Allison, K.C., Ahima, R.S., O'Reardon, J.P., Dinges, D.F., Sharma, V., Cummings, D.E., Heo, M., Martino, N.S., Stunkard, A.J. (2005) Neuroendocrine profiles associated with energy intake, sleep and stress in the night eating syndrome. *J Clin Endocrinol Metab., 90,* 6214–6217.

Allison, K.C., Crow, S., Reeves, R.R., West, D.S., Foreyt, J.P., DiLillo, V.G., Wadden, T.A., Jeffery, R.W., Van Dorsten, B., Stunkard, A.J. (2007) The prevalence of binge eating disorder and night eating syndrome in adults with type 2 diabetes mellitus. *Obesity, 15,* 1285–1291

Allison, K.C., Engel, S.G., Crosby, R.D., de Zwaan, M., O'Reardon, J.P., Wonderlic, h S.A., Mitchell, J.E., Smith West, D., Wadden, T.A., Stunkard, A.J. (2008) Evaluation of diagnostic criteria for night eating syndrome using item response theory analysis. *Eat Behav., 9,* 398-407.

Allison, K.C., Latzer, Y., Tzischinsky, O., Vinai, P. (2008) What is Night Eating Syndrome? New Directions Toward a Unified Definition. *International Journal of Child and Adolescent Health, 2,* 175-184

Allison, K.C., Lundgren, J.D., O'Reardon, J.P., Geliebter, A., Gluck, M.E., Vinai, P., Mitchell, J.E., Schenck, C.H., Howell, M.J., Crow, S.J., Engel, S., Latzer, Y., Tzischinsky, O., Mahowald, M.W., Stunkard, A.J. (2010) Proposed diagnostic criteria for night eating syndrome. *Int J Eat Disord., 43*, 241-7.

Allison, K.C., Wadden, T.A., Sarwer, D.B., Fabricatore, A.N., Crerand, C.E., Gibbons, L.M., Stack. R.M., Stunkard, A.J., Williams, N.N. Night eating syndrome and binge eating disorder among persons seeking bariatric surgery: prevalence and related features. *Obesity 2006, 4*, 77S–82S

American Sleep Disorders Association. (1990) *International Classification of Sleep Disorders: Diagnostic and Coding Manual.* Rochester, MN. American Sleep Disorders Association.

Andersen, G.S, Stunkard A.J., Sorensen, T.I.A., Pedersen, L., Heitman, B.L. (2004) Night eating and weight change in middle-aged men and women. *Int J Obes*, *28*, 1138–1143.

Birketvedt, G., Florholmen, J., Sundsfjord, J., Osterud, B., Dinges, D., Bilker, W., Stunkard, A.J. (1999) Behavioral and neuroendocrine characteristics of the night-eating syndrome. *JAMA*, *282*, 657–663.

Birketvedt, G., Sundsfjord, J., Florholmen, J.R. (2002) Hypothalamicpituitary-adrenal axis in the night eating syndrome. *Am J Physiol Endocrinol Metab*, *282*, E366–E369.

Cerú-Björk, C., Andersson, I., Rossner, S. (2001). Night eating and nocturnal eating. Two different or similar syndromes among obese patients?. *International Journal of Obesity and Related Metabolic Disorders, 25*, 365-372.

Clifton, P.G., Kennett, G.A. (2006) Monoamine receptors in the regulation of feeding behavior and energy balance. *CNS Neurol Disord Drug Targets*, *5*, 293–312.

Colles, S.L., Dixon, J.B., O'Brien, P.E. (2007) Night eating syndrome and nocturnal snacking: association with obesity, binge eating and psychological distress. *Int J Obes., 31,* 1722–1730.

Dallman, M.F., Warne, J.P., Foster, M.T., Pecoraro, N.C. (2007) Glucocorticoids and insulin both modulate caloric intake through actions on the brain. *J Physiol*, *583*, 431–436.

de Zwaan, M., Roerig, D.B., Crosby, R.D., Karaz, S., Mitchell, J.E. (2006) Nighttime eating: a descriptive study. *Int J Eat Disord., 39,* 224-32.

Frazer, A. (1997). Pharmacology of antidepressants. *J Clin Psychopharmacol., 17*, 2S–18S

Friedman, S., Even, C., Thuile, J., Rouillon, F., Guelfi, J.D. (2006) Night eating syndrome and winter seasonal affective disorder. *Appetite, 47,* 119-22.

Geliebter, A., Gluck, M.E., Yahav, E. (2002) Cortisol following a stress test and dexamethasone suppression test (DST) in relation to psychopathology in the night eating syndrome. *Appetite*, *39*, 77. (Abstract)),

Gluck, M.E., Geliebter, A., Satov, T. (2001). Night Eating Syndrome is associated with depression, low self esteem, reduced daytime hunger, and less weight loss in obese outpatients. *Obesity Research, 9*, 264-267.

Gluck, M.E., Venti, C.A., Salbe, A.D., Krakoff, J. (2008) Nighttime eating: commonly observed and related to weight gain in an inpatient food intake study. *Am J Clin Nut*, *88*, 900–905.

Goel, N., Stunkard, A.J., Rogers, N.L., Van Dongen, H.P., Allison, K.C., O'Reardon, J.P., Ahima, R.S., Cummings, D.E., Heo, M., Dinges, D.F. (2009) Circadian rhythm profiles in women with night eating syndrome. *J Biol Rhythms., 24,* 85-94.

Goel, N., Stunkard, A.J., Rogers, N.L., Van Dongen, H.P.A., Allison, K.C., O'Reardon, J.P., Ahima, R.S., Cummings, D.E., Moonseong, H., Dinges, D. (2009) Circadian rhythm profiles in women with night eating syndrome. *J Biol Rhythms, 24,* 85.

Goncalves, M.D., Moore, R.H., Stunkard, A.J., Allison, K.C. (2009) The treatment of night eating: the patient's perspective. *Eur Eat Disord Rev*, *17*, 184–190.

Grilo, C.M., Masheb, R.M. (2004) Night-time eating in men and women with binge eating disorder. *Behav. Res. Ther., 42,* 397-407.

Huszar, D., Lynch, C.A., Fairchild-Huntress, V., Dunmore, J.H., Fang, Q., Berkemeier, L.R., Gu, W., Kesterson, R.A., Boston, B.A., Cone, R.D., Smith, F.J., Campfield, L.A., Burn, P., Lee, F. (1997) Targeted disruption of the melanocortin-4 receptor results in obesity in mice. *Cell*, *88*, 131–141.

Jeanrenaud, B., Rohner-Jeanrenaud, F. (2000) CNS-periphery relationships and body weight homeostasis: influence of the glucocorticoid status. *Int J Obes Relat Metab Disord*, *24,* S74–S76.

Kuldau J.M., Rand C.S.W. (1986). The night eating syndrome and bulimia in the morbidly obese. *Int. J. Eat. Disord., 5,* 143-148,

Lamerz, A., Kuepper-Nybelen, J., Bruning, N., Wehle, C., Trost-Brinkhues, G., Brenner, H., Hebebrand, J., Herpertz-Dahlmann, B. (2005) Prevalence of obesity, binge eating and night eating in a cross sectional field survey of 6-year-old children and their parents in a German urban population. *J Child Psychol Psychiatry 46,* 385–393.

Lu, X.Y., Kim, C.S., Frazer, A., Zhang, W. (2006) Leptin: a potential novel antidepressant. *Proc Natl Acad Sci U.S.A., 103*, 1593–1598.

Lundgren, J.D., Allison, K.C., Crow, S., O'Reardon, J.P., Berg, K.C., Galbraith, J., Martino, N.S., Stunkard, A.J. (2006) Prevalence of the night eating syndrome in a psychiatric population. *Am J Psychiatry, 163*, 156–158.

Lundgren, J.D., Rempfer, M.V., Brown, C.E., Goetz, J., Hamera, E. (2010) The prevalence of night eating syndrome and binge eating disorder among overweight and obese individuals with serious mental illness. *Psychiatry Res., 28,* 233-6.

Lundgren, J.D., Newberg, A.B., Allison, K.C., Wintering, N.A., Plossel, K., Stunkard, A.J. (2008) SPECT imaging of serotonin transporter binding in patients with night eating syndrome. *Psychiatry Res, 162,* 214–220.

Marshall, H.M., Allison, K.C., O'Reardon, J.P., Birketvedt, G., Stunkard, A.J. (2004) Night eating syndrome among non obese persons. *Int J Eat Disord., 35,* 217-22.

Morse, S.A., Ciechanowski, P.S., Katon, W.J., Hirsch, I.B. (2006) Isn't this just bedtime snacking? The potential adverse effects of night-eating symptoms on treatment adherence and outcomes in patients with diabetes. *Diabetes Care, 29,* 1800-4.

Napolitano M.A., Head S., Babyak M.A., Blumenthal J.A. (2001). Binge eating disorder and night eating syndrome: Psychological and behavioral characteristics. *International Journal of Eating Disorders, 30,* 193-203.

O'Reardon, J.P., Ringel, B.L., Dinges, D.F., Allison, K.C., Rogers, N.L., Martino, N.S., Stunkard, A.J. (2004); Circadian eating and sleeping patterns in the night eating syndrome. *Obes Res., 12*, 1789–1796.

Pawlow, L.A., O'Neil, P.M., Malcolm, R.J. (2003) Night eating syndrome: effects of brief relaxation training on stress, mood hunger and eating patterns. *Int J Obes Relat Metab Disord., 27,* 970-978.

Powers P.S., Perez, A., Boyd, F. Rosemurgy, A. (1999) Eating Pathology before and after Bariatric Surgery: A Prospective Study. *Int J Eat Disord., 25*, 293-300.

Rand, C.S., Macgregor, A.M., Stunkard, A.J. (1997). The night eating syndrome in the general population and among postoperative obesity surgery patients. *International Journal of Eating Disorders, 22*, 65-69.

Rasmussen, F., Tholin, F., Tynelius, P.O. (2007) Importance of genes and environmental factors for symptoms of night eating among 5209 pairs of twins from Sweden. *Int J Obes*; *4*: PO.21.

Rogers, N.L., Dinges, D.F., Allison, K.C., Maislin, G., Martino, N., O'Reardon, J.P., Stunkard, A.J. (2006) Assessment of sleep in women with night eating syndrome. *Sleep, 29,* 814–819.

Sassaroli, S., Ruggiero, G.M., Vinai, P., Cardetti, S., Carpegna, G., Ferrato, N., Vallauri, P., Masante, D., Scarone, S., Bertelli, S., Bidone, R, Busetto L, Sampietro S (2009) Daily and nightly anxiety among patients affected by night eating syndrome and binge eating disorder. *Eat Disord., 17*, 140-5.

Spaggiari, M.C., Granella, F., Parrino, L., Marchesi, C., Melli, I., Terzano, M.G. (1994) Nocturnal eating syndrome in adults. *Sleep, 17*, 339-344.

Striegel-Moore, R.H., Dohm, F.A., Hook, J.M., Schreiber, G.B., Crawford, P.B., Daniels, S.R. (2005) Night eating syndrome in young adult women: prevalence and correlates. *Int J Eat Disord., 37*, 200-6.

Striegel-Moore, R.H., Franko, D.L., May, A., Ach, E., Thompson, D., Hook, J.M. (2006) Should night eating syndrome be included in the DSM? *Int J Eat Disord., 39*, 544-9. Review.

Striegel-Moore, R.H., Franko, D.L., Thompson, D., Affenito, S., Kraemer, H.C. (2006) Night eating: prevalence and demographic correlates. *Obes Res*, *14,* 139–147.

Stunkard, A.J., Grace, W.J., Wolff, H.G. (1955). The night-eating syndrome; a pattern of food intake among certain obese patients. *American Journal of Medicine, 19,* 78-86.

Stunkard, A.J., Allison, K.C., Lundgren, J.D., O'Reardon, J.P. (2009) A biobehavioural model of the night eating syndrome. *Obes Rev., 10*, 69-77.

Stunkard, A.J., Allison, K.C., O'Reardon, J.P. (2005). The night eating syndrome: a progress report. *Appetite, 45,* 182-6.

Stunkard, A.J., Berkowitz, R., Wadden, T., Tanrikut, C., Reiss, E., Young, L. (1996) Binge eating disorder and the night-eating syndrome. *Int J Obes Relat Metab Disord., 20*, 1-6.

Sutton, G.M., Perez-Tilve, D., Nogueiras, R., Fang, J., Kim, J.K., Cone, R.D., Gimble, J.M., Tschop, M.H., Butler, A.A. (2008). The melanocortin-3 receptor is required for entrainment to meal intake. *J Neurosci.*, *28*, 12946–12955.

Tholin, S., Lindroos, A.K., Tynelius, P., Akerstedt, T., Stunkard, A.J., Bulik, C. (2009) Prevalence of night eating in obese and non-obese twins. *Obesity*; *17,* 1050–1055.

Tzischinsky, O., Latzer, Y., Epstein, R., Tov, N. (2000) Sleep-wake cycles in women with binge eating disorder. *Int J Eat Disord., 27*, 43-8.

Tzischinsky, O., Latzer, Y. (2004) Nocturnal eating: prevalence, features and night sleep among binge eating disorder and bulimia nervosa patients in Israel. *Eur Eat Disorders Rev*, *12,* 101-9.

Zakrzewska, K.E., Cusin, I., Stricker-Krongrad, A., Boss, O., Ricquier, D., Jeanrenaud, B., Rohner-Jeanrenaud, F. (1999) Induction of obesity and hyperleptinemia by central glucocorticoid infusion in the rate. *Diabetes*, *48*, 365–370.

In: Pathways to Obesity and Main Roads to Recovery
Editor: Piergiuseppe Vinai
ISBN: 978-1-61122-740-6

Chapter VII

Sleep-related Eating Disorder

Mauro Manconi[1,2] and Matteo Mario Anelli[1]
Sleep Center, Department of Neuroscience, Scientific Institute and University Ospedale San Raffaele, Milan, Italy.
Sleep Center, Neurocenter (EOC) of Southern Switzerland, Ospedale Civico, Via Tesserete, Lugano, Switzerland.

Abstract

The Sleep-related eating disorder (SRED) belongs to the parasomnias, which are unusual and undesirable daytime behavioral phenomena occurring during the sleep period. It is characterized by recurrent episodes of nocturnal eating in a variable, usually reduced, state of alertness, which are not linked to waking eating disorders such as bulimia, binge-eating and anorexia nervosa. The absence of full awareness can induce the occasional intake of inedible food and injuries during food preparation. These are the main features that distinguish SRED from nocturnal eating syndrome (NES), but the distinction between these two syndromes is still a controversial matter.

Introduction

Although unusual, at least sometimes in a lifespan, almost every human being will experience nocturnal food intake. When nocturnal eating behavior occurs frequently and interferes with the health and quality of life, it becomes a medical problem, and hence may be encountered in the clinical practice of general and specialists physicians.

According to the International Classification of Sleep Disorders (ICSD-2), (Table 7.1), Sleep-related eating disorder (SRED) belongs to the parasomnias, which are an unusual and undesirable behavioral phenomena occurring almost exclusively during the sleep period.[1] Central to parasomnias, such as sleep-talking, sleepwalking, and SRED, is the atypical emergence of regular daytime behavior in the normal quiescent state of sleep during a partial and variable state of consciousness (Kryger, Roth & Dement, 2005).

Table 7.1. Diagnostic criteria for sleep-related eating disorder (American Academy of Sleep Medicine 2005)[1]

A. Recurrent episodes of involuntary eating and drinking occur during the main sleep period
B. One or more of the following must be present with the recurrent episodes of involuntary eating and drinking: a. Consumption of peculiar forms or combinations of food or inedible or toxic substances b. Insomnia related to sleep disruption from repeated episodes of eating, with a complaint of nonrestorative sleep, daytime fatigue, or somnolence c. Sleep-related injury d. Dangerous behaviors performed while in pursuit of food or while cooking food e. Morning anorexia f. Adverse health consequences from recurrent binge eating of high-caloric foods
C. The disturbance is not better explained by another sleep disorder, medical or neurological disorder, mental disorder, medication use, or substance use disorder

According to this point of view, SRED and some other parasomnias may be considered as arousal disorders, triggered by an incomplete awakening. Probably, they are a consequence of an abnormal central nervous compartmentalization of the three main states of being: wakefulness, non-rapid eye movement (NREM) sleep and rapid eye movement (REM) sleep. Therefore, these states of dissociation often occur during the transition between wakefulness and sleep, in both directions, or during shifts in sleep stages. Moreover, SRED is often associated with other sleep disorders such as sleep apnea or periodic leg movements that favor abnormal nocturnal behavior by increasing the number and intensity of arousals.

SRED is characterized by recurrent episodes of nocturnal eating during a variable, usually reduced, state of alertness, occurring after the sleep onsets, which are not linked to waking eating disorders such as bulimia, binge-eating and anorexia nervosa (Howell et al., 2009). The absence of full conscious awareness, the consequent occasional intake of inedible food and injuries during food preparation, are the main features that distinguish SRED from nocturnal eating syndrome (NES). Indeed, the distinction between SRED and NES is still a controversial matter, and some authors consider these diseases to be positioned at opposite poles of a continuum clinical spectrum of eating disorders, mainly characterized by different levels of consciousness during eating (Howell et al., 2009; Vetrugno et al., 2006).

Historical Notes

Eating disorders may also occur, and in some cases almost exclusively, during the nocturnal period. Indeed, this problem only first received attention in 1955, when physician Albert Stunkard described the so-called NES (Stunkard et al., 1955). The perspective of Stunkard was that of an eating disorder specialist, so his description mainly focused on eating behavior, to the detriment of details concerning awareness and sleep in general. Therefore, the fundamental clinical features chose to identify patients affected by NES consisted of: morning anorexia, evening hyperphagia (25% of daily food intake after 7 pm, before bedtime), insomnia, lower mood and emotional distress. Since that moment, the issue of nocturnal eating was repeatedly revised and, when later neurologists, psychiatrics and sleep specialists took an interest in the matter, the syndrome was partially, and then completely, separated into two apparently distinct nosological entities.

It was 1990, when the sleep scientific community decided to include a new parasomnia in the International Classification of Sleep Disorder (ICSD-1, 1990). The disorder was named Night Eating and Drinking Syndrome (NEDS); it was probably the same disorder described by Stunkard, but the aspects concerning sleep were more thorough, going beyond details of food intake. Without paying attention to the period of wakefulness after dinner and prior to sleep-onset, and to a specific amount of food required for the diagnosis, NEDS was defined as "frequent and recurrent awakenings to eat and normal sleep onset following ingestion of the desired food."

What was at the beginning only a divergence under the nosological profile soon became a real problem of the uniqueness of the syndrome. This occurred four years later, when Schenck and Mahowald first observed patients who ate during night without, or with a low grade, of awareness, in a state of incomplete consciousness and without the ability to recall the episodes the following morning (Schenck et al., 1993;` Schenck & Mahowald, 1994). This nocturnal behavior resembled that of other classic parasomnias such as sleep-walking or sleep-talking, except for the type of automatic activity that regarded the food ingestion. To reinforce that a poor level of awareness is central to the phenomenon, the eating of non-edible objects or the injuries during preparing or cooking the food were reported by these patients. The authors named this disturbance as SRED and specified that it was often triggered or associated with other sleep disorders such as other parasomnias, periodic limb movements disorder and sleep apnea.

Based on this fundamental description, the second edition of the ICSD (2005) was updated so that NES was recognized as an eating disorder and subsequently removed (American Academy of Sleep Medicine, 2005). At the same time, the term SRED was first introduced, incorporating part of criteria that were previously used to define NEDS. Herein, SRED was defined as the presence of "recurrent episodes of involuntary eating and drinking occurring during the main sleep period." The episodes could be accompanied by "consumption of strange items, insomnia, sleep-related injury, occurrence of dangerous behaviors in the search for food, morning anorexia, and adverse health consequences related to nocturnal eating."

Except for the amount of nocturnal food intake and for its consumption also in the pre-sleep period, the main feature that distinguishes the NES from SRED is the level of consciousness of the subject during his nocturnal eating episodes. Patients with NES usually reported to be fully awake during eating, while patients affected by SRED report to be "half asleep, half awake" or even fully asleep while eating and may be unable to recollect the nocturnal episodes. The possibilities that episodes with different grade of consciousness may coexist in the same patients makes this distinction still controversial and suggests the idea that NES and SRED represent the opposite extremities of a continuum range of alertness of the same night eating disorder.

Clinical Features and Diagnostic Criteria

SRED consists of recurrent episodes of involuntary eating and drinking during arousals from nocturnal sleep, with problematic consequences (for complete diagnostic criteria, see the Table 1). (Winkelman, 1998) The episodes of eating are described as occurring in an involuntary or "out-of-control" manner during any time in the sleep cycle after an interval of sleep and typically during partial arousals from sleep with subsequent partial recall (Schenck & Mahowald, 1994). Frequently, patients cannot be easily brought to full consciousness during an episode of eating or drinking, and consequently, they may not remember what they ate during the night. For this, SRED and somnambulism seem to match partially. However, some patients seem to maintain a certain level of activation and conscience, and therefore bear the memory of episode in the morning.

By a self-administered questionnaire, Winkelman et al., (1999) found a prevalence rates of 16.7% of night eaters in a series of patients affected by eating disorder during the day, 8.7% in an outpatient eating disorder group, and 4.6% in a healthy group students. SRED is preponderant in the female population, with a prevalence ranging between 60 and 80% (Howell et al., 2009). Although follow-up studies on the syndrome are poor, SRED seems to be a chronic condition, which usually occurs nightly or more times in a single night period. Similar to NES and other parasomnia, SRED may have a genetic predisposition. Sometimes, patients reported the occurrence of the same disorder in other member of family (de Ocampo et al., 2002).

Patients usually consume peculiar forms or combinations of food or inedible or toxic substances. Subjects often report to prefer high caloric food such as carbohydrates and fats, and show less preference for healthful foods like vegetables and fruits. The most commonly foods consumed by patients are: bread, pie and dairy products such as ice cream, peanut butter, chocolate and other sweets. It was noted that patients do not complain of being hungry, and foods are often preferred in the night are not during the day (Vetrugno et al., 2006; Winkelman, 1998). During an episode, there may occur different consumption of food or combination of food, including non-edible or use of toxic substances such as frozen or uncooked foods, buttered cigarettes, animal food and salt sandwiches, unpalatable foods such as raw bacon, coffee grounds and eggs shell, sunflower shells, glue, and cleaning solutions (Schenck & Mahowald, 1994; Winkelman, 1998; Schenck, 2006). In some cases, food can be prepared and consumed in a strict food and hot meals or cold, simple or entire; however, injuries can occur inside or outside during the preparation and consumption of food, including activities such as hazardous drinking excessively hot liquids, choking on thick foods, and lacerations from careless food preparation (Howell et al., 2009). Patients may ingest poisonous substances or food that they are allergic. Two of our patients needed an urgent intervention after having ingested significant amounts of bleach.

Adverse consequences, besides consumption of peculiar combinations of food or non-edible substances and dangerous food preparation behavior, include: morning anorexia, sleep-related injury and weight gain and obesity (American Academy of Sleep Medicine, 2005; Howell et al., 2009; Schenck & Mahowald, 1994; Winkelman, 1998; Schenck, 2006). Studies have demonstrated that SRED is associated with weight gain and obesity. Some patients with SRED restrict their daytime and evening food consumption or start or increase physical activity in order to halt or slow down the progressive weight gain from their sleep-related eating. Schenck & Mahowald (1994) observed that nearly half of their patients met the criteria for being considered overweight, and that 44% of patients declared that more than 20% of their excess weight gain was determined from eating at night.

Insomnia related to sleep disruption from repeated episodes of eating, with a complaint of non-restorative sleep, daytime fatigue, or somnolence, may be associated with SRED. Most of the patients complain that without nocturnal food intake, they are not able to fall asleep again. Sleep macrostructure between nocturnal eating episodes is usually normal, and sleep insomnia is proportional to the number of the episodes and the duration of them (Vetrugno et al., 2006). Morning anorexia, sometimes associated with abdominal distension, is often reported by these patients.

Video-polysomnographic Findings

The gold standard for the instrumental investigation of SRED is represented by the video-polisomnography (V-PSG) (Vetrugno, 2006; American Academy of Sleep Medicine, 2005). In this case, the sleep lab should be equipped with a food-and-drink dinner table positioned at the bedside with staples chosen and brought in by the patients themselves. Sleep recordings and scoring should be done according to standard methods and include electroencephalogram (EEG) (C3-A2; C4-A1, O2-A1); right and left electrooculogram; chin superficial electromyogram (EMG); and EKG. Other possible informative muscles to record are represented by the tibialis anterior, facial/masticatory muscles such as orbicularis oculi, orbicularis oris, masseter, temporalis and sternocleidomastoideus. Oro-nasal airflow, thoracic and abdominal respiratory efforts with a strain gauge, and oxygen saturation (SaO2), are useful to exclude sleep-related breathing disorders. V-PSG can give information on the EEG activity and on the behavior of the patient during the nocturnal eating episodes. Moreover, a technician may test the level of awareness of the patient during eating and may assess the morning recall of the nocturnal episode.

Different from the NES, patients affected by SRED usually do not eat before the sleep onset. One or more eating episodes per night might be recorded. The majority of the episodes arouse after awakening from NREM sleep, either during stage N_2 or slow wave sleep (SWS) (Howell et al., 2009; Vetrugno et al., 2006; Winkelman, 1998). Less frequently, eating episodes might emerge from REM sleep. The latency between the awakening and the food intake may vary widely, from few seconds to more than one hour, but usually ranges between seconds and few minutes (Figure 7.1) (Vetrugno et al., 2006).

This delay is shorter for episodes that occur during SWS than those from stage 2 NREM sleep. Also, the duration of eating episodes is variable, ranging between seconds and more than 20 to 30 minutes, but usually ends in few minutes. Co-morbidity with other sleep disorders, such as restless legs syndrome (RLS) or obstructive sleep apnea syndrome (OSAS), may prolong the duration of the eating episodes. The sleep onset after eating is usually short, ranging between few seconds and few minutes (Figure 7.2).

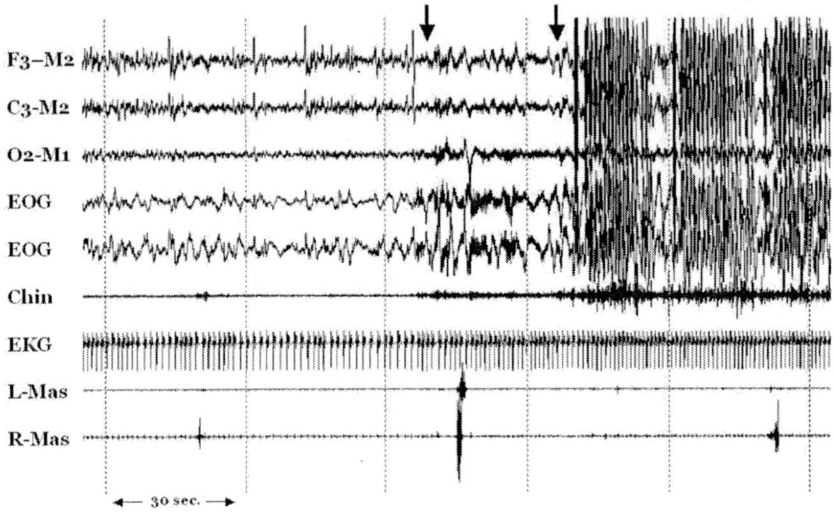

Figure 7.1. Nocturnal Polysomnographic sample. Eating episode emerging from stage 2 NREM sleep. Arrows indicate the 23 seconds of latency between awakening and eating onset. EEG (F3, C3, O2); M mastoid; Chin sub-mental muscle; EKG electrocardiography; L-Mas and R-Mas left and right masseter muscles.

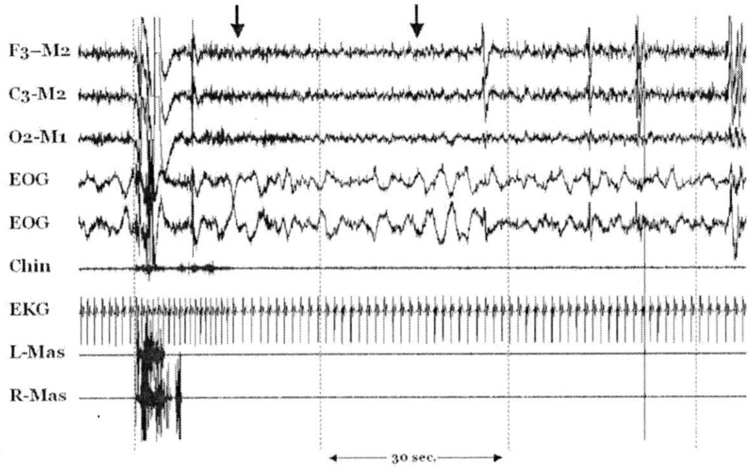

Figure 7.2. Nocturnal Polysomnographic sample. Eating episode emerging from stage 2 NREM sleep. Arrows indicate the 29 seconds of latency between the end of eating and sleep onset. EEG (F3, C3, O2); M mastoid; Chin sub-mental muscle; EKG electrocardiography; L-Mas and R-Mas left and right masseter muscles.

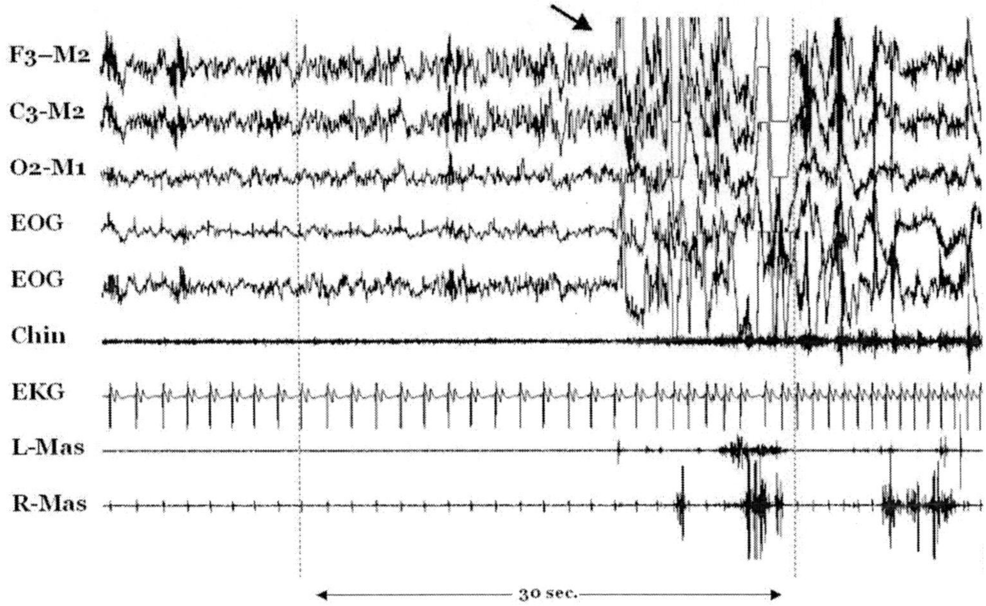

Figure 7.3. Nocturnal Polysomnographic sample. Eating episode emerging from stage 2 NREM sleep. Arrow indicates the arousal follows by an awakening, occurring before the onset of eating. EEG (F3, C3, O2); M mastoid; Chin sub-mental muscle; EKG electrocardiography; L-Mas and R-Mas left and right masseter muscles.

The EEG recorded during the episodes is usually characterized by normal alpha activity, also with electrooculogram, heart and breathing rates typical of wakefulness (Figure 7.3 and 7.4) (Vetrugno et al., 2006).

The level of consciousness may vary among patients and in the same patient depending on the single episode. The better way to establish the level of awareness during eating is to interrogate directly the patient while he is eating and to match the response with the EEG activity. Under this point of view, the available data in the literature are controversial. While Vetrugno et al., (2006) reported a full consciousness during the nocturnal eating episodes in a series of 35 polysomnographic patients, the percentage of patients with full consciousness represents only 21% and 9% of the casistic series described respectively by Schenck et al., (1994) and Winkelman et al., (1998). Spaggiari et al., (1994) agreed with a good level of vigilance during the episodes, but the authors reported to deal with patients affected by NES rather than SRED (Spaggiari et al., 1994). This discrepancy might be explained in different ways: the concomitant use of psychotropic drugs, which can decrease the level of consciousness; the psychiatric presence of a co-morbidity; the heterogeneity of the method to assess the vigilance (direct question during episodes, EEG activity, presence of morning amnesia, occurring of injury or ingestion of inedible food); or simply, the authors described two different population of patients. Obviously, also in the same patient, the level of awareness might be influenced by the sleep inertia, so it is lower when episodes emerge from SWS than from Stage 2 NREM, and when the delay between the awakening and the eating onset is short.

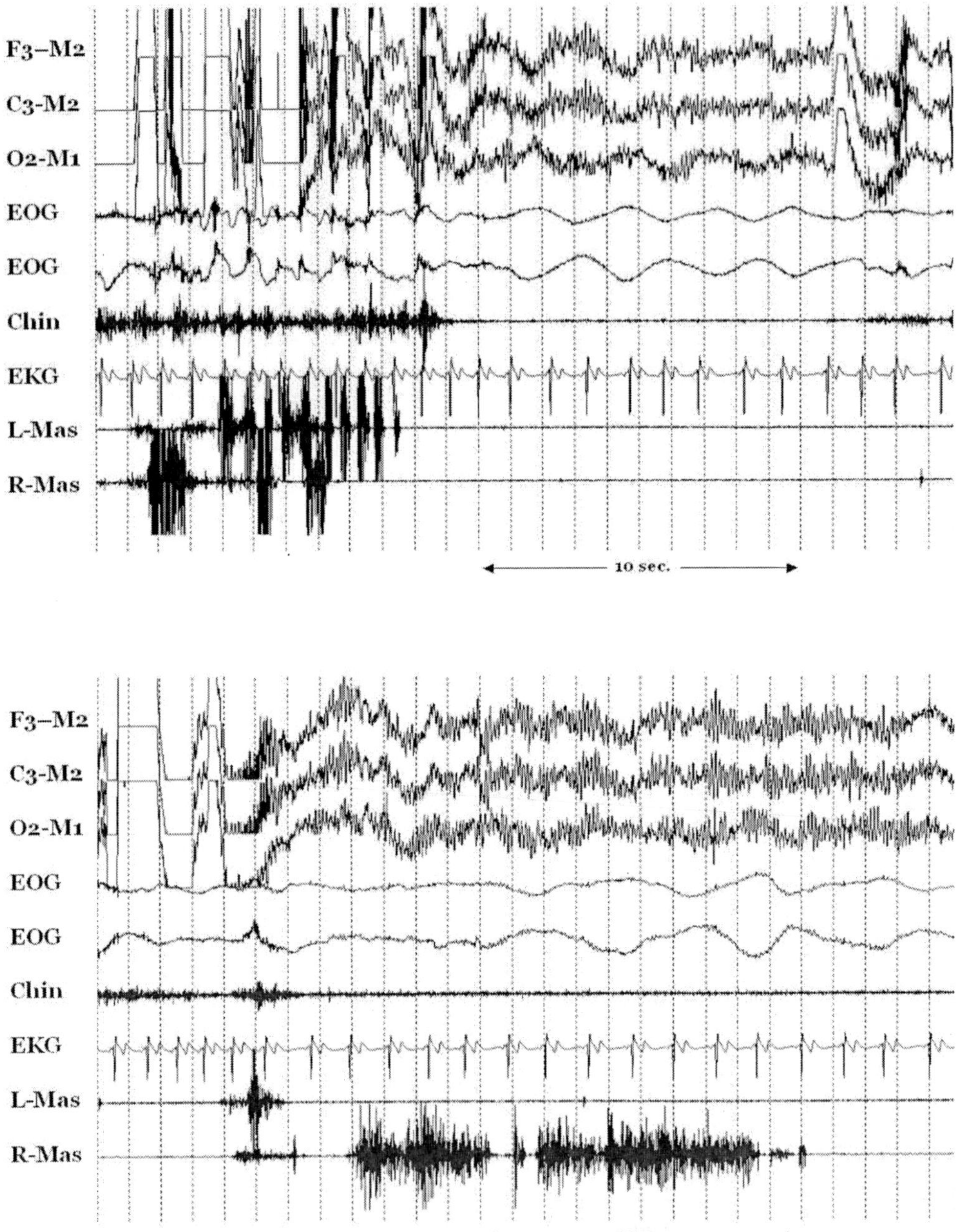

Figure 7.4. Nocturnal Polysomnographic samples. The EEG parameters show the presence of alpha activity during eating. EEG (F3, C3, O2); M mastoid; Chin sub-mental muscle; EKG electrocardiography; L-Mas and R-Mas left and right masseter muscles.

Although the polysomnographic data in the literature are scanty, on average, the sleep structure outside of the episodes is described as quietly normal (Howell et al., 2009; Vetrugno et al., 2006). A mild increase in percentage of the stages 1 and 2 NREM, together with a mild decreasing of SWS and an unchanged REM sleep, are usually described. The co-occurrence of SRED with other sleep disorders, such as RLS, OSAS and parasomnia are frequently reported, and in these cases a greater sleep disruption and a significant reducing of the sleep efficiency might be met (Provini et al., 2009; Eveloff & Millman, 1993; Horiguchi et al., 1999; Eiber et al., 2001). In the original series of 38 patients, sleepwalking was noted in 23 subjects (Schenck & Mahowald, 1994). Sleepwalking and other parasomnias without eating often precedes SRED in the medical history. This led many researchers to consider SRED a "'sleepwalking variant disorder,'" or an arousal disorder that can be triggered by a variety of sleep disorders (Howell et al., 2009).

Other frequent polysomnographic features are represented by periodic limb movements (PLM), and by various facial muscle activations during sleep (Vetrugno et al., 2006; Provini et al., 2009). In these patients, the positioning of surface electrodes on different facial muscles during the polysomnography often disclose repetitive chewing movements during NREM sleep and after arousals from both NREM and REM sleep. Part of this muscular activity may be classified as swallowing (Figure 7.5) and repetitive/rhythmic masticatory (Figure 7.6) behaviors.

Jatrogenic Form

Several drugs, mainly the sedative psychotropic ones, may cause confusional arousal, overall during the first part of the night and during slow wave sleep. The sleep inertia associated with these partial awakening may trigger unusual behavior and involuntary eating episodes looking like those described in SRED.

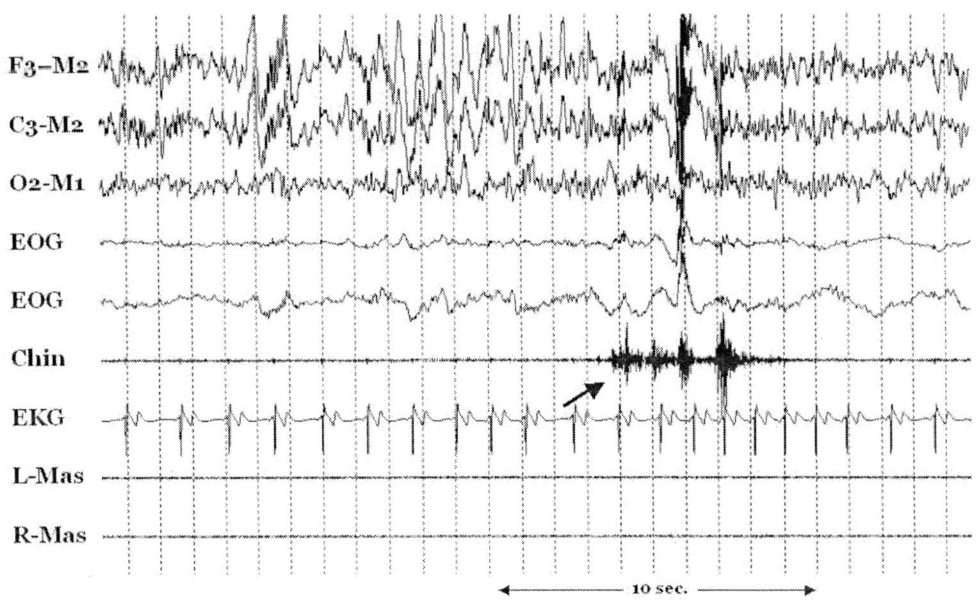

Figure 7.5. Nocturnal Polysomnographic sample. Arrow indicates a swallowing activity occurring during stage 2 NREM sleep in patient affected by SRED. EEG (F3, C3, O2); M mastoid; Chin submental muscle; EKG electrocardiography; L-Mas and R-Mas left and right masseter muscles.

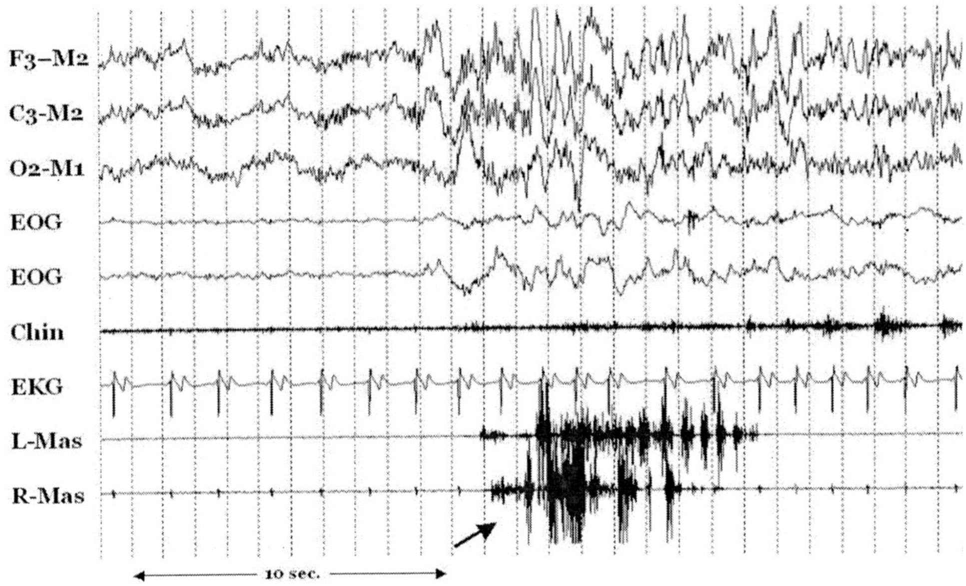

Figure 7.6. Nocturnal Polysomnographic sample. Arrow indicates a rhythmic mascticatory activity occurring during stage 2 NREM sleep in patient affected by SRED. EEG (F3, C3, O2); M mastoid; Chin sub-mental muscle; EKG electrocardiography; L-Mas and R-Mas left and right masseter muscles.

Parasomnias such as sleepwalking, SRED and sleep-driving, have been reported to be triggered by zolpidem (a non-benzodiazepine hypnotic with short half-life, agonist of GABA-A receptors, indicated for the short-term insomnia) (Dang et al., 2009; Morgenthaler et al., 2002; Najjar 2007). Chiang et al., (2008) reported two cases in which SRED was induced by the extended-release zolpidem but not with the immediate-release formulation.

Different neuroleptics, such as risperidone (Lu et al., 2004) and olanzepine, (Paquet et al., 2002) have been described as possible inductors of acute forms of SRED. Horiguchi et al., (1999) described a case of SRED secondary to neuroleptic-induced RLS and PLM in a schizophrenic male patient, provoked by low-dosage haloperidol, and completely inhibited by clonazepam treatment.

SRED episodes usually recovery after the withdrawal of the incriminated drugs.

Differential Diagnosis

Except for the overlap between SRED and NES, which needs to be further elucidated, SRED should be mainly differentiated from the other eating behavior disorders such as bulimia nervosa, binge eating disorder and anorexia (Winkelman, 2006). The co-existence of the above-mentioned disorders and SRED can be observed, but inappropriate compensatory phenomena, such as laxative, self-induced vomiting, diuretics or other purging activities should lack at least during the night time. Patients with SRED and excessive weight gain may increase eventually fast during the day or increase the physical activity to prevent obesity; however, they usually do not incur in the inappropriate behaviors listed above.

The presence of Kleine-Levin syndrome should be always excluded in SRED patients. Subjects affected by this syndrome are usually male adolescents, who present a clinical entity occurring periodically one to five times per year, lasting days or weeks, characterized by hypersomnia, hypersexuality and hyperphagia (Ortega-Albas & Entrambasaguas-Barreto 2003; Arnulf et al., 2005; Arnulf et al., 2008; Arnulf et al., 2008a).

Other medical conditions presenting possible nocturnal eating episodes, which need to be excluded before to establish a SRED diagnosis, are: hypoglycemic states, peptic ulcer disease, reflux esophagitis and Kluver-Bucy syndrome (placidity, bulimia, hyperorality, hypersexuality, visual agnosia).

References

American academy of sleep medicine. (2005) *The international classification of sleep disorders. Diagnostic and coding manual.* Westchester. IL

American academy of sleep medicine. *The international classification of sleep disorders.* Westchester: 1990.

Arnulf, I., Lecendreux, M., Franco, P., Dauvilliers, Y. (2008) Kleine-levin syndrome: state of the art. *Rev. neurol., 164,* 658-68.

Arnulf, I., Lin, L., Gadoth, N., File, J., Lecendreux, M., Franco, P. et al., (2008) Kleine-levin syndrome: a systematic study of 108 patients. *Ann. neurol, 63,* 482-93.

Arnulf, I., Zeitzer, J.M., File, J., Farber, N., Mignot, E. (2005) Kleine-levin syndrome: a systematic review of 186 cases in the literature. *Brain, 128,:*2763-76.

Chiang, A., Krystal, A. (2008) Report of two cases where sleep-related eating behavior occurred with the extended-release formulation but not the immediate-release formulation of a sedative-hypnotic agent. *J clin. sleep med, 4,* 155-6.

Dang, A., Garg, G., Rataboli, P.V. (2009) Zolpidem induced nocturnal sleep-related eating disorder (nsred) in a male patient. *Int. j eat. disord., 42,* 385-6.

De ocampo, J., Foldvary, N., Dinner, D.S., Golish, J. (2002) Sleep-related eating disorder in fraternal twins. *Sleep med., 3,* 525-6.

Eiber, R., Friedman, S. (2001) Correlation between eating disorders and sleep disturbances. *Encephale, 27,* 429-34.

Eveloff, S.E., Millman, R.P. (1993) Sleep-related eating disorder as a cause of obstructive sleep apnea. *Chest, 104*, 629-30.

Horiguchi, J., Yamashita, H., Mizuno, S., Kuramoto, Y., Kagaya, A., Yamawaki, S. et al., (1999) Nocturnal eating/drinking syndrome and neuroleptic-induced restless legs syndrome. *Int. clin. psychopharmacol., 14,* 33-6.

Howell, M.J., Schenck, C.H., Crow, S.J. (2009) A review of nighttime eating disorders. *Sleep med rev., 13,* 23-34.

Kryger, M. H., Roth, T., Dement W. (2005) *Principles and practice of sleep medicine.* Philadelphia. Elsevier Saunders.

Lu M.L, Shen, W.W. (2004) Sleep-related eating disorder induced by risperidone. *J clin. psychiatry, 65,* 273-4.

Morgenthaler, T.I., Silber, M.H. (2002) Amnestic sleep-related eating disorder associated with zolpidem. *Sleep med., 3,* 323-7.

Najjar, M. Zolpidem and amnestic sleep-related eating disorder. (2007) *J clin. sleep med, 3,* 637-8.

Ortega-Albas, J.J, Entrambasaguas-Barreto, M. (2003) Kleine levin syndrome and sleep-related eating disorder. *Rev.neurol, 37,* 200.

Paquet, V., Strul, J., Servais, L., Pelc, I., Fossion, P. (2002) Sleep-related eating disorder induced by olanzapine. *J clin.psychiatry, 63,* 597.

Provini, F., Antelmi, E., Vignatelli, L., Zaniboni, A., Naldi, G., Calandra-Buonaura, G. et al., (2009) Association of restless legs syndrome with nocturnal eating: a case-control study. *Mov disord.*, 24, 871-7.

Schenck, C.H. (2006) A study of circadian eating and sleeping patterns in night eating syndrome (NES) points the way to future studies on NES and Sleep-Related Eating Disorder. *Sleep med., 7,* 653-6.

Schenck, C.H., Hurwitz, T.D., O'connor, K.A., Mahowald, M.W. (1993) Additional categories of sleep-related eating disorders and the current status of treatment. *Sleep, 16,* 457-66.

Schenck, C.H., Mahowald, M.W. (1994). Review of nocturnal sleep-related eating disorders. *Int.j.eat.disord., 15,* 343-56.

Spaggiari, M.C., Granella, F., Parrino, L., Marchesi, C., Melli, I., Terzano, M.G. (1994) Nocturnal eating syndrome in adults. *Sleep, 17,* 339-44.

Stunkard, A.J., Grace, W.J., Wolff, H.G. (1955) The night-eating syndrome; a pattern of food intake among certain obese patients. *Am. j med, 19,* 78-86.

Vetrugno, R., Manconi, M., Ferini-Strambi, L., Provini, F., Plazzi, G., Montagna, P. (2006) Nocturnal eating: sleep-related eating disorder or night eating syndrome? A videopolysomnographic study. *Sleep, 29,* 949-54.

Winkelman, J.W. (1998) Clinical and polysomnographic features of sleep-related eating disorder. *J clin. psychiatry, 59,* 14-9.

Winkelman, J.W. (2006) Sleep-related eating disorder and night eating syndrome: sleep disorders, eating disorders, or both? *Sleep, 29,* 876-7.

Winkelman, J.W., Herzog, D.B., Fava, M. (1999) The prevalence of sleep-related eating disorder in psychiatric and non-psychiatric populations. *Psychol.med., 29,* 1461-6.

In: Pathways to Obesity and Main Roads to Recovery
Editor: Piergiuseppe Vinai
ISBN: 978-1-61122-740-6

Chapter VIII

Assessment of Obese Patients

Piergiuseppe Vinai[1], Silvia Cardetti[1], Gabriella Carpegna[1], Noemi Ferrato[1], Loriana Murciano[2], Elena Ponzio[3] and Paola Vallauri[1]
[1]Gnosis: N profit research group, Cuneo; Studi Cognitivi Post Graduate Psychotherapy Cognitive School research group, Milan, Italy
[2]Ville Turina e Amione clinic, San Maurizio Canavese, Turin, Italy
[3]Studi Cognitivi Post Graduate Psychotherapy Cognitive School, Milan; DSM Franco Basaglia ASL Torino 2, Turin Italy

Abstract

This chapter is a sort of flow chart useful for deciding how to treat different "obesities," including a summary of factors that could influence the choice of a specific therapy. In it are suggested instruments useful in highlighting medical and psychopathological co-morbidities and summarized diagnostic criteria of eating disorders frequently related to obesity.

Introduction

Many factors can play a role in onset and maintenance of obesity. The principal are shown in Table 8.1. All of them have to be explored during the assessment in order to evaluate not only which are the most relevant for each patient, but more importantly, which ones are still active and how much they could interfere with the patient's attempts to lose weight.

Table 8.1. Factors involved in weight gain

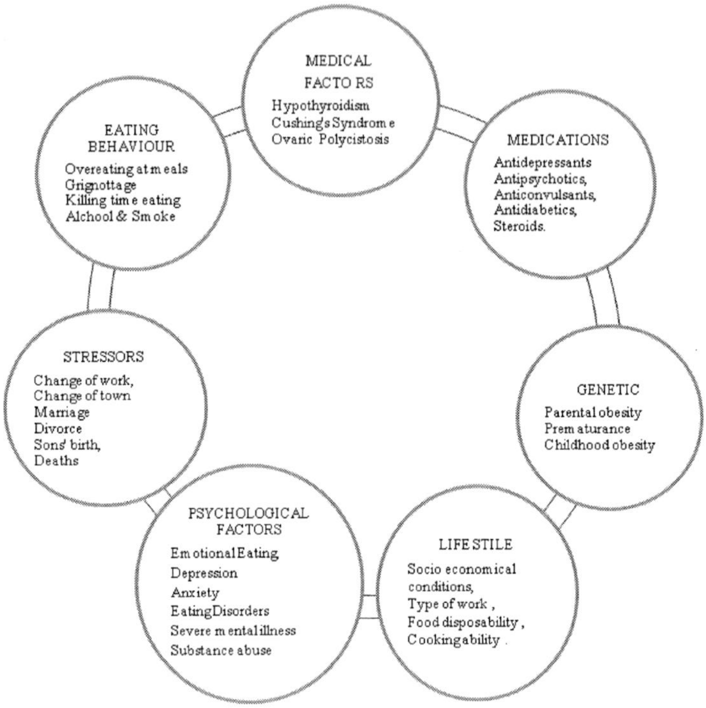

In exploring the factors indicated in Table 8.1, we suggest to avoid a predefined order, starting from those that the patient sees as the most relevant in his personal history of weight gain, gradually widening the observation to the others. This is to make sure the patients understand that we want to explore their own personal pathways that led them to obesity. In our opinion, it is very important to know not only how they gained weight (their lifestyles and eating behaviors), but also their opinions on the causes of weight gain. Only knowing them we can propose a change they can accomplish. This is why the first step has to be the definition of the patient's naive theories regarding his weight gain.

The medical and the psychological assessments are illustrated separately in this chapter, but the best chance is to find a therapist able to assess both.

Assessment of Naive Theories on Obesity

The first session is a very important step and heavily influences patient's decision to follow the proposed therapy. As obese people are frequently exposed to social criticism and judgment, it is particularly important to avoid a judging conduct in approaching the weight history. The first aim of the clinician is to understand the patients' opinions regarding their obesity and their convictions as to the way to recovery, in order to—if necessary—discuss with them to find out the real reasons of weight gain and the best way to deal with them. For example, a patient who is convinced that his obesity is only due to genetic causes will be less willing to accept a change in his alimentary habits and will rather expect a pharmaceutical or surgical solution, whereas a person justifying his excessive weight with difficulties in dealing with stress will expect the clinician to solve his emotional problems rather than engage actively in following a diet.

Brody, Masheb and Grilo (2005) reported that obese patients with BED may have treatment preferences that are independent of variability in their clinical presentations. Treatment preferences were related to patients' perceptions of their primary problems. The patients who preferred Cognitive Behavioral Therapy appear to base their treatment selections more on their problem perception than on their primary treatment goals, whereas the patients who preferred Behavioral Weight Loss programs seem to select treatments based more on their primary treatment goals (weight loss) than on their problem perceptions.

If the patient's and therapist's opinions regarding the reasons of obesity onset and the therapeutic approach are too far apart, it will be difficult for the patient to follow the proposed treatment. Consequently, the therapist's first task is to close the gap between the two positions. This style of assessment can, hence, already be a therapeutic instrument, helping the patients to reformulate their own theories and, therefore, opening them more towards the treatment. The following box shows the first questions we ask all of our patients.

- "Which is your problem?"
- "In your opinion, why did you gain and maintain your weight?"
- "What do you expect from the therapy?"

The clinicians have clearly to ask the patients to report their own convictions on the topic, not what they have learnt from previous specialists. In fact, we are at this point not interested in the level of their knowledge about obesity but in their deep convictions on the matter. Only knowing these can we adjust our style of treatment without battling their theories on causes and cure of obesity.

If the patient doesn't indicate spontaneously which factors were the most important ones in his process of gaining weight, it might be useful helping him by prompting to put in order of importance the factors shown in Table 8.2.

It is also helpful to know the relative importance that the patient attributes to each factor. For this task, it might be useful asking the patient to highlight the importance percentage for each one on a pie chart.

The order of importance given to each factor by the patient influences the chronological order in which we are going to work out the assessment of each factor that could be involved in the weight gain. For example, for a patient, who is convinced that his obesity is mainly due to genetic reasons, the order will be GEN MED DRUG LIFE EAT STRESS PSY; for someone who believes that the stress-related factors are responsible for their obesity, one can use the approach of STRESS- PSY –EAT—LIFE—MED—DRUG—GEN; for patients who believe that their obesity is secondary to medical pathologies, we would suggest the approach of MED—DRUG—GEN—EAT—LIFE—STRESS—PSY and so on. In the next pages, the order of the of assessment's steps will follow the naive hypothesis of a patient thinking that his weight gain is mainly due to psychological reasons independent from himself: "*I overeat because my life is so horrible; I cannot follow a diet in these conditions!*" In this case, the order of the assessment's steps will be STRESS-PSY–EAT—LIFE—MED—DRUG—GEN.

Table 8.2. Assessing patient's naive theories on his weight gain

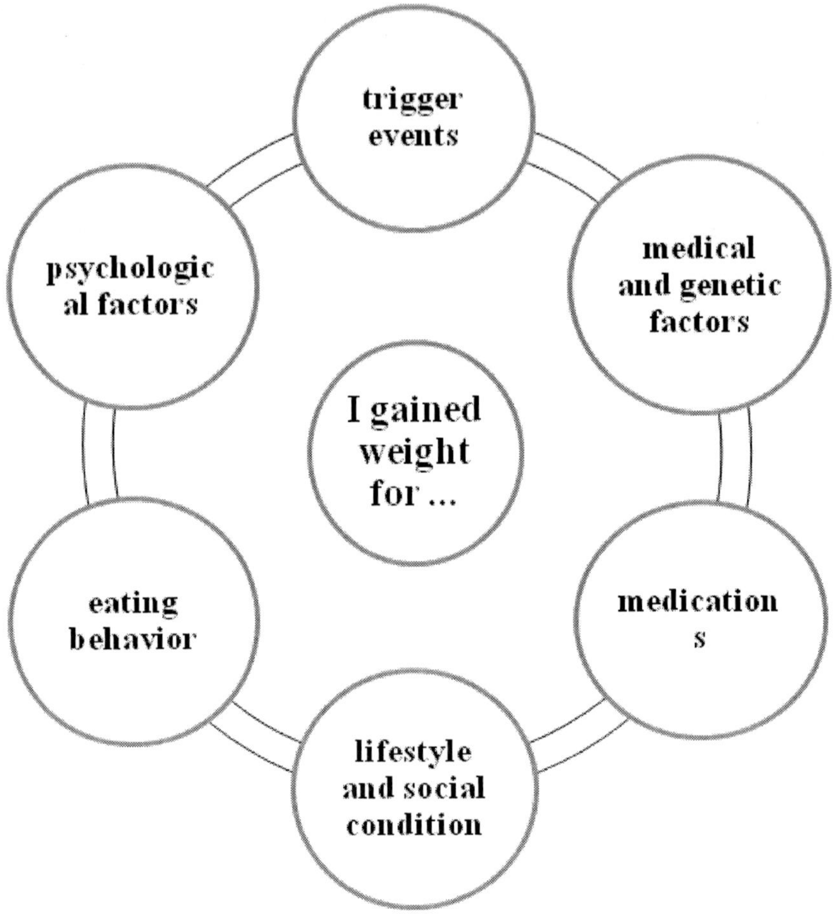

Obviously, the naive theories of the patient influence only the order in which the various subjects are handled. It will be the clinician's experience to guide him in deciding how much time dedicate to each step, but it is important not to pass on to the next step without being reasonably certain that all preceding points have been clarified. Table 8.2 might be used as a check list to be sure to have explored all areas. If, as often happens, the patient has already and without success undergone other therapies in order to lose weight, it is important to explore their theories regarding their failure as to confute them whenever they don't correspond to the real data or to not repeat the same mistakes.

The interview goes on evaluating the patient's motivation for losing weight even if it is possible that several aspects of their motivation have already emerged during the examination of his naive theories.

Motivation to Change

Two of the most important problems of the clinicians dealing with obesity are the high dropout rate and the weight-maintaining problem. Many studies indeed refer the drop out as the main failing cause in obesity therapies (Richman et al., 1992), which ranges between 10% and 80%. In fact, many studies (Mc Guire et al., 1999; Wing & Hill, 2001; Wing & Phelan, 2005) report that only about 20% of subjects have maintained the weight reached or have still lost weight a year after the end of the therapy,.

It is then essential to evaluate the patient's motivation for the treatment: in fact, undertaking the obesity therapy with a badly motivated patient increases the drop out possibility, risking, especially with patients who already tried many times to lose weight, to expose them to a further failure and to strengthen the self-conceived idea of being incapable or to enhance the vision of the treatment as too hard for them.

The clinician, according to his sensitivity and preparation, decides whether either to use specific questionnaires or only a clinical interview to assess the motivation of the patient. During the interview, the sense of self-efficiency (Bandura, 1977, 1991, 1995) and the locus of control (Rotter, 1966) have to be deeply analyzed.

A way of evaluating the motivation is drawing up a balance sheet with expected benefits through weight loss, with costs (in terms of effort, money, time, emotional costs…) that the patient thinks to have to pay, and with resources he believes he has at his disposal. It could be useful writing down a real balance sheet, which will be modified as the patient and the therapist analyze and discuss every single point.

The Expected Benefits

During the evaluation of benefits, the therapist will study in depth the positive consequences the patient imagines to gain from weight loss. Obese patients do not expect only aesthetic advantages (Cheskin & Donze, 2001; Brink & Ferguson, 1998; Levy & Heaton, 1993) (which seem to be the most important among women) and health-related returns (i.e., to get less tired during physical activities, to sweat less, to reduce the risk of chronic pathologies…). They also hope to obtain psychological and social rewards (i.e., feeling more self-confident and determined, being loved, respected, to get a better job, etc.). Even though these are often the patient's fundamental objectives, they are frequently revealed only after a deeper examination, while initially, more culturally and socially acceptable motivations are given.

Once the pro and con list has been worked out, it will be possible to ask the patient to rate every expected advantage, in order to better understand the secondary advantages of weight loss. It is important to discuss with the patient which of these objectives are realistically related to weight loss and which are unconnected. It often happens that the patient realizes that his primary objective (i.e., a major assertiveness) is not related with weight: this fact can contribute to his serenity; on the other hand, it can also weaken his motivation for weight loss treatment. However, if the patient will be able to lose weight, without reaching the secondary advantages he expects, he could be disappointed, stop the diet and begin to gain weight again. It is, therefore, important to understand the value of each single secondary advantage to downsize the unrealistic ones (being loved by everyone, becoming assertive, etc.) and to reinforce those functional to the treatment (i.e., health, well-being, physical fitness, etc.).

It is also useful to evaluate the expected benefits related to dropping out from the treatment (avoiding the possibility of failing the diet, avoiding intimate relationships with the other sex, that patients feel unable to face…). These factors, being connected to cognitive constructs related with self-image, relationships with others and image of the world, are often the greatest obstacles to the success of the treatment. For example, a person who strongly wishes to be thin can see as devastating for the self-image the risk of failing a diet. On the other hand, a person who feels himself incapable of managing an affective relationship could maintain his "*protective shell of fat*" as a deterrent for people of the other sex.

The Expected Costs

One of the factors that most influence the motivation of the patient is the renunciation. Patients are often mistakenly convinced that to get fit, it is necessary to completely cut out certain foods (often the most liked ones) and focus on what they cannot eat, not considering all those aliments they can choose. In this way, sensations and emotions caused by the renunciation become unacceptable. In the analysis of patient's motivation, it is very important to explore these naïve theories to correct them. This part of the assessment plays a very important role the dietician that can explain how to lose weight doesn't mean completely renounce to the pleasure of the food.

Another great effort for the patient is to do a regular physical activity. In this case, it is necessary to evaluate the presence of feelings of inadequacy or shame connected to their body image. Once these factors are considered, it should be easier to deal with dysfunctional ideas related to the patient's physical aspect or to help them to choose an activity compatible with the uneasiness they feel in exposing their body (i.e., the swimming pool is unlikely to be easily accepted).

The Resources

To make an objective exam of the real possibilities of succeeding, it is useful to make a list of the resources (personal, material, affective, environmental, etc.) that the patient has at his disposal: ability in preparing dietetic foods, opportunities to exercise and/or emotional and practical support of friends and partners. Past successful attempts to lose weight, even if only briefly, have to be assessed. It is also essential to investigate the perception the patient has of his own self-efficacy in changing his lifestyle. The patient would begin to lose weight if he thinks to have few possibilities to reach this goal.

Another essential element of the motivation that has to be carefully investigated is the amount of the expected weight loss. It is not sufficient to ask the patient how many kilos he expects to lose, because his thin self-image frequently does not correspond with the expressed number of kilos, being much smaller.

A way of understanding the real expected amount of the weight loss is ask the patient to visualize and describe how he imagines himself after having lost weight, which clothes he hope to use and which size he intends to reach. If the expectations are too far from the reality, the first aim of the treatment will be the re-definition of the expectations both related to the number of kilos he can lose and to his thin self-image. A discrepancy between the patient's expectations and the weight loss that can be pursued without causing health risks; if not considered, it can expose the patient to the risk of being disappointed and then to the abandonment in case of losses little inferior to what he expected, or of having changes in the physical aspect much more slower than he desired. A research of Foster et al., (1997) found that the ideal weight loss for the patients was equivalent to the 38% of the body weight at the beginning of the treatment; an acceptable weight loss, not the ideal, was around the 30% and the minimum acceptable weight loss was of the 25%. A weight loss of the 17% was considered unacceptable. For the clinicians, a 10% of weight loss is the recommended one. The motivation has to be monitored also during the treatment having a peculiar attention to the signs of scarce involvement into the therapy: delays, boredom, forgetting homework, claiming the futility of the treatment or his own inability to perform it, etc.

Psychological Assessment

Steps of Psychological Assessment

If naive theories focus on psychological factors influencing obesity onset, the interview will continue with the assessment of those factors. Being directly connected to their theories, the evaluation will be more reasonable and acceptable. In assessing psychological aspects of obesity, we should never forget that these are subjects looking for a therapy for obesity, not for the treatment of a psychopathology.

Possible indicators of eating disorders—binge eating, excessive weight loss, emotional eating and nocturnal eating—need a special attention by the clinician. If the pathology is confirmed, the patient has to be treated using the specific protocols described in the third part of this book.

During the clinical interview, other traces of psychopathologies may emerge: alexithymic traits, dysfunctional body perception, depression, anxiety and obsessive symptoms. In these cases, even deeper and less easily revealed areas of the patient's personality have to be explored to exclude the presence of a psychosis or a personality disorders. These patients need to be treated following the indications of chapter XX.

If no eating disorders or severe psychiatric pathologies emerge, probably we are dealing with a patient who might have gained weight for reasons mainly connected to bad eating habits or dysfunctional psychological mechanisms, which cannot be classified as true and proper psychopathologies. With these patients, the cognitive behavioral technique of the ABC is helpful to explore their dysfunctional beliefs, the impulsivity, the level of self-esteem and the presence of emotional eating. and possible cognitive biases.

This final step of the assessment will allow the clinician to determine those patients who could benefit from a self-help program and the ones who will need the intervention of psychological support, focusing on their specific difficulties.

Is the Psychological Assessment always Useful?

Not all the patients consider obvious the implication of psychological factors in the weight gain and sometimes they do not react positively if the clinician is interested in psychological aspects of their lives. So, before starting the psychological assessment, it is necessary to explain the reasons that move us to investigate areas apparently far away from the problem that brought them to the therapist. If this does not happen, our anamnesis could induce the patient to think that we consider him affected by a psychiatric problem. If an oculist asks a patient to strip naked without justifying his behavior, he couldn't be surprised for patient's awkwardness or reluctance to do that

The connection between psychopathology and obesity is a controversial subject, and some questions still haven't had univocal answer. Is it always useful to evaluate the obese patient's psychopathological functioning? Is it possible to defer if there are no signs of eating disorders or serious psychopathologies? A severe mental illness requires a specific approach, but what changes in our therapeutic approach if the subject is also affected by anxiety or dysthimia?

We justify the time employed in the psychological assessment of every obese patient by asking other questions: "Don't we have to know why the patient failed the preceding diets? Is it useless for the therapist to know in advance the patient's way of thinking? Is it useful to know how he usually reacts to failures, how he faces difficulties, which are his motivations to lose weight, which expectations he has from his new body image?"

If the heightened presence of psychopathology and eating disorders (Simon & Arterburn, 2009; Larrañaga Vidal & García-Mayor, 2009) amongst the patients affected by obesity is a consolidated datum, it is not so evident which is the correlation between the two statuses. It is unclear whether there is only a frequent co-morbidity, or if psychopathology contributes to gaining weight, or if the obesity is a predisposing factor to the onset of a psychological distress due to social stigmatization and/or for the interiorization of prejudices obese people value: lack of will, incapacity of taking control, gluttony, etc. Moreover, it is not completely clear if the presence of a psychopathology influences the outcome of a diet, or how the strategy should be modified for the weight loss dealing with patients affected by a psychopathology. For these reasons, the psychological evaluation we propose is not only psychiatric, to exclude the presence of a psychopathology, but also psychological, to know the patient's way of thinking that can interfere with the weight loss program and/or lead to a regain of the lost weight. It is not only a diagnostic process, but also a deep exploration of emotions, convictions, motivations and aims, no matter if pathological or not, that lead that patient's behavior in his weight gain, loss and maintaining.

What Is the Relationship between Obesity and Psychopathology?

Many studies reported that the presence of psychopathologies among obese patients is significantly more frequent than in the normal-weight population. Carpiniello et al., (2009) found among 150 obese patients a lifetime prevalence of 58% of Axis I disorders and a 28% of Axis II disorders, while the 23% of patients were affected by both an Axis I and Axis II disorders. The highest prevalence rate was found for Anxiety Disorders (about 35%), followed by Mood disorders (30%) and Eating Disorders (18%). The results were confirmed by another study (Carpiniello et al., A, 2009) including 293 obese subjects.

Algul et al., (2009) suggest a multimodal approach to obesity, including psychiatric evaluation and intervention as a routine practice. They found that Class II obese patients had a significantly worse psychological status than control group and need to be treated in a bio-psycho-social manner, including the management of their psychopathologies. Castellini et al., (2008) found in a sample of 397 consecutive overweight/obese patients an high rate of depressive (38%) and anxious (71.5%) symptoms. A positive association between severe eating disorder psychopathology and clinical depression was observed, but neither the level of psychopathology nor the presence of an eating disorder were associated with the severity of being overweight.

Kasen and coll. (2008) collected three waves of data over three decades in order to evaluate the prospective associations between elevations in BMI, generalized anxiety disorder (GAD) and major depressive disorder (MDD) in a sample of 544 women. They found a evidence of the mental health consequences of obesity: a baseline BMI > or =30 significantly increased the odds for subsequent GAD and MDD by 6.27 and 5.25 times, respectively, after adjusting for other significant risk factors. Odds of GAD also increased significantly, given a baseline BMI > or =25 (by 2.44 times); however, this association was not independent of other significant risk factors.

Pickering et al., (2007) suggest that treatment guidelines for psychiatric disorders need to address the management of co-morbid overweight and obesity, and treatment guidelines for obesity need to address the management of co-morbid psychopathology. Hasler et al., (2004) performed a prospective community-based cohort study including 591 subjects between ages 19 and 40, followed over twenty years through six subsequent semi-structured diagnostic interviews. They found that generalized anxiety disorder was negatively associated with being overweight while atypical depression and binge eating were positively associated with both increased weight gain and being overweight. Aggressive personality traits also were positively associated with being overweight, but not related to the rate of weight change. These results persisted after controlling for substance use, levels of physical activity, demographic variables and family history of weight problems.

Assessment of Eating Disorders

Binge Eating Disorder and Night Eating Syndrome are the most frequent eating disorders amongst obese patients; both the disturbances play an important role in onset and maintenance of obesity. They have, therefore, to be excluded during the assessment.

Binge Eating Disorder (BED)

Diagnostic criteria for Binge Eating Disorder: (DSM-IV-TR; APA 2000) include:

Recurrent episodes of binge eating, defined by both the following characteristics:

1. Eating in a defined time period (e.g., in the course of two hours) a doubtlessly bigger quantity of food than what most people would eat during the same time period and under the same circumstances.

2. Feeling of loss of control over eating during these episodes (e.g., feeling of not being able to stop eating or of not being able to control what or how much is eating).

> WARNING
>
> *Not all of those who eat too much are to be considered binge eaters. The aspect that defines bingeing beyond the consumption of a large quantity of food is in fact the loss of control with regard to food intake: the subject has to be aware of an incapacity of controlling their alimentary behavior during bingeing even though they are not hungry any more and/or a feeling of unpleasant satiety.*

Bingeing is associated with at least three of the following symptoms:

- Eating much faster than normal;
- Eating until a feeling of unpleasant satiety is reached;
- Eating large quantities of food without a feeling of physical hunger;
- Eating alone due to a feeling of embarrassment over how much food is being consumed;
- Feeling disgusted with oneself, depression and feeling of guilt after each episode.

The bingeing occurs on average for at least two days per week over a period of six months.

> WARNING
>
> *In the next edition of DSM, BED should be included amongst eating disorders, and some of the diagnostic criteria indicated here should be subject to variation; in particular, it is expected that the number of bingeing episodes will be reduced from currently twice to once a week and for the diagnosis it will be enough that the symptoms persist for at least three months, to be consistent with anorexia nervosa and bulimia nervosa.*

The regular occurrence of inappropriate compensatory behaviors (vomit, laxatives, fasting and strenuous physical exercise) are not associated with bulimic episodes and happen exclusively in the course of anorexia nervosa and bulimia nervosa.

In clinical practice, BED patients may present other psychopathological features not connected with the main diagnosis that have to be treated as well. For this reason, when a patient is diagnosed as affected by BED, it is very important to investigate both specific and general psychopathologies (Todisco & Vinai P, 2008). Initial evaluation has to include a complete examination of the mental status including conscience, mood, anxiety and psychotic spectrum, and a detailed personal and familiar anamnesis.

Specific Psychopathology of BED Patients

de Zwaan M, (2001) reported that BED is more common among overweight people seeking treatment for obesity than among overweight people in a community sample. This could suggest that people with BED are more concerned about their physical problems and tend more to seek treatment. BED patients control their food intake less than other obese people and also have a greater dissatisfaction towards their physical shapes that sometimes leads to disgust. They tend to worry about weight loss and strategies to quickly lose weight. This leads them to a deeper gap between expectations and reality that has negative consequences on self-esteem, sense of inadequacy and mood. Binge is perceived as strongly ego dystonic and represents a hard and painful experience (Ricca et al., 2009).

Eating behaviors, such as speed and amount of food intake, binge, compensatory conducts, abstain from food, vomiting, abuse of laxatives or diuretics and exercise must be investigated. A central characteristic of a binge episode is a sense of loss of control while eating that very often brings the patient to the difficulty or impossibility to stop once started.

According to de Zwaan (2001), about half of the patients with BED start binge eating first in the absence of dieting. It seems that bingeing is more connected to disinhibition rather than to dietary restraint. Often negative emotional states such as anger and frustration, depression and anxiety trigger a binge episode. After the binge episode, other emotions of a negative type such as guilt, disgust, regret and self-loathing often occurs (de Zwaan M, 2001). Body image disturbances and other ED diagnosis may be present and need to be accurately evaluated, too.

General Psychopathology and BED

The relationship between BED and other psychiatric syndromes has been the target of several studies. Psychological characteristics of BED patients such as negative self-evaluation and low self-esteem, reward dependence, loss of autonomy, external locus of control, alexithymia and poor interpersonal relationships may expose patients, on the other hand, to a major risk for other psychiatric disorders. In particular, many investigators found that overeating is strictly connected to emotional stress and represents what is commonly called "emotional eating" (Brewerton T, 1997). Some studies have shown that BED patients have an increased lifetime rate of other eating disorders, in particular bulimia Nervosa. De Zwaan (2001) suggests the "possibility of some shared vulnerability across a range of eating disorders."

Obese BED patients tend to have higher psychiatric co-morbidity compared to other obese patients. In particular, several studies show that BED patients have a lifetime prevalence of major depressive disorder, anxiety disorder or depressive symptoms in almost 50% of the cases (de Zwaan, 2001), and frequently a dysphoric state can be found among these patients.

Clinical evaluation should include also a particular attention to those aspects of personality that can influence the life of the patient and could affect the treatment or contribute to the onset of the symptoms. Higher rates of impulsive behaviors (such as kleptomania or compulsive buying) and higher rates of personality disorders of cluster B and C have been reported in BED patients, and some authors suggest that BED lays in a continuum between compulsive-impulsive disorders and affective spectrum disorders (Brewerton, 1997). In many cases, impulsiveness can expose the patient to a major risk for bingeing but also for dangerous impulsive acts such as alcohol and substances abuse (Todisco, Vinai, 2008).

Finally, as for any other patient seeking psychiatric evaluation, it is very important to evaluate the global functioning in any area of life: family, friends and social relationships, work, studies and so on. Parental depression and adverse childhood experiences have also to be investigated since many patients with BED often report histories of significant family dysfunction (Todisco, Vinai, 2008; Brewerton, 1997).

Assessment's Instruments

There are many psychometric tools to investigate the specific psychopathology of BED, as well as the general one (Anderson et al., 2004). The most commonly used are:

- Structured or semi-structured clinical interviews;
- Questionnaires of self-evaluation;
- Self-monitoring tools.

Eating Disorder Examination (EDE) (Cooper, Fairburn, 1987; Fairburn, Cooper, 1993).

It is a semi-structured interview that allows examination of the specific psychopathology of eating disorders, it is considered the "gold standard" for the diagnosis of these pathologies. It allows to evaluate two behavioral indexes during the last 28 days: the excessive food consumption (based on quantity of food and on the presence of control loss) and the compensatory behaviors (vomit, laxatives, diuretics, excessive physical activity).

The EDE has four subscales:

1. restriction,
2. worry about food,
3. worry about physical forms,
4. worry about weight.

The interviewer attributes point for the severity of the symptoms from 0—non existence of the pathology to 6—severe pathology.

PRO The interviewer and the interviewee set up a sort of calendar of significant events of the previous month, which helps the subject to pay attention to his eating behavior (Bartholome et al., *2006).*

CONS It requires a specific training to be used and it takes about an hour. It cannot be used in groups or when anonymity is requested (Garner, 2002).

Alternatives to the EDE for diagnosis and monitoring of BED are the *Yale-Brown-Cornell Eating Disorder Scale (YBC-EDS)* (Mazure et al., 1994), the *Interview for the Diagnosis of Eating Disorders-IV (IDED-IV)* (Kutlesic et al., 1998) and the dedicated selection of eating disorders of the *Structured Clinical Interview for DSM-IV (SCID)* (First et al., 1996a, 1996b), but it requires much time and a specific training and, therefore, is only used for patients with particularly severe co-morbidity.

Self-report

The scales of self-evaluation (tests, questionnaires, lists of symptoms) compiled by the patient are valid instruments of screening non-clinical populations or in the context of research. They can give valid indications for a multidimensional assessment of the patient but it is not advisable to base diagnoses or decisions as to treatment only upon them.

> *PRO completely standardized, no training is required, they are economic, fast to carry out and to analyze and administrable in groups (Anderson, 2004). Further, they reduce errors of the interviewer and their interaction with the subject.*
>
> *CONS possibility of false responses, involuntary or deliberate, of responses given in series (the patient always tends to give affirmative, negative or socially more accepted responses) (De Giacomo* et al., *2005) or of receiving more pathological responses than those obtained through interviews (Peterson, Miller, 2005).*

There are scales for the evaluation of the specific psychopathology of BED, as well as for the general one. The specific questionnaires have often revealed certain weak points, such as unspecified time period evaluated, the terminology utilized (e.g., "binge episode") and no direct exploration of frequency of symptoms (Carter et al., 2004).

Between those we suggest:

The *Questionnaire On Eating And Weight Patterns (QEWP)* (Nangle et al., 1994; Spitzer et al., 1992) and its revised version, the *Questionnaire On Eating And Weight Patterns-Revised (QEWP-R)* (Spitzer, Yanovski, Marcus, 1993), the first instrument appropriately developed to diagnose BED, which measures the method and quantity of binge episodes and supplies information on patient's history of diet and weight.

The *Eating Disorder Examination-Questionnaire (EDE-Q) (*Fairburn, Beglin, 1994*)*. The version in form of questionnaire developed by Fairburn and colleagues consists of 36 items; it refers to a period of 28 days and examines in a direct way the frequency of the peculiar behaviors of the eating disorder. The EDE questionnaire is capable of distinguishing between obese patients with this particular disorder and those without (Wilson et al., 1993). It corresponds directly to the questions of EDE and uses the same scoring method. Studies evaluating the correspondence between EDE and the EDE questionnaire report contrasting results. Peterson and colleagues (2007) demonstrated acceptable levels of internal consistency for the global score and the subscales of the EDE-Q (worries about food intake, worries about physical form, worries about weight). They still underlined the necessity to further investigate the factorial structure of this instrument (Peterson et al., 2007). Elder and his colleagues (2006) compared the EDE questionnaire with the QEWP-R, using a sample of obese subjects candidates for bariatric surgery. They found that both are useful in identifying patients affected by clinically significant binge eating. The EDE questionnaire, however, seems to differentiate better between those who do not binge or binge rarely and those who regularly binge.

The *Binge Eating Scale (BES)* (Gormally et al., 1982). This is a scale specifically studied for obese patients, useful to examine in depth the severity of binge episodes and the life events and emotions connected to them. It consists of 18 items and although it does not allow a BED diagnosis, it supplies valid elements to suspect its presence (Dalle Grave, 2001).

The *Obesity-Related Well-Being Questionnaire (Orwell-97).* The body weight has a large impact on the quality of life. The evaluation of the quality of obese is possible using the ORWELL-97 (Mannucci et al., 1999). It is an 18-item questionnaire, which explores the impact of symptoms due to obesity on physical well-being, emotional status and relationships.

The *Impact of Weight on Quality of Life (IWQOL)* can be alternatively used (Kolotkin et al., 1995), but it evaluates only the presence of symptoms related to obesity, not how they impact on the subject's quality of life.

Self-monitoring

The self-monitoring process requires the use of a diary in which are recorded the caloric consumption, the weight control methods and thoughts and emotions related to food intake. (Garner, 2002).

> *PRO Undoubtedly, it is an optimal method for obtaining information.*
>
> *CONS The use of this instrument is somewhat inflated so several patients could have already used it in previous attempts (failed) to lose weight. This can induce them to refuse it as a useless tool. Several patients*
>
> *CAVEAT The ability to adequately estimate their food consumption varies from patient to patient. Frequently, obese subjects have alexithymic traits and fail in recording their emotions.*

To help clinicians not particularly expert in eating disorders to diagnose BED according to the criteria of DSM IV TR, our research group developed the BED Questionnaire (BED-Q), a structured self-administered interview following all these criteria.

BED Questionnaire

1. Does it happen that in a short space of time you eat quantities of food much larger than those you normally eat?
   Never At least once a week At least twice a week Practically daily
2. Are you following a strict diet for at least three months?
   YES NO
3. Have you had extended periods of fasting during the last three months?
   Never Sometimes Frequently Very frequently
4. Do the binges follow exasperate diets or prolonged periods of fasting?
   Never Rarely Sometimes Often
5. Did/do the binges occur exclusively in periods when you were/are judged very underweight?
   Yes No
6. Since when did the binges occur?
   At least a month / at least three months / at least six months / at least one year
7. With which frequency do you eat in a short period of time more food than you would normally eat?

Never / Once a week / at least twice a week / Practically every day.

8. Do you induce vomiting after the binges?
   Never Sometimes Systematically Always
9. Do you use laxatives to make up for the effects of the binges?
   Never Sometimes Systematically Always
10. Do you practice intense physical activity to make up for the effects of the binges?
    Never Sometimes Systematically Always
11. During the binges, does it happen that you have a unpleasant sensation of not being able to control your alimentation?
    Never Sometimes Often Always
12. Does the difficulty controlling your alimentation consequently create discomfort or worries?
    Not at all A little Quite a bit Very much
13. How long do the binges usually last?
    Less than 15 minutes/Between 15 minutes and 1 hour/About 2 hours/More than 2 hours
14. With regard to your normal alimentary conduct, during the binges do you eat
    Slower than usual As usual Faster than usual Much faster than usual
15. When you binge, do you eat until you feel:
    Just satiated Full Very full Full to bursting
16. On average, how hungry do you feel before the binges?
    Not at all A little Quite a bit Very much
17. Does it happen that you binge alone due to the embarrassment for what you are doing?
    Never Sometimes Often Always
18. Does it happen that you feel depressed after the binges?
    Never Sometimes Often Always
19. Does it happen that feels disgusted with yourself after the binges?
    Never Sometimes Often Always
20. Does it happen that you feel guilty after the binges?
    Never Sometimes Often Always
21. Do you feel ashamed after the binges?
    Never Sometimes Often Always

Scoring

Give one point for answer No at questions 2, 3, 4, 5.
Give one point for answers c or d at questions 1, 6, 10, 11.
Give one point for answers a or b at questions 7, 8, 9, 12.
Give one point for answers c or d at questions 13, 14, 15, 16, 17, 18, 19, 20.

The necessary score for a BED diagnosis is 12 points for the first twelve questions and at least three points for questions 13 to 20.

Assessment of Binge Eating Disorder in Children

A retrospective study of obese women with BED showed that early onset of binge eating is associated with an earlier onset of obesity, more eating disorder psychopathology and a tendency for more mood disorders (Marcus et al., 1995). However, BED criteria developed for adults may not be appropriate for use with children. So Marcus and Kalarchian (2003) proposed provisional criteria for measuring BED in children based on a review and synthesis of findings from epidemiological and community-based studies in pediatric populations, researches focusing on the development of eating behavior in children and studies of binge eating in overweight children and adolescents.

The criteria include recurrent episodes of binge eating not linked to the regular use of inappropriate compensatory behaviors (purging, fasting, excessive exercise), characterized by both food seeking in absence of hunger (e.g., after a full meal) and a sense of lack of control over eating. Binge episodes have to be associated with food seeking in response to negative affect (e.g., sadness, boredom, restlessness) or as a reward or to episodes of sneaking or hiding food. Symptoms must persist over a period of three months. The episodes do not occur exclusively during the course of anorexia nervosa or bulimia nervosa. (Marcus and Kalarchian, 2003).

A variety of methods has been used to diagnose binge eating behavior or BED in children. These included unstructured interviews as well as instruments such as the Kids' Eating Disorders Survey (KEDS) (Childress, 1993) and the Eating Symptoms Inventory (ESI) (Whitaker, 1989), but both do not assess loss of control, that is particularly difficult to measure in children, given the difficulties that they may have understanding the definition of loss of control. (Shapiro et al., 2007) Morgan et al., (2002) suggested using queries to explain loss of control (e.g., "when you start to eat, and you eat and eat and eat, and you just can't stop").

Shapiro et al., (2007) developed a structured interview for use with children to test the Marcus & Kalarchian's provisional BED criteria, the Children's Binge Eating Disorder Scale (C-BEDS).

The authors suggest that C-BEDS may be a better screening instrument as it is more sensitive in capturing binge eating behaviors than the SCID threshold diagnosis, but may be too restrictive as a screening instrument for children. If children answer affirmatively to the C-BEDS questions, then the assessor may follow-up with additional questions or perform a more extensive interview using other measures. Specificity may be improved by amending the interview so that question two is a follow-up of question one or by using a Likert scale for questions one to five instead of a yes/no response (Shapiro et al., IJED, 2007).

Assessing Night Eating Syndrome and Sleep-related Eating Disorder

Differential Diagnoses

The first step with a patient who complains about episodes of night eating symptoms is the differential diagnosis between NES and SRED. While the first is an eating disorder that can be treated through a specific psychotherapy (see chapter XVIII), the latter is a parasomnia requiring a pharmaceutical treatment (see chapter XIX). In Table 8.3, the diagnostic criteria of both syndromes are summarized.

Table 8.3. Compared diagnostic criteria of Night Eating Syndrome and Sleep-Related Eating Disorder

Proposed research diagnostic criteria for Night Eating Syndrome

I. The daily pattern of eating demonstrates a significantly increased intake in the evening and/or nighttime, as manifested by one or both of the following:
   A. At least 25% of food intake is consumed after the evening meal
   B. At least two episodes of nocturnal eating per week
II. Awareness and recall of evening and nocturnal eating episodes are present.
III. The clinical picture is characterized by at least three of the following features:
   A. Lack of desire to eat in the morning and/or breakfast is omitted on four or more mornings per week
   B. Presence of a strong urge to eat between dinner and sleep onset and/or during the night
   C. Sleep onset and/or sleep-maintenance insomnia are present four or more nights per week
   D. Presence of a belief that one must eat in order to initiate or return to sleep
   E. Mood is frequently depressed and/or mood worsens in the evening
IV. The disorder is associated with significant distress and/or impairment in functioning.
V. The disordered pattern of eating has been maintained for at least three months.
VI. The disorder is not secondary to substance abuse or dependence, medical disorder, medication, or another psychiatric disorder

(Allison et al., 2010)

Diagnostic criteria for Sleep-Related Eating Disorder

A. Recurrent episodes of involuntary eating and drinking occur during the main sleep period
B. One or more of the following must be present with the recurrent episodes of involuntary eating and drinking:
   a. Consumption of peculiar forms or combinations of food or inedible or toxic substances
   b. Insomnia related to sleep disruption from repeated episodes of eating, with a complaint of nonrestorative sleep, daytime fatigue, or somnolence
   c. Sleep-related injury
   d. Dangerous behaviors performed while in pursuit of food or while cooking food
   e. Morning anorexia
   f. Adverse health consequences from recurrent binge eating of high-caloric foods
C. The disturbance is not better explained by another sleep disorder, medical or neurological disorder, mental disorder, medication use, or substance use disorder.

(American Academy of Sleep Medicine, 2005).

Both pathologies share some symptoms

- *Nocturnal eating*
- *Morning anorexia*
- *Sleep onset and/or sleep-maintenance insomnia.*

- *The disorder is not secondary to substance abuse or dependence, medical disorder, medication, or another psychiatric disorder*

but there are substantial differences between them.

- *Consumption of inedible food or toxic substances and dangerous behaviors performed while in characteristics of SRED patients,*
- *Awareness and recall of nocturnal eating episodes, presence of a belief that one must eat in order to initiate or return to sleep and depressed mood are characteristics of NES patients.*

Furthermore, there are several sleep pathologies frequently associated with SRED: *Restless Legs Syndrome and Obstructive Sleep Apnea,* and SRED itself has been linked with sedating medications (see Table 8.4). In particular, the widely prescribed benzodiazepine receptor agonists such as zolpidem (Morgenthaler & Silber, 2002) can induce the symptoms of the syndrome.

Table 8.4. Medications frequently related to onset of SRED

- Midazolam
- Olanzapine
- Risperidone
- Triazolam
- Zolpidem
- Zopiclone

Assessment Instruments

Specific instruments have been adjusted in order to carry out the diagnosis of NES. (Geliebter Gluck et al., 2001; Allison et al., 2004).

Night Eating Diagnostic Questionnaire (NEDQ) (Gluck et al., 2001)

It consists of 21 questions that examine the relative habits at the moment of going to bed, nocturnal awakenings, waking up in the morning, the caloric value taken on in the evening hours, morning anorexia, beliefs on alimentation and sleep and the presence of depression or depressive moods.

Night Eating Questionnaire (NEQ) (Allison et al., 2004)

It is structured into 14 finalized questions to underline the presence of symptom combinations, corresponding to diagnostic criteria of NES.

PRO It can be self-administered and quickly executable and can give the patient a better awareness of his disorder

CONS The actual form of the questionnaire does not permit making a diagnosis of NES according to the criteria suggested by the 1st International Symposium on NES but only underlines the presence of behavioral characteristics which can lead to suspect the diagnosis of NES.

The first five items examine the nocturnal eating habits; the following questions refer to variation of mood, the possible difficulties connected with falling asleep and the presence of nocturnal awakenings. The authors perceive a score of 25 as sufficient to classify the presence of NES, whereas lower scores following qualitative analysis can shed light on possible dysfunctional areas.

Assessment of Psychiatric Disorders

During the clinical interview, other psychopathological traits (e.g., alexithymia, body image disturbances, depression, anxiety, obsessive disturbances) can emerge; on these will focus the psychiatric assessment.

The relationship between obesity and psychiatric syndromes has been the target of several studies. In particular, many investigators found that binge eating is strictly connected to emotional stress and represents what is commonly called "emotional eating" (Brewerton T, 1997).

There are many tools to evaluate general and specific psychopathology according to the different needs and settings (clinical investigations or treatment), but, in our opinion, in the daily practice, the clinical interview is one of the best ways to collect information. In order to standardize the collected data, the semi-structured interviews are useful tools.

A battery of tests can include:

- *Beck Depression Inventory (BDI)* (Beck, 1978). A cut off of 17 identifies the presence of a Major Depression.
- *Body Uneasiness Test (BUT)* (Cuzzolaro et al., 1999) to asses alterations of body image frequently connected to eating disorders
- *Eating Disorder Examination, 12th edition (EDE)* (Cooper, Fairburn, 1987; Fairburn, Cooper, 1993), a standardized interview designed to assess the specific psychopathology of anorexia nervosa, bulimia nervosa and binge eating disorder. It contains four clusters of items: restraint of eating, warring about food, warring about body shape, warring about weight and can be also useful to evaluate the outcome of the therapies.
- *Symptom Checklist 90 (SCL-90)* (Derogatis et al., 1997), another very commonly used test to check psychiatric comorbidity with 90 items and 9 subscales.
- *State Trait Anxiety Inventory (STAI)* (Spielberg et al., 1970) to evaluate anxiety.
- *Structured Clinical Interview for DSM-IV (SCID-IV),* a structured interview useful to identify psychiatric diagnoses. The diagnostic modules are formulated in accordance with the diagnostic categories of the DSM-IV.
- *Three Factor Eating Questionnaire (TFEQ)* (Stunkard, Messick, 1985), an interview designed to assess three dimensions of eating behavior: cognitive restraint of eating, disinhibition, and hunger. This test is very useful to explore reasons connected to restraint of eating and gives important hints about the risk of drop out.

Assessment of Personality Traits

The last part of our psychological assessment includes the analysis of personality characteristics of the patient.

Table 8.6. Beliefs and emotions related to a binge episode

A (Activating event)	B (beliefs about A)	C (consequences)
"I've eaten out of the meal"	"I will never lose weight" "I'm a loser"	Interruption of the diet. "I feel bad" (depress mood)

Following the theories of cognitive behavioral psychotherapy, we assess patients' cognitive stile, their way of thinking, the contents of their thoughts and their typical ideation, such as their ability in recognizing and managing their own emotions.

The most known cognitive models investigate the presence of cognitive biases, automatic or recurrent thought scheme (Beck, 1975; Ellis, 1977; Kelly) (with the related emotional background) and the metacognitive strategies used by patients to face negative emotions.

Cognitive and emotional functions are strictly connected and reciprocally influenced. This is the reason why it is essential to find out, during the assessment, pathological maintaining circles of patients' symptoms. For example, subjects affected by emotional eating frequently use a ruinous strategy (to snack, overeat, etc.) to front a negative emotion; this can reinforce their negative self-evaluation, worsening their emotional conditions.

Treating obese patients, frequently multi-treated, it is essential to understand the vicious circles at the base of the relapses before undertaking a further treatment to avoid the risk of another failure. First of all, it is essential to individuate which are the patient's core beliefs concerning his weight problem and his related emotions. One of the most used in the cognitive behavioral therapy practice is the ABC technique (Ellis, 1977) (Table 8.5), helping the patient in recognizing his thoughts and emotions related to that specific event.

Obese patients often have a fragile self-esteem *"I've eaten out of the meal again; I'm feeling so bad. If I go on this way, I will never lose weight. I'm a loser"* and need to be frequently confirmed about their value; but to reach this objective they tend to impose to themselves difficult tasks, so they frequently fail confirming their sense of low value.

Other patients have a hypertrophic sense of duty and personal responsibility *"I must not eat, but I just can't, I don't have enough will power,"* sustained by the belief that keeping weight under control is not so difficult and can be done without any effort. These beliefs can induce depressive symptoms and difficulties in engaging themselves in healthy behaviors *"I don't even start the diet; I already know I will fail...I messed everything up eating this biscuit, so I can eat the whole packet."*

Several subjects are frightened by thoughts connected to the terrible consequences of failing in their attempt to lose weight. *"If I will fail the diet again, I would feel very badly, I don't think I could tolerate it."* These thoughts can induce anxiety in front of the food, a situation that they consider at risk. Other patients think they cannot face negative emotions, so just they perceive them immediately have to placate, and food is one of the elective modalities to calm down unpleasant emotions. A lapse during a diet can arouse negative emotions not easily tolerable, which will enhance the probability of episodes of emotional eating to calm down anxiety. During the assessment of all obese subjects, it is necessary to exclude the presence of these pathological thoughts and behaviors.

Alexithymia

Obese patients frequently have a low ability in discriminating and labeling their emotions. For this reason, they can label an unpleasant emotion (sadness, anger) as a physical states such as hunger or "desire of a palatable food."

To assess patients' ability in recognizing their emotions the *Toronto Alexithymia Scale (TAS-20)* can be useful (Bagby, Parker,. & Taylor, 1994). It is a 20-item self-report scale rated using a 5-point Likert scale. It has three subscales: *Difficulty Identifying Feeling subscale* (*DIF*), measuring difficulty in identifying emotions and in distinguishing them from bodily sensations; *Difficulty Describing Feelings subscale (DDF),* measuring difficulty in describing emotions to other people; and *Externally Oriented Thinking subscale (EOT),* measuring the tendency to focus the attention externally thinking or a preoccupation with the details of external events. TAS-20 uses cut-off scoring: equal to or less than 51 = non-alexithymia, equal to or greater than 61 = alexithymia. Scores of 52 to 60 = possible alexithymia. (Bagby, Parker & Taylor, 1994).

Cognitive Biases

Cognitive bias and dysfunctional thought processes often sustain patients' beliefs and consequent emotions that have to be recognized and discussed during the assessment. One of the most frequent is the overestimation of benefits related to the weight loss.

Many patients think that only by losing weight they will find a partner; if they fail, they will be alone forever. This can induce them to renounce engaging in a diet, frightened by the dramatic consequences of a failure. This cognitive rigidity is associated with a tendency to the dichotomous thinking, for which can only be true a condition (i.e., full reaching of the objective) or it's opposed (the total failure), any other condition (i.e., a weight loss minor then the desired one) is not acceptable. Another effect of this way of thinking is the idea that the not recommended foods immediately become "prohibited" foods, generating a frustration, due to the renouncement, becoming more and more constrictive and hard to tolerate.

Furthermore, the tendency to characterize foods as "prohibited," frequently activates a selective attention *"I cannot eat this food, but I like it so much,"* inducing worry about food and generating obsessive thoughts; a very dysfunctional construct in patients with impulsive traits. To evaluate impulsivity, it can be useful to employ the *Barrat Impulsiveness Scale (BIS),* designed to measure three, a priori defined, sub traits, labeled: cognitive impulsiveness, motor impulsiveness and non-planning impulsiveness (Barratt, 1985; Patton, Stanford, & Barratt, 1995).

The perfectionism is another factor making it difficult to follow a diet. To lose weight requires time, commitment and trust in the possible results: if the patient does not tolerate the possibility of an error (i.e., the eventuality of surrender to some alimentary temptation) and thinks that these tumbles will inevitably lead to a total failure, he will risk giving up to the first mistake. These thoughts, in addition to making the exposition to any palatable food a cause of anxiety, can induce depressive feelings due to the fear of failing the diet.

Moreover, frequently patients tend to minimize the results they reach if they don't need a big effort, so a correct diet, not too restrictive, so easy to follow but needing a long time to lose weight is frequently considered of scarce value.

Another common tendency is to attribute only to their own weakness their failures *"I won't never lose weight, I like eating too much,"* without considering the role of metabolic and physiologic factors playing against an obese person attempting to lose weight. In this case, it is useful evaluate if the patient uses a selective abstraction, recalling exclusively episodes that confirm a negative vision of himself; events that could disconfirm his thesis are not considered.

Obese patients generally consider the body modification an objective to achieve through the weight loss, but their weight loss expectations are frequently unrealistic. Learning to accept their own aspect is functional to the adherence to the treatment. The assessment of body image can help the clinic to evaluate if it is necessary to deal with these problematic areas (Williamson et al., 2000). *The Body Uneasiness Test (BUT)* (Marano et al., 2007) can be a valuable multidimensional tool for the clinical assessment of body uneasiness in obesity.

If obese patients are affected by chronic pathologies (diabetes, cardiovascular problems, etc.), it is important to explore their thoughts regarding the illness. In several patients, the onset (usually unexpected) of this kind of problem can contribute to develop the idea of being weak and frail or powerless facing the destiny. These kinds of considerations worsen their sense of efficacy in influencing their own health. In other cases, instead, the fear of illness or death can be a highly motivating factor. For these reasons, patients' naive theories regarding their own illnesses have also to be careful assessed.

Table 8.6. Lifestyle assessment check list

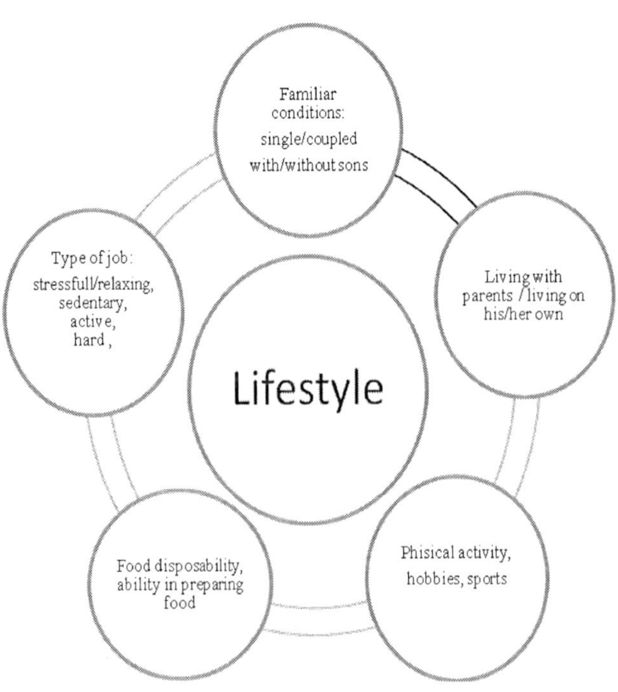

Behavioral and Lifestyle Assessment

Lifestyle

Patient's lifestyle is an important factor in onset and maintenance of obesity. (Table 8.6) Weight gain is not only due to excessive caloric intake but also to scarce expenditure, so a sedentary work and a tendency to be "a sitting sportsman" influence the outcome of a diet. Assessing the daily physical activity, the clinician can already disconfirm the conviction that it is necessary to partake in a strong physical exercise to lose weight, while it is more useful to walk quietly 30 minutes a day. For further information on this topic, see the chapter XI.

Familiar conditions also play an important role in a diet: it is not the same to eat alone or to be part of a family where persons usually overeat at meals. Several female patients claim their difficulty in following a diet because they are surrounded by junk-food that they "*have to prepare*" for their sons: "*I cannot deprive them, in the past I eat as I would, now they have not to suffer for my diet.*"

They have the dysfunctional conviction that a good parent has to offer everyday a lot of food to the sons. In these cases, it can be useful to underline the importance of obesity prevention since from childhood, moreover, frequently obese people are also affected by metabolic disorders such as diabetes or hypercholesterolemia, that have a genetic component, so also their sons are at risk for them.

Eating Behavior

To perform an efficient dieting program, it is not sufficient to know what the patient eats but also where and when he does it and who prepares the meals. (Table 8.7) It is not the same to follow a diet for a lorry driver eating the most part of the days in fast foods services, for a cook of a restaurant or for a single (unable also to cook an egg) living with his Italian, obese, mother.

Table 8.7. assessment of eating behavior

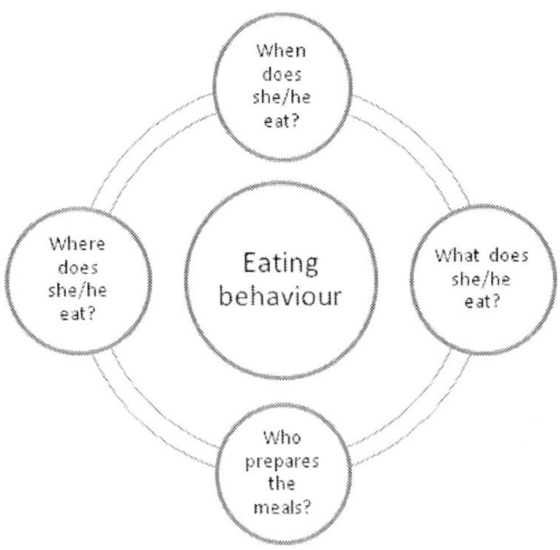

When Does The Patient Eat?

Frequently, obese subjects skip breakfast, "*I begin a new diet every day*." This can induce overeating at lunch or having a snack, usually of unhealthy foods, later in the morning. Other subjects eat high-caloric food between the meals, reducing their food intake at meals, so in front of a diet, they claim that they currently do not eat so much. In this case, it is important, using a food diary, to assess all the calories they introduce in a day. Moreover, the tendency to frequent eating can be a sign of impulsivity, emotional eating and loss of control with food. All these factors play a negative role on the outcome of a diet and need further investigation to find out if they are only caused by unhealthy habits or if they are symptoms of a sub-threshold eating disorder. On the other hand. several subjects skip lunch for job reasons, having only a large meal at dinner. This can reduce their sense of guilt for overeating at dinner time.

What Does He Really Eat?

It is important to avoid generic description of foods but instead to find out the real content of every dish of the patient. In our experience, the description of an apparently healthy eating habit: *"I eat meat and vegetables for lunch and a vegetable soup with a fruit for dinner*," became with a deeper interview: "*for lunch 200 grams of beefsteak cooked in Milanese stile* (coated with scrambled egg and bread crumbs and then fried in generous olive oil) *and a portion of French fries*." For dinner, the patient eats a typical Italian dish: a soup of beans with bacon, and a banana for fruit.

In other cases, the subjects don't eat large amounts of food but gain weight because they introduce an excessive number of calories, being completely unaware of the caloric content of foods they usually chose, so it has to be explored the patient's knowledge regarding this topic.

As already stated elsewhere, the assessment style is very important; the clinicians have to avoid every judgment on patient's behavior, the only goal is to understand if there are dietary mistakes that we can help to correct. To enhance the sense of collaboration with the patient, we ask them to photograph all the food they eat in a day. During the assessment, we ask the patient to describe what he eats and then we see the photographs together; in this way, if there is a discrepancy between the photo and the recall, we can say to the patients: *"If you would like to hide something to me you don't photograph that food, but you have take a photo so there is no attempt to take in me, you were really convinced of having eat what you said, but the reality was different: we have found a first reason in your gaining weight!"*

A further factor that can induce a difficulty in evaluating food intake is the under-estimation of the amount of food—that is a characteristic widespread among general population, including children, as found by our research group (Vinai et al., 2008). This tendency can induce unawareness of overeating, representing a protective factor in case of shortage of food, but a risk factor for obesity in case of food abundance.

Where does she/he eat?

Frequently diets fail for the low compliance of the subjects, but also because they have not the possibility (without spending too much time or money) of choosing healthy foods, so have to be assessed the real possibilities of each patient to find easily an healthy food. E.g., patients usually eating in a fast food cannot easily follow the suggestions of a dietician. They have to be trained to recognize the healthy foods they can find there. Those having their lunch into their office could choose aliments as cheese, bread, pizza, cakes, that are easier to maintain, without a refrigerator, and more palatable, than a cold dish of cooked vegetables, if there is not the possibility of heating food. Unfortunately all those foods have a high concentration of calories. Other subjects in the same situation could decide of skipping lunch to avoid an excessive caloric intake but this fact could induce an overeating at dinner. All these factors have to be known by the clinician to avoid the risk of proposing an impossible diet to the patients.

Last but not least has to be assessed who is the person usually preparing the meals for the patient. It is quite unnecessary improve patient's skills in managing caloric content of food and in preparing low caloric dishes if somebody else usually prepares his meals.

Diet History

The history of previous diets followed by the patients has to be also assessed. which factors mainly contributed to their failure? Was it due to an incongruous eating behavior (excessive caloric restriction, low palatability and/or variety of suggested foods...), or to subjective factors (magic expectations, scarce compliance, lack of information on strategies to maintain the weight loss). Moreover have to be cleared the chronology of the failure of previous diets. Was the biggest difficulty in starting the diets, in following them or in maintaining the weight loss?

Restitution

At the end of the assessment, the clinician will fill in a check list of factors influencing weight gain of that specific patient, (Table 8.8) a sort of graph of his personal pathway to obesity.

Table 8.8. Patient's pathway to obesity

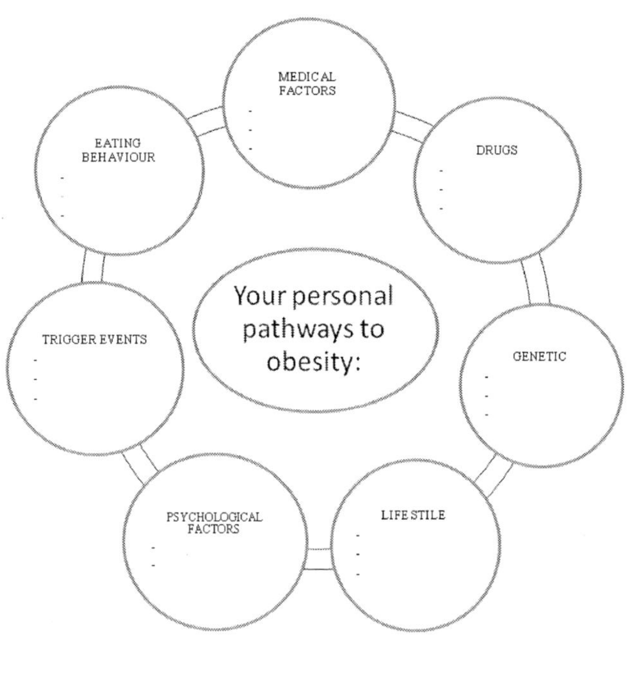

Then it will be filled in with the patient an analogous graph showing the factors that he can modify to lose weight: the best roads he can follow to recovery. (Table 8.9).

Table 8.9. Patient's main roads to recovery

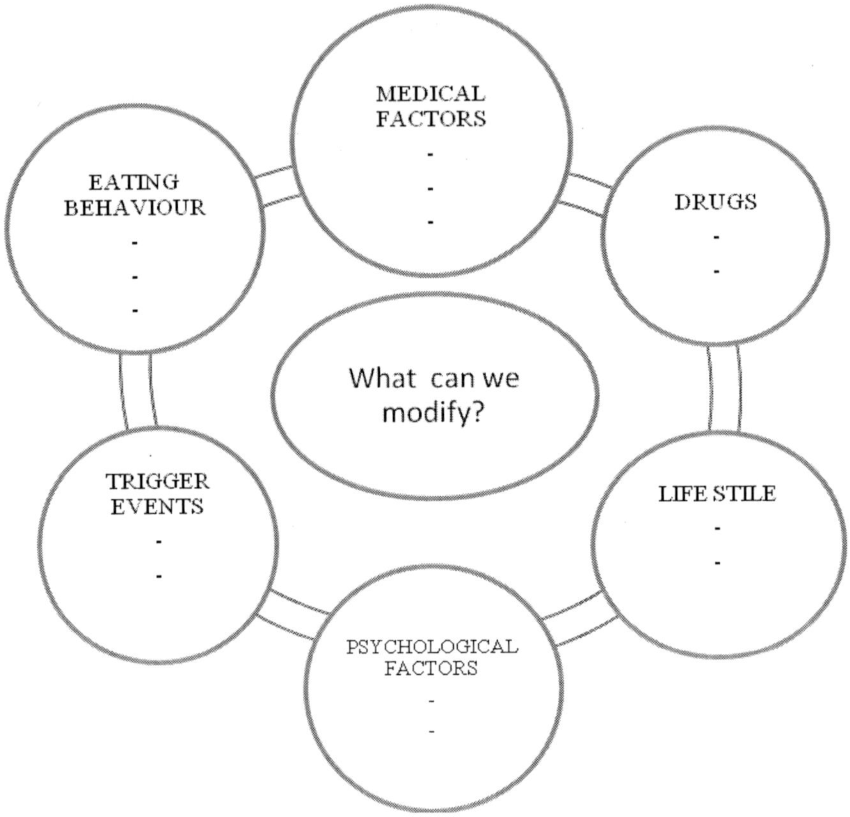

Medical Assessment

Following the World Health Report 2000, obesity is a major risk factor for the development of chronic diseases and mortality so it is not surprising that frequently, the first step in patients' assessment is the evaluation of their medical condition (Mokdad et al., 2000; Flegal et al., 2005).

The risk of cardiovascular events rises with increasing Body Mass Index (BMI) (Manson et al., 1990), and World Health Organization recommends measurement of the BMI as a universal criterion of overweight (≥25) and obesity (≥30). BMI is calculated as weight in kilograms (kg) divided by the square of height in meters (m2). It provides an estimation of total body fat based on height and weight that applies to adult subjects (National Heart, Lung, and Blood Institute (NHLBI) and North American Association for the Study of Obesity (NAASO), 2000; World Health Organization, 2000; American Medical Association, 2003). Using the BMI value, patients can be classified as *Underweight BMI* < 18.5 *Normal* BMI ranging from 18.5 to 24.9 *Overweight* BMI ranging from 25.0 to 29.9 *Obesity* Class I (Mild obesity) BMI ranging from 30.0 to 34.9, Class II (Moderate obesity) BMI ranging from 35.0 to 39.9 II, Class III (Severe obesity) BMI > 40.

> WARNING
>
> *Patients frequently fail in reporting their height and weight so BMI have to be calculated measuring and weighting the patients.*

In rare cases, BMI is not useful to predict body fat content because it does not distinguish the composition of lean versus fat tissue, so, for example, a bodybuilder may have a high score of BMI due to excessive muscularity and by contrast, an old woman may be obese, having a normal BMI, due to a lean body mass. In these cases, estimation of body fat can be also done by *Skin Fold Thickness Measurement (SFTM)*. From three to nine different standard anatomical sites around the body can be used for this purpose. The tester pinches a double layer of skin and the underlying adipose tissue, but not the muscle. The calipers are then applied 1 cm below and at right angles to the pinch, and a reading in millimeters is taken.

Bioelectrical impedance analysis and dual energy x-ray absorptiometry are also available for assessing patients' proportions of lean and fat mass. However, these techniques are not currently recommended for office use (De Lorenzo et al., 2006).

The *Bioelectrical Impedance Analysis (BIA)* method is a more affordable but less accurate way to estimate body fat percentage. The general principle behind BIA is that the resistance to electricity varies between adipose, muscular and skeletal tissue: fat-free mass is a good conductor, as it contains a large amount of water and electrolytes, while fat is a poor conductor. Two conductors are attached to the body, typically on the feet, and a small electrical current is sent through; it is sent up one leg, across the abdomen and down the other leg. The resistance between the conductors will provide a measure of body fat. Factors that affect the accuracy of the method include instrumentation, the prediction equation formulated to estimate the Fat Free Mass, the subject's hydration level and the amount of liquid consumed before the test. As electricity travels more easily through water, a large amount of water consumed can result in a measure of a lower body fat percentage.

Recently, *Dual Energy X Ray Absorptiometry (DEXA)*, a technique developed for the determination of bone mineral content but capable of measuring three body components—bone mineral mass, fat mass and lean mass—has expanded its application to the analysis of body fat mass but given the cost of the method, it is not used in daily clinical practice.

Measures of abdominal fat distribution such as *Waist Circumference (WC)* measured at the level of the iliac crest, or *Waist to Hip Ratio (WHR)* are also encouraged by World Health Organization (2000) because the health risks of overweight and obesity are independently associated with excess abdominal fat (Lean, Han, Seidell, 1998; Han, Van Leer, Seidell, Lean, 1995) clinically defined as a waist circumference >102 cm in men and >88 cm in women. Population studies have shown that people with excess abdominal fat have an excess burden of impaired health and increased cardiovascular risk compared to those with normal waist circumferences. (Larsson et al., 1984; Lapidus et al., 1984; Ducimetiere, Richard, Cambien, 1986; Yusuf et al., 2005). The WC has also correlated well with area of visceral fat mass assessed with magnetic resonance imaging (Valsamakis et al., 2004). In addition, data from the National Health and Nutrition Examination Survey (Janssen, Katzmarzyk, 2002), indicated that within the categories of healthy weight, overweight and Class I (mild) Obesity, adults with high waist circumference values were increasingly likely to have hypertension, diabetes, dyslipidemia and the metabolic syndrome compared with those with normal waist circumference values. Following Schneider et al., (2007), the waist circumference appears to be better indicators of cardiovascular risk than the BMI.

WARNING

The measure of waist circumference have to be taken at level of the iliac crests the end of a normal expiration; to speak with the patient during the measure is useful to avoid the risk of underestimation of WC due to excessive expiration.

Obese patients need a complete physical evaluation to investigate if they are affected by pathologies that can induce a secondary obesity; moreover, they are at higher risk to develop several illnesses than normal-weight subjects. The link between obesity, metabolic diseases (gout and diabetes) hypertension and cardiovascular diseases is well known, but obesity is a risk factor also for other illness that couldn't be immediately linked to weight excess (Table 8.10).

Table 8.10. Pathologies frequently linked to obesity

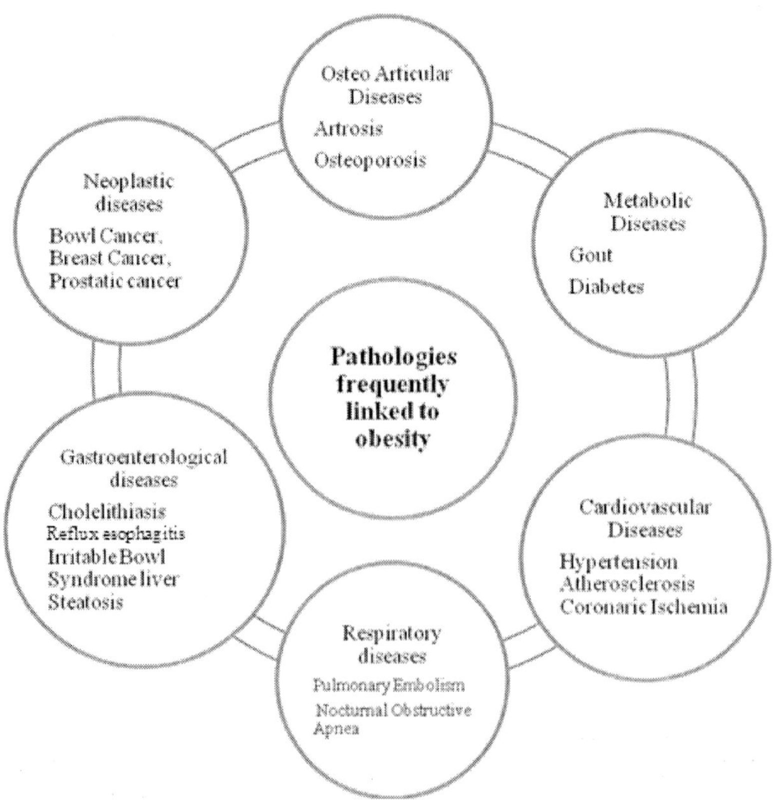

It is useful also to perform a laboratory blood analysis including blood cell count; hematocrit, hemoglobin, sodium, potassium, chloride, calcium bicarbonate, blood urea nitrogen (BUN), magnesium, protein electrophoresis, creatinine, and glucose, lipidic profile (including total cholesterol, High density lipoprotein cholesterol (HDL-C), Low density lipoprotein cholesterol (LDL-C) and triglycerides), a liver profile (including alanine transaminase (ALT), aspartate transaminase (AST), alkaline phosphatase (ALP), albumin, gamma glutamyl transpeptidase (gGT) and total bilirubin) and a urinalysis. To exclude a malfunctioning of the thyroid, we also dose the serum's level of the Thyroid Stimulating Hormone (TSH). An electrocardiogram (ECG) is also included in our medical assessment to evaluate if the patient is affected by any heart pathology related to obesity: left ventricular hypertrophy, coronary disease, etc. Further examinations could be necessary if the results of medical visits and laboratory analysis suggest the possible presence of specific co-morbidities. Furthermore, obese patients require a follow-up of their medical condition during the time.

Contrary to patients' frequent opinions, obesity induced by medical diseases is a very rare condition. Only few pathologies can induce it (hypothyroidism, Cushing's syndrome and ovaric polycistosis), and they are quite infrequent. Moreover, the possibility of an early diagnosis and an adequate treatment usually prevent the onset of a secondary obesity due to these diseases. In 25 years of clinical practice, we only found a very few patients affected by a secondary obesity.

Pharmacological Assessment

Frequently, patients claim that their being overweight is due to drug side effects. Vossenaar et al., (2004) found that 9% of adults attributed weight gain to drugs they were prescribed.

Table 8.11. Drugs that can influence the weight of a person

Anti Epyleptics: Valproate	**Antipsychotics:** Risperidone Clozapine Olanzapine	**Corticosteroids:** Prednisone
Anti diabetics: Insulin Glipizide Glimepiride Glibenclamide Pioglitazone	**Anti ipertensives beta-blockers:** Atenolol Metoprolol Propranolol	**Antidepressants:** Nortriptyline Doxepin Amitriptyline

This percentage sounds unrealistic, but several drugs prescribed on a long-term basis in the treatment of chronic disease are consistently associated with weight gain. This effect can arise from an increased appetite (corticosteroids) or a reduced metabolic rate (beta-adrenoceptor blockers) (Pijl H, Meinders AE, 1996). In Table 8.11, there is a list of medications that can induce weight gain divided on the basis of their indications. In 2007 Leslie, Hankey & Lean reviewed 43 randomized controlled studies involving more than 25,000 patients to determine the real effect on weight of drugs usually believed to induce weight gain. In our knowledge, this is the most comprehensive review on this topic; we strongly suggest reading it for further information on the matter.

All the mentioned drugs are widely used (Ness-Abramof & Apovian, 2005) in the general population; e.g., Valproate is one of the first-line treatments for epilepsy. Moreover, several categories of these medications—beta-blockers anti-diabetics and antidepressants—play a prominent role in the management of pathologies that frequently affect obese patients, respectively hypertension, diabetes mellitus and depression, so their use has to be carefully researched by the clinicians. For the involvement of anti psychotic drugs (Allison DB et al., 1999, Álvarez-Jiménez et al-2008) in weight gain, also see Chapter XX.

References

Algul, A., Ates, M.A., Semiz, U.B., Basoglu, C., Ebrinc, S., Gecici, O., Gülsün, M., Kardesoglu, E., Cetin, M. (2009) Evaluation of general psychopathology, subjective sleep quality, and health-related quality of life in patients with obesity. *Int J Psychiatry Med.*, *39,* 297-312.

Allison, D.B., Mentore, J.L., Moonseong, H., Chandler, L.P., Cappelleri, J.C., Infante, M.C., Weiden, P.J. (1999) Antipsychotic-Induced Weight Gain: A Comprehensive Research Synthesis. *Am J Psychiatry, 156*, 1686–96.

Álvarez-Jiménez, M., Hetrick, S.E., Gonzáles-Blanch, C., Gleeson, J.F., & McGorry, P.D. (2008). Non-pharmacological management of antipsychotic-induced weight gain: systematic review and meta-analysis of randomized controlled trials. *The British Journal of Psychiatry, 193*, 101-107.

AMERICAN PSYCHIATRIC ASSOCIATION (2000), *Manuale diagnostico e statistico dei disturbi mentali, ed. rivista* (DSM-IV-TR). Tr. it. Masson, Milano 2002.

American Medical Association. (2003) Roadmaps for Clinical Practice Case Studies In *Disease Prevention and Health Promotion Assessment and Management of Adult Obesity: A Primer for Physicians.*

Anderson, D.A., Lundgren, J.D., Shapiro, J.R., Paulosky, C.A. (2004), "Assessment of eating disorder. Review and recommendations for clinical use." *Behavior Modification, 11,* 763-782.

Anonymous (2000) Obesity: preventing and managing the global epidemic: report of a WHO consultation. *World Health Organ Tech Rep Ser 894*, 1–253.

Bagby, R. M., Parker, J. D. A. & Taylor, G. J: (1994) The Twenty-Item Toronto Alexithymia Scale-I. Item Selection and Cross-Validation Of The Factor Structure. *Journal of Psychosomatic Research, 38,* 23-32.

Bandura, A. (1977) Self-efficacy: toward a unifying theory of behavioral change. *Psychol Rev. 84,* 191-215.

Bandura, A. (1991). Self-efficacy mechanism in physiological activation and health-promoting behavior. In J. Madden, IV (Ed.), *Neurobiology of learning, emotion and affect* (pp. 229-270). New York: Raven.

Bandura, A. (1995). Self-efficacy. In A. S. R. Manstead & M. Hewstone (Eds.), *Blackwell encyclopedia of social psychology* (pp. 453-454). Oxford: Blackwell

Barratt, E. S. (1985). Impulsiveness subtraits: Arousal and information processing. In J. T. Spence and C. E. Izard (Eds.), *Motivation, Emotion and Personality* (137-146). Elsevier Science, North Holland.

Bartholome, L.T., Raymond, N.C., Lee, S.S., Peterson, C.B., Warren, C.S. (2006) Detailed analysis of binges in obese women with binge eating disorder: Comparisons using multiple methods of data collection. *Int J Eat Disord., 39*, 685-93.

Beck, A.T. (1975) *Cognitive Therapy and the Emotional Disorders*. International Universities Press Inc.

Beck, A.T., Steer, R.A., Brown, G.K. (1987), *Beck Depression Inventory-2nd Edition*. The Psychological Corporation, Harcourt Brace & Company, San Antonio.

Brink, P.J., Ferguson, K. (1998) The decision to lose weight. *West J Nurs Res., 20,* 84-102.

Brody ML, Masheb RM, Grilo CM. (2005) Treatment preferences of patients with binge eating disorder. *Int J Eat Disord., 37*,:352-6.

Carpiniello, B., Pinna, F., Pillai, G., Nonnoi, V., Pisano, E., Corrias, S., Orrù, M.G., Orrù, W., Velluzzi, F., Loviselli, A. (2009) Psychiatric comorbidity and quality of life in obese patients. Results from a case-control study. *Int J Psychiatry Med, 39*, 63-78.

Carter, J.C., Mcfarlane, T.L., Olmsted, M.O. (2004). Psychometric assessment of eating disorders. In Brewerton, T.D, *Clinical Handbook of Eating Disorders. An Integrated Approach*. (pp. 21-46). New York-Basel. Marcel Dekker.

Morgenthaler, T.I., Silber, M.H. (2002) Amnestic sleep-related eating disorder associated with zolpidem. *Sleep Med.,* 3, 23-327.

Castellini, G., Lapi, F., Ravaldi, C., Vannacci, A., Rotella, C.M., Faravelli, C., Ricca, V. (2008) Eating disorder psychopathology does not predict the overweight severity in subjects seeking weight loss treatment. *Compr Psychiatry., 49,* 359-63.

Cheskin, L.J., Donze, L.F. (2001) Appearance vs. health as motivators for weight loss. *JAMA,* 286, 2160.

Childress AC, Brewerton TD, Hodges EL, Jarrell MP. (1993).The Kids' Eating Disorders Survey (KEDS): A study of middle school students. *J Am Acad Child Adolesc Psychiatry, 32*, 843–850.

Cooper, Z., Fairburn, C.G. (1987), The Eating Disorder Examination: a semistructured interview for the assessment of the specific psychopathology of eating disorder. *International Journal of Eating Disorders, 6,* 1-8.

Cuzzolaro, M., Vetrone, G., Marano, G. (1999), "BUT: una nuova scala per la valutazione del disagio relativo all'immagine del corpo. *Psichiatria dell'infanzia e dell'adolescenza, 66*, 417-428.

Dalle Grave, R. (2001), *Terapia cognitivo comportamentale dell'obesità.* Positive Press, Verona.

De Giacomo, P., Renna, C., Santoni Rugiu, A. (2005) La diagnosi e la valutazione. In De Giacomo, P., Renna, C., Santoni Rugiu, A. *Manuale sui Disturbi dell'Alimentazione.*

Anoressia, Bulimia, Disturbo da Alimentazione Incontrollata. (pp. 94-97). Milano. Franco Angeli.

De Lorenzo, A., Maiolo, C., D'Agostino, G., Arcudi, G. (2006) Guidelines and malpractice in obesity treatment *Clin Ter., 157,* 143-52.

de Zwaan M (2001) Binge eating disorder and obesity. *Int J Obes Relat Metab Disord., 25* Suppl, S51-5.

Derogatis, L.R. (1977), *Symptoms Check-List 90-R (SCL 90-R), Scoring and Procedures Manual-I for the Revised Version*. Johns Hopkins School of Medicine, Goldbeck.

Ducimetiere, P., Richard, J., Cambien, F. (1986) The pattern of subcutaneous fat distribution in middle-aged men and the risk of coronary heart disease: the Paris Prospective Study. *Int J Obes, 10*, 229–240.

Elder, K.A., Grilo, C.M. (2007) The Spanish language version of the Eating Disorder Examination Questionnaire: comparison with the Spanish language version of the eating disorder examination and test-retest reliability. *Behav Res Ther., 45,* 1369-77.

Ellis A., Russell G. et al., (1977) *Handbook of Rational-Emotive Therapy*, NY: Springer.

Fairburn, C.G., Beglin, S.J. (1994). Assessment of eating disorders: interview or self-report questionnaire?. *International Journal of Eating Disorders, 16,* 363–370.

Fairburn, C.G., Cooper, Z. (1993), The Eating Disorder Examination-12th edition. In Fairburn, C.G., Wilson, G.T, *Binge Eating. Nature, Assessment, and Treatment.* Guilford Press, New York, pp. 317-360.

First, M.B., Gibbon, M., Spitzer, R.L., Williams, J.B. (1996), *User's Guide for the Structured Clinical Interview for DSM-IV Axis I Disorders*. Biometrics Research, New York.

First, M.B., Gibbon, M., Spitzer, R.L., Williams, J.B., Benjamin, L.S. (1997), *User's Guide for the Structured Clinical Interview for DSM-IV Axis II Personality Disorders.* American Psychiatric Press, Washington, DC.

Flegal, K.M., Graubard, B.I., Williamson, D.F., Gail, M.H. (2005) Excess deaths associated with underweight, overweight, and obesity. *JAMA, 293*, 1861–1867.

Foster, G.D, Wadden, T.A., Vogt, R.A., Brewer, G. (1997) What is a reasonable weight loss? Patients' expectations and evaluations of obesity treatment outcomes. *J Consult Clin Psychol., 65,* 79-85.

Garner, D.M. (2002), Measurement of eating disorder psychopathology. In FAIRBURN, C.G., BROWNELL, K.D. (a cura di), *Eating Disorders and Obesity. A Comprehensive Handbook.* Guilford Press, New York, 141-146.

Gormally, J., Black, S., Daston, S., Rardin, D. (1982). The assessment of binge eating severity among obese persons. *Addictive Behaviors, 7,* 47-55.

Han, T.S., Van Leer, E.M., Seidell, J.C., Lean, M.E.J. (1995) Waist circumference action levels in the identification of cardiovascular risk factors: prevalence study in a random sample. *British Medical Journal, 311*, 1401–1405.

Hasler, G., Pine, D.S., Gamma, A., Milos, G., Ajdacic, V., Eich, D., Rössler, W., Angst, J. (2004) The associations between psychopathology and being overweight: a 20-year prospective study. *Psychol Med., 34,* 1047-57.

Janssen, I., Katzmarzyk, P.T., Ross, R. (2002) Body mass index, waist circumference, and health risk. Evidence in support of current National Institutes of Health guidelines. *Arch Intern Med., 162*, 2074–2079.

Kasen, S., Cohen, P., Chen, H., Must, A. (2008) Obesity and psychopathology in women: a three decade prospective study. *Int J Obes, 32*, 558-66.

Kolotkin, R.L., Head, S., Hamilton, M., Tse, C.J. (1995), Assessing impact of weight on quality of life, *Obesity Research, 3,* 49-56.

Kutlesic, V., Williamson, D.A., Gleaves, D.H., Barbin, J.M., Murphy-Eberenz, K.P. (1998). The Interview for the Diagnosis of Eating Disorders-IV: application to DSM-IV diagnostic criteria. *Psychological Assessment, 10*, 41-48.

Lapidus, L., Bengtsson, C., Larsson, B., Pennert, K., Rybo, E., Sjostrom, L. (1984) Distribution of adipose tissue and risk of cardiovascular disease and death: a 12-year follow up of participants in the population study of women in Gothenburg, Sweden. *British Medical Journal, 289,* 1257–1261.

Larrañaga Vidal, A-, García-Mayor, R.V. (2009) High frequency of non-specific eating disorders in obese persons] *Nutr Hosp, 24*, 661-6.

Larsson, B., Svardsudd, K., Welin, L., Wilhelmsen, L., Bjorntorp, P., Tibblin, G. (1984) Abdominal adipose tissue distribution, obesity, and risk of cardiovascular disease and death: 13 year follow up of participants in the study of men born in 1913. *British Medical Journal, 288*, 1401–1404.

Lean, M.E.J., Han, T.S., Seidell, J.C. (1998) Impairment of health and quality of life in people with large waist circumference. *Lancet, 351*, 853–856.

Leslie WS, Hankey CR, Lean ME. (2007) Weight gain as an adverse effect of some commonly prescribed drugs: a systematic review. *QJM.*100, 395-404

Levy, A.S., Heaton, A.W. (1993) Weight control practices of U.S. adults trying to lose weight. *Ann Intern Med.,119,* 661-6.

Manson, J.E., Colditz, G.A., Stampfer, M.J., Willett, W.C., Rosner, B., Monson, R.R., Speizer, F.E., Hennckens, C.H. (1990) A prospective study of obesity and risk of coronary heart disease in women. *N Engl J Med., 322,* 882–889.

Marano, G., Cuzzolaro, M., Vetrone, G., Garfinkel, Pe., Temperilli, F., Spera, G., Dalle Grave, R., Calugi, S., Marchesini, G.; QUOVADIS Study Group (2007) validating the Body Uneasiness Test (BUT) in obese patients. *Eat Weight Disord., 12,* 70-82.

Marcus MD, Kalarchian MA. (2003) Binge eating in children and adolescents. *Int J Eat Disord*, *34,* S47–S57.

Marcus, M., Moulton, M., Greeno, C. (1995) Binge eating onset in obese patients with binge eating disorder. *Addict Behav, 20,* 747–755.

Mazure, C.M., Halmi, K.A., Sunday, R.A., Romano, S.J., Einhorn, A.M. (1994), The Yale-Brown-Cornell Eating Disorder Scale: development, use, reliability and validation. *Journal of Psychosomatic Research*, 28, 425-445.

McGuire, M.T., Wing, R.R., Klem, M.L., Hill, J.O. (1999) Behavioral strategies of individuals who have maintained long-term weight losses. *Obes Res,. 7,* 334-41.

Mokdad, A.H., Marks, J.S., Stroup, D.F., Gerberding, J.L. (2000) Actual causes of death in the United States,. *JAMA, 291,* 1238–1245.

Morgan, C., Yanovski, S., Nguyen, T., McDuffie, J., Sebring, N., Jorge, M., et al., (2002) Loss of control over eating, adiposity, and psychopathology in overweight children. *Int J Eat Disord, 31,* 430–441.

Nangle, D.W., Johnson, W.G., Carr-Nangle, R.E., Engler, L.B. (1994). Binge eating disorder and the proposed DSM-IV criteria: psychometric analysis of the Questionnaire on Eating and Weight Patterns. *International Journal of Eating Disorders, 16,* 147-157.

National Heart, Lung, and Blood Institute (NHLBI) and North American Association for the Study of Obesity (NAASO). Practical Guide to the Identification, Evaluation, and

Treatment of Overweight and Obesity in Adults. Bethesda, Md: National Institutes of Health; 2000.

Ness-Abramof R, Apovian CM. (2005) Drug Induced Weight Gain. *Drugs* Today, 8, 547–55.

Patton, J. H., Stanford, M. S. & Barratt, E. S. (1995). Factor structure of the Barratt impulsiveness scale. *Journal of Clinical Psychology, 51,* 768-774.

Peterson CB, Crosby RD, Wonderlich SA, Joiner T, Crow SJ, Mitchell JE, Bardone-Cone AM, Klein M, le Grange D. (2007) Psychometric properties of the eating disorder examination-questionnaire: factor structure and internal consistency. *Int J Eat Disord, 40,* 386-9.

Peterson, C.B., Miller, K.B. (2005). Assessment of eating disorder. In Wonderlich, S., Mitchell, J., De Zwaan, M., Steiger, H., *Eating Disorders Review: Part I.* (pp. 105-126). Oxford. Radcliffe Publishing.

Pickering, R.P., Grant, B.F., Chou, S.P., Compton, W.M. (2007) Are overweight, obesity, and extreme obesity associated with psychopathology? Results from the national epidemiologic survey on alcohol and related conditions. *J Clin Psychiatry., 68,* 998-1009.

Pijl H, Meinders AE. (1996) Bodyweight change as an adverse effect of drug treatment. *Drug Safety, 14,* 329–42.

Mannucci, E., Ricca, V., Barciulli, E., Di Bernardo, M., Travaglini, R., Cabras, P.L., Rotella, C.M. (1999) Quality of life and overweight: the obesity related well-being (Orwell 97) questionnaire. *Addict Behav.,24*, 345-57.

Ricca, V., Castellini, G., Lo Sauro, C., Ravaldi, C., Lapi, F., Mannucci, E., Rotella, C.M., Faravelli, C. (2009) Correlations between binge eating and emotional eating in a sample of overweight subjects. *Appetite, 53,* 418-21.

Richman, R.M., Steinbeck, K.S., Caterson, I.D. (1992) Severe obesity: the use of very low-energy diets or standard kilojoule restriction diets. *Med J Aust.,156*, 768-70.

Rotter, J.B. (1966) Generalized expectancies for internal versus external control of reinforcement. *Psychol Monogr., 80*, 1-28.

Schneider, H.J., Glaesmer, H., Klotsche, J., Böhler, S., Lehnert, H., Zeiher, A.M., März, W., Pittrow, D., Stalla, G.K., Wittchen, H.U., for the DETECT Study Group. (2007). Accuracy of Anthropometric Indicators of Obesity to Predict Cardiovascular Risk *The Journal of Clinical Endocrinology & Metabolism, 92,* 589-594

Shapiro, J.R., Woolson, S.L., Hamer, R.M., Kalarchian, M.A., Marcus, M.D., Bulik, C.M. (2007) Evaluating binge eating disorder in children: development of the children's binge eating disorder scale (C-BEDS). *Int J Eat Disord., 40*, 82-9.

Simon, G.E., Arterburn, D.E. (2009) Does comorbid psychiatric disorder argue for or against surgical treatment of obesity? *Gen Hosp Psychiatry. 31*, 401-2.

Spielberg, C., Gorsuch, R., Lushene, R. (1970) *Manual for the State-Trait Anxiety Inventory.* Palo Alto. Consulting Psychologists Press.

Spitzer, R.L., Devlin, M., Walsh, B.T., Hasin, D., Wing, R., Marcus, M.D., Stunkard, A., Wadden, T.A., Yanovski, S., Agras, S.W., Mitchell, J., Nonas, C. (1992). Binge Eating Disorder: a multisite field trial of the diagnostic criteria. *International Journal of Eating Disorders, 11,* 191-203.

Spitzer, R. L., Yanovski, S. Z., Marcus, MD. (1993) *The Questionnaire on Eating and Weight Patterns-Revised (QEWP-R)*. New York State Psychiatric Institute: New York.

Stunkard, A.J., Messick, S. (1985), The three-factor eating questionnaire to measure dietary restraint, dishinibition, and hunger. *Journal of Psychosomatic Research*, *29,* 71-83.

Todisco, P,. Vinai, P., (2008) *La fame infinita.* Torino Centro Scientifico Editore.

Valsamakis, G., Chetty, R., Anwar, A., Banerjee, A.K., Barnett, A., Kumar, S. (2004) Association of simple anthropometric measures of obesity with visceral fat and the metabolic syndrome in male Caucasian and Indo-Asian subjects. *Diabet Med., 21*, 1339–1345.

Vinai, P., Carpegna, G., Cardetti, S., Ferrato, N., Vallauri, P., Masante, D., Meister, A., Ruggiero, G.M., Sassaroli, S. (2008) Food is never enough: nature and nurture's influence on children's food dose evaluation. *Eating Disorders., 16,* 128-35.

Vinai, P., Todisco, P. (2007). *Q uando le emozioni diventano cibo.* Milano. Libreria Cortina

Vossenaar, M., Anderson, A., Lean, M., Ocke, M. (2004) Perceived reasons for weight gain in adulthood. *Int J Obes 28,* S67

Whitaker, A., Davies, M., Shaffer, M., Johnson, J., Abrams, S., Walsh, B., et al., (1989) The struggle to be thin: A survey of anorexic and bulimic symptoms in a non-referred adolescent population. *Psychol Med., 9,* 143–163.

Williamson, D.A., Womble, L.G., Zucker, N.L., Reas, D.L., White, M.A., Blouin, D.C., Greenway, F. (2000) Body image assessment for obesity (BIA-O): development of a new procedure. *Int J Obes Relat Metab Disord., 24,* 1326-32.

Wilson, G.T., Nonas, C.A., Rosenblum, G.D. (1993). Assessment of binge eating in obese patients. *International Journal of Eating Disorders, 13,* 25-33.

Wing, R.R., Hill, J.O. (2001) Successful weight loss maintenance. *Annu Rev Nutr, 21,* 323-41.

Wing, R.R., Phelan, S. (2005) Long-term weight loss maintenance. *Am J Clin Nutr, 82,* 222S-225S.

World Health Organization. Obesity: Preventing and Managing the Global Epidemic. Geneva, Switzerland: World Health Organization; 2000.WHO Technical Report Series 894.

Yusuf, S., Hawken, S., Ounpuu, S., Bautista, L., Franzosi, M.G., Commerford, P., Lang, C.C., Rumboldt, Z., Onen, C.L., Lisheng, L., Tanomsup, S., Wangai, Jr P., Razak, F., Sharma, A.M., Anand, S.S. INTERHEART Study Investigators (2005) Obesity and the risk of myocardial infarction in 27,000 participants from 52 countries: a case-control study. *Lancet, 366,* 1640–1649.

In: Pathways to Obesity and Main Roads to Recovery
Editor: Piergiuseppe Vinai
ISBN: 978-1-61122-740-6

Chapter IX

Selecting and Preparing Patients for Bariatric Surgery: The Preoperative Psychological Consultation

Anthony N. Fabricatore[1] *and Joseph A. Giorgio*[2]

[1] Center for Weight and Eating Disorders, Department of Psychiatry, University of Pennsylvania School of Medicine, PA, USA

[2] Department of Psychology, La Salle University, PA, USA

Abstract

Bariatric surgery is the treatment of choice for extremely obese individuals who are unable to achieve long-term weight control with lifestyle modification and/or pharmacotherapy. The complexity of surgical procedures, as well as the associated risks and expense, warrants careful selection and preparation of candidates. However, whether the preoperative evaluation and selection process should always include a mental health component has been the subject of some debate. In the following sections, we briefly review the literature on the presence of psychopathology in obese and extremely obese persons, and the relationship between preexisting psychiatric disorder and the outcomes of bariatric surgery. Subsequently, we describe approaches to the preoperative psychological consultation and the outcomes of these clinical interactions.

Introduction

Extreme Obesity and Bariatric Surgery

The World Health Organization has called obesity a "global epidemic" (World Health Organization, 1998). The development and spread of this epidemic have been especially apparent in the United States, where the prevalence of obesity (i.e., a body mass index > 30 kg/m^2) more than doubled, from 15% to over 30%, in the last two decades of the 20th century (Flegal, Carroll, Ogden, & Johnson, 2002; Ogden, Carroll, Curtin, McDowell, Tabak, & Flegal, 2006). Increases in prevalence also have been noted in other developed countries, as well as in several developing nations (World Health Organization, n.d.). The health ramifications of this disorder are well documented and include increased risk of early death, type 2 diabetes, cardiovascular disease, some forms of cancer, sleep apnea, and arthritis (National Institutes of Health/National Heart, Lung, and Blood Institute [NIH/NHLBI], 1998). Persons with extreme obesity, characterized by a body mass index (BMI) > 40 kg/m^2, are at particular risk of these complications, as well as psychological distress and impaired quality of life (NIH/NHLBI, 1998; Adams et al., 2006; Onyike, Crum, Lee, Lyketsos, & Eaton, 2003; Kolotkin, Crosby, & Williams, 2002). Unfortunately, the prevalence of extreme obesity is growing even more rapidly than that of obesity per se. In the time it took for the U.S. prevalence of obesity to double, extreme obesity increased five-fold (Sturm, 2003).

Bariatric surgery is the treatment of choice for extremely obese individuals who are unable to achieve long-term weight control with lifestyle modification and/or pharmacotherapy (NIH/NHLBI, 1998). Roux-en-Y gastric bypass (RYGB) and laparoscopic adjustable gastric banding (LAGB) are the most commonly used procedures (Buchwald & Williams, 2004). Others include biliopancreatic diversion with or without duodenal switch, vertical banded gastroplasty, and vertical sleeve gastrectomy. With RYGB, a small pouch (i.e., 15 to 30 ml) is isolated on the lesser curvature of the stomach to restrict food intake, and a limb of the small intestine is joined to the pouch. This significant alteration of the gastrointestinal anatomy results in nutrients bypassing the distal stomach and 80 to 150 cm of small intestine. By contrast, LAGB restricts food intake without altering the digestive tract. With LAGB, the gastric pouch (of ~30 ml) is created by placing a ring around the upper portion of the stomach. The ring is lined with an inflatable band so that the stoma between the upper and lower sections of the stomach can be constricted (or dilated) by increasing (or removing) saline through an infusion port that is placed subcutaneously in the abdomen.

Results of a meta-analysis indicated that patients who underwent RYGB and LAGB achieved mean weight reductions of 43.5 kg and 30.1 kg, respectively, at one year, and 41.5 kg and 34.8 kg, respectively, after at least three years' follow-up (Maggard et al., 2005). The Swedish Obese Subjects (SOS) study found that patients maintained a 25% reduction in initial body weight with RYGB and 14% with adjustable banding procedures (similar to LAGB) at an average of ten years postoperatively (Sjöström et al., 2007). The same study, however, also found that a significant minority (i.e., 25% of banding patients and 9% of bypass patients) failed to maintain more than a 5% reduction in initial weight at ten years (Sjöström et al., 2004).

Limitations notwithstanding, both procedures are associated with significant improvement in, or resolution of, a variety of comorbid conditions (e.g., Maggard et al., 2005; Tice, Karliner, Walsh, Petersen, & Feldman, 2008). Furthermore, bariatric surgery is associated with significant reductions in risk of early death, compared with matched nonsurgical controls (Sjöström et al., 2007; Adams et al., 2007; Peeters et al., 2007). There are, however, risks associated with bariatric surgery. Early (< 30 days) and late (> 30 days to two years) mortality rates have been estimated at 0.1% and 0.0%, respectively, for laparoscopic banding procedures, and 0.2 to 0.4% and 0.1 to 0.7%, respectively, for gastric bypass (Buchwald, Estok, Fahrbach, Banel, & Sledge, 2007). Complications, which include infection, deep vein thrombosis, malnutrition, and reoperation, are estimated in 20% of cases (Maggard et al., 2005).

Improvements in mental health and quality of life frequently accompany the broad improvements in physical health and longevity that patients achieve with bariatric surgery. A number of reviews have found reductions in depression and eating pathology, as well as increased social and occupational function following bariatric surgery (e.g., Herpertz et al., 2003; Sarwer, Wadden, & Fabricatore, 2005; van Hout, Boekestein, Fortuin, Pelle, & van Heck, 2006; Wadden et al., 2007). Resolution of psychopathology, however, is not universal and exceptions are notable. One study found a trend toward greater risk of suicide and other non-disease related death among bariatric surgery recipients, compared with untreated controls (Adams et al., 2007). In addition, there have been reports of alcohol addiction and other problematic compulsive behaviors in a minority of patients after surgery. The prevalence of this phenomenon, however, is unknown, as are the mechanisms that may explain it (see Sogg, 2007).

Patient Selection

The complexity of bariatric surgery, as well as the associated risks and expense, warrants careful selection and preparation of candidates. A National Institutes of Health (NIH) Consensus Conference Statement set the first eligibility criterion at a BMI $\geq$ 40 kg/m^2, or $\geq$ 35 kg/m^2 in the presence of severe obesity-related comorbidities (NIH, 1991). We note that some groups advocate lowering the BMI threshold to 30 kg/m^2 (e.g., O'Brien et al., 2006; Kakoulidis, Karringer, Gloaguen, & Arvidsson, in press), but this movement has not yet gained widespread acceptance.

The 1991 NIH statement indicated that patients under consideration for surgery should be "selected carefully after evaluation by a multidisciplinary team with medical, surgical, psychiatric, and nutritional expertise." Whether the preoperative evaluation and selection process should, as a matter of course, include a mental health component has been the subject of some debate. In a 2004 update to the 1991 NIH statement, the American Society for Metabolic and Bariatric Surgery (ASMBS, formerly American Society for Bariatric Surgery) concluded that evaluation by a mental health professional (as well as by other specialists) "is not routinely needed but should be available if indicated" (Buchwald & Consensus Conference Panel, 2005). Cases in which such consultations are indicated are not specified. Furthermore, there is no empirically derived algorithm, analogous to the guidelines for the treatment of obesity (NIH/NHLBI, North American Association for the Study of Obesity, 1998), that instructs practitioners in the conduct of preoperative psychological evaluations and the conclusions that can be drawn from them. Although best practice guidelines have been published (e.g., Greenberg, Sogg, & Perna, 2009), the limitations of their evidence bases preclude specific recommendations to clinicians about what to do with the patient seated across from them.

In the following sections, we briefly review the literature on the presence of psychopathology in obese and extremely obese persons, and the relationship between preexisting psychiatric disorder and the outcomes of bariatric surgery. Subsequently, we describe approaches to the preoperative psychological consultation and the outcomes of these clinical interactions.

Psychopathology in Obesity and Extreme Obesity

Whether obese individuals are at increased risk of psychological disorder has been the subject of numerous investigations (for reviews, see Wadden & Stunkard, 1985; Friedman & Brownell, 1995; Berkowitz & Fabricatore, 2005). Early studies typically were limited by small or non-representative samples or by the use of non-validated instruments to assess psychopathology. Several examinations have not only corrected these methodological issues, but also have sought to identify moderators of the relationship between body weight and distress. Furthermore, the focus has expanded to include anxiety, substance use, and personality disorders, whereas many previous investigations have been limited to depressive disorder or symptoms.

Results of several recent epidemiological investigations suggest that obese persons have increased odds of having a lifetime history of major depressive disorder, bipolar disorder, and anxiety disorders, compared with individuals in the normal-weight range (i.e., BMI 18.5 to 24.9 kg/m^2) or with non-obese individuals (i.e., BMI < 30 kg/m^2; Simon et al., 2006; Barry, Pietrzak, & Petry, 2008; Petry, Barry, Pietrzak, & Wagner, 2008; Mather, Cox, Enn, & Sareen, 2009). As shown in Tables 9.1a & 9.1b, these relationships are typically stronger in women versus men, and they increase with the severity of obesity. Mechanisms that account for the higher risk of psychopathology in obese women and extremely obese individuals may include greater quality of life impairment, weight-related stigma, and body image dissatisfaction experienced by people in those groups (Kolotkin, Meter, & Williams, 2001; Kolotkin, Crosby, & Williams, 2002; Carr, Jaffe, & Friedman, 2008; Puhl & Brownell, 2001; Sarwer, Thompson, & Cash, 2005). Findings regarding lifetime substance use disorders are less consistent than what has been observed for mood and anxiety disorders. Whereas one study showed that obese persons had significantly lower odds of ever having met criteria for a substance use disorder (Simon et al., 2006), another showed significantly greater odds (Petry et al., 2008). We note that because these studies have been cross-sectional, they do not allow us to draw conclusions about whether causation exists or in which direction.

Given that extreme obesity is associated with greater psychopathology and that distress is generally greater in clinical than in general populations (Fitzgibbon, Stolley, & Kirschenbaum, 1993), it is reasonable to expect a high prevalence of psychological disorders among patients seeking bariatric surgery. However, investigations that used rigorous diagnostic interviews to assess bariatric surgery candidates are rare. Two examples are summarized in Table 2. Kalarchian and colleagues (2007) reported on 288 bariatric surgery candidates who were evaluated using the Structured Clinical Interview for DSM-IV (SCID; First et al., 2002) and SCID-II (to diagnose personality disorders; First et al., 1997), independently of the preoperative screening process. Two-thirds of the sample was found to have met criteria for at least one Axis I mental disorder sometime during their lives, and 38% met criteria at the time of the evaluation. In a similar study, Mauri et al. (2008) evaluated 282 bariatric surgery candidates using the SCID and SCID-II (along with other interview-based tools). The sample was less obese than that in the Kalarchian study (mean BMI = 43.5 vs. 52.2 kg/m^2), and a smaller percentage had at least one current Axis I disorder (21%). The pattern of results, however, was similar.

Table 9.1a. Odds ratios (95% confidence intervals) of meeting criteria for psychiatric disorders in one's lifetime: findings from four epidemiological studies that used structured diagnostic interviews

Disorder or Category	Simon et al., 2006*			Mather et al., 2009**			Barry et al., 2008***		Petry et al., 2008****	
	Obese	Obese Men	Obese Women	Obese	Obese Men	Obese Women	Obese Men	Obese Women	Obese	Extremely Obese
Any Mood Disorder	1.27 (1.15-1.41)	1.21 (.99-1.46)	1.29 (1.11-1.50)	1.29 (1.12- 1.49)	1.17 (.91-1.50)	1.38 (1.16-1.64)	1.39 (1.21-1.60)	1.79 (1.63-1.28)	1.56 (1.44-1.69)	2.00 (1.74-2.31)
Major Depressive Disorder	1.21 (1.09-1.35)			1.41 (1.22-1.64)	1.38 (1.05-1.81)	1.43 (1.21-1.68)	1.35 (1.14-1.59)	1.58 (1.43-1.75)	1.53 (1.41-1.67)	2.02 (1.74-2.35)
Bipolar Disorder/ Mania	1.47† (1.12-1.93)			1.53 (1.17-2.00)	1.39 (.88-2.18)	1.67 (1.23-2.28)	1.20 (.93-1.55)	2.24 (1.80-2.78)	1.55 (1.29-1.86)	2.70 (2.00-3.66)
Any Anxiety Disorder	1.28 (1.05-1.57)	1.17 (.82-1.67)	1.34 (1.09-1.64)	1.22 (1.10-1.36)	1.25 (1.06-1.46)	1.20 (1.05-1.38)	1.35 (1.18-1.53)	1.76 (1.58-1.96)	1.54 (1.41-1.68)	1.97 (1.67-2.31)
Any Substance Use Disorder	.78 (.65-.93)	.75 (.60-.93)	.88 (.65-1.18)							
Alcohol Use Disorder									1.21 (1.11-1.33)	1.33 (1.12-1.58)
Drug Use Disorder									1.06 (.94-1.19)	1.41 (1.07-1.85)

Table 9.1b. Odds ratios (95% confidence intervals) of meeting criteria for psychiatric disorders in the past year: findings from four epidemiological studies that used structured diagnostic interviews

Disorder or Category	Simon et al., 2006*	Mather et al., 2009**			Barry et al., 2008***		Petry et al., 2008****	
	Obese	Obese	Obese Men	Obese Women	Obese Men	Obese Women	Obese	Extremely Obese
Any Mood Disorder	1.19 (1.00-1.42)	1.20 (.98-1.46)	1.05 (.73-1.52)	1.30 (1.04-1.63)	1.33 (1.20-1.59)	1.75 (1.52-2.01)	1.52 (1.35-1.70)	1.91 (1.58-2.31)
Major Depressive Disorder	1.09 (.89-1.34)	1.24 (1.02-1.52)	1.21 (.82-1.80)	1.27 (1.02-1.58)	1.31 (1.03-1.67)	1.49 (1.25-1.76)	1.45 (1.28-1.63)	1.95 (1.57-2.42)
Bipolar Disorder/ Mania	1.61† (1.07-2.43)	1.91 (1.33-2.73)	1.45 (.82-2.56)	2.44 (1.52-3.91)	1.15 (.80-1.64)	2.41 (1.84-3.17)	1.63 (1.24-2.14)	2.58 (1.74-3.81)
Any Anxiety Disorder	1.34 (1.07-1.66)	1.29 (1.11-1.48)	1.45 (1.14-1.84)	1.19 (1.00-1.42)	1.36 (1.16-1.61)	1.79 (1.58-1.96)	1.56 (1.40-1.73)	2.08 (1.73-2.50)
Any Substance Use Disorder	.65 (.40-1.06) -	.88 (.66-1.16)	.87 (.62-1.24)	.88 (.55-1.41)				
Alcohol Use Disorder		1.05†† (.80-1.39)					.87 (.75-1.01)	.88 (.64-1.20)
Drug Use Disorder		.53†† (.31-.89)					.82 (.64-1.05)	1.01 (.61-1.69)

Note: Cells contain odds ratios (95% confidence intervals).

* Participants were 9,125 US adults in National Comorbidity Survey-Replication study. Mental disorders were assessed using the World Mental Health–Composite International Diagnostic Interview (WMH-CIDI). BMI was calculated using self-reported height and weight. Odds ratios calculated using nonobese persons (BMI $\leq$ 29.9 kg/m^2) as the reference group.

** Participants were 36,984 Canadians, aged $\geq$ 15 years. Sample was nationally representative. Diagnoses made based on face-to-face (86%) or telephone (14%) assessments using the World Mental Health–Composite International Diagnostic Interview (WMH-CIDI) [26]. Odds ratios were calculated using nonobese persons (BMI $\leq$ 29.9 kg/m^2) as the reference group and analyses were adjusted for age, gender (when possible), education, other psychiatric disorders, and medical comorbidities.

*** Participants were 40,790 US adults in National Epidemiologic Survey on Alcohol and Related Conditions (NESARC). Mental disorders were assessed using the NIAAA Alcohol Use Disorder and Associated Disabilities Interview Schedule–DSM-IV Version (AUDADIS-IV). Odds ratios were calculated using normal weight persons (BMI = 18.5-24.9 kg/m^2) as the reference group and analyses were adjusted for age, education, race/ethnicity, income, marital status, region of country, and urban vs. rural residence.

**** Data from 41,654 participants in NESARC. Odds ratios were calculated using normal weight persons (BMI = 18.5-24.9 kg/m^2) as the reference group and analyses were adjusted for age, gender, ethnicity, education, income, marital status, region of country, and urban vs. rural residence.

† Includes Bipolar I and Bipolar II.

†† Includes substance dependence only.

In both studies, the most common current Axis I conditions were binge eating disorder and major depressive disorder, and the most common diagnoses on Axis II were avoidant and obsessive-compulsive personality disorders. While these findings suggest high rates of psychopathology in bariatric surgery candidates, the lack of a control group precludes comparisons with non-obese, less obese, or non-treatment-seeking individuals.

Table 9.2. Percentage of bariatric surgery candidates meeting criteria for psychiatric disorders: results of two investigations that employed diagnostic interviews

Disorder or Category	Kalarchian et al., 2007		Mauri et al., 2008	
	Lifetime	Current	Lifetime	Current
Any Axis I Disorder	66.3	37.8	37.6	20.9
Any Mood Disorder	45.5	15.6	22.0	6.4
Major Depressive Disorder	42.0	10.4	19.1	4.6
Bipolar Disorder (I or II)	3.5	1.7	2.2	1.1
Dysthymic Disorder	—	3.8	1.1	1.1
Any Anxiety Disorder	37.5	24.0	18.1	12.4
Panic Disorder	19.4	5.9	8.5	4.6
Agoraphobia	3.5	1.0	2.1	
Social Phobia	9.4	9.0	3.2	2.8
Specific Phobia	8.0	7.3	5.3	5.0
Obsessive-Compulsive Disorder	3.8	2.1	2.8	2.1
Post-traumatic Stress Disorder	11.8	2.8	1.8	1.1
Generalized Anxiety Disorder	—	6.3	1.1	1.1
Any Substance Use Disorder	32.6	1.7	1.1	
Any Eating Disorder	29.5	16.3	12.8	7.1
Bulimia Nervosa	3.5	0.3	1.8	0.4
Binge Eating Disorder	27.1	16.0	11.0	6.7
Any Axis II Disorder	66.3	37.8	37.6	20.9
Paranoid Personality Disorder		5.6		.7
Schizoid Personality Disorder		2.1		—
Schizotypal Personality Disorder		0.4		—
Antisocial Personality Disorder		2.8		—
Borderline Personality Disorder		4.9		1.8
Histrionic Personality Disorder		0		—
Narcissistic Personality Disorder		0.7		0.4
Avoidant Personality Disorder		17.0		6.8
Dependent Personality Disorder		1.7		0.4
Obsessive-Compulsive Personality Disorder		7.6		13.9

Psychopathology and the Outcomes of Bariatric Surgery

The ability of preoperative psychopathology and other psychological variables to predict weight loss and other outcomes of bariatric surgery has been a frequent subject of empirical study and debate. As summarized in several reviews (Bocchieri, Meana, & Fisher, 2002; Herpertz et al., 2003; van Hout, Boekestein, Fortuin, Pelle, & van Heck, 2006; Wadden et al., 2007), findings have been mixed. Whereas some studies have shown that higher depression scores at baseline are related to less weight loss, others suggest a relationship in the opposite direction. The same is true of preoperative binge eating. In general, it appears that preoperative psychosocial variables are better predictors of postoperative psychosocial variables than they are of weight loss or complications.

In a follow-up of a study described above, Kalarchian and colleagues (2008) reported six-month outcomes for 207 patients who completed preoperative SCID and SCID-II assessments. Controlling for initial BMI, age, race, and gender, a lifetime history of a mood disorder or anxiety disorder was associated with significantly less weight loss. Whereas patients with no history of any Axis I disorder lost 30% of their initial weight (57% of their excess weight) at six months, those with a history of a mood or anxiety disorder lost 25% of their initial weight (46 to 47% of their excess weight) at that time. Neither lifetime history of substance use or eating disorders, nor any current Axis I or Axis II disorders were significantly related to weight loss at six months.

Before concluding that preoperative psychopathology does or does not constitute a contraindication to bariatric surgery, two points require consideration. First, even when a diagnosis was related to less weight loss (Kalarchian et al., 2008), the average reduction in the affected group (i.e., 25% of initial weight) could not be considered treatment failure. Second, the six-month follow-up may not have been sufficient to allow differences to be observed. The SOS study showed that weight loss peaks, on average, at 12 to 18 months postoperatively, at which time regain may begin (Sjöström et al., 2004, 2007). It is possible that the potency of the surgery at six months overwhelmed any potential influence of psychopathology. Longer-term follow-up in studies that rigorously applied diagnostic criteria at baseline is needed.

Is the Preoperative Psychological Consultation Worthwhile? Is it Harmful?

As noted earlier, the ASMBS concluded that not all bariatric surgery candidates require evaluation by a mental health professional. The value of the preoperative psychological evaluation was further questioned by Ashton and colleagues (Ashton, Favretti, & Segato, 2008). These authors eloquently examined the availability and quality of evidence for four premises: 1) some patients will fail to lose a significant amount of weight with bariatric surgery; 2) preoperative psychological screening will identify some candidates as abnormal; 3) preoperative psychological abnormality will predict poor weight loss outcomes; and 4) identification of at-risk patients will reduce failure or enhance targeted support. Lack of support for the third premise (on which the fourth is predicated) led the authors to ultimately reject the conclusion that psychological screening should be part of the preoperative evaluation of bariatric surgery candidates. Moreover, Ashton et al. concluded that such screening amounts to a "form of prejudice" against obese individuals.

Our reading of the literature leads us to agree with Ashton and colleagues' (2008) statement that there is insufficient evidence to support the claim that preexisting psychopathology portends failure of bariatric surgery. Does it follow, however, that the preoperative psychological evaluation is (at best) useless or (at worst) prejudicial, as Ashton and colleagues contend?

First, we believe that the potential value and justness of the preoperative psychological consultation depend on its nature, as well as the knowledge base and biases of the consultant. A mere search for psychopathology—regardless of its type, determinants, or influence—followed by a statement that the affected patient is an inappropriate candidate for bariatric surgery is irresponsible and unethical. We review alternative approaches below.

Second, we note that the scientific process does not allow us to accept a null hypothesis; we may only reject it or fail to reject it. Because a relationship or effect has not been found, we cannot conclude that it does not exist. As Aston et al. (2008) stated, "myriad methodological problems...have been such a conspicuous feature of previous studies and...have consistently undermined attempts to reach reliable, evidence based conclusions." Some of those problems include poor or inconsistent definitions of the psychological variables of interest, high rates of attrition, and non-experimental design. Study design is of particular concern. No randomized controlled trials have compared outcomes between patients who were or were not required to undergo a preoperative psychological consultation. Until findings of more rigorous studies become available, bariatric surgery programs are left to decide whether to continue or to cease the practice of preoperative psychological evaluation. Pertinent to this decision are beliefs about the likelihood and magnitude of potential benefits and risks. That is, can we provide a service that may be useful in some way without causing harm?

Our position is that the preoperative preparation process should include a psychological consultation. Note our use of the terms "psychological" (vs. "psychiatric") and "consultation" (vs. "evaluation"). Whereas psychiatry is the science and practice of diagnosing and treating mental disorders, psychology is the study of mental processes and behaviors. The latter includes not only psychopathology, but also "normal" affects, cognitions, and behaviors. Certainly, determining whether a patient meets criteria for a mental disorder is an important component of the evaluation; a significant minority of patients have an Axis I disorder and may benefit from a referral for treatment. Diagnosing disorders, however, should not be the sole focus. Likewise, the nature of the contact should not be solely evaluative. As others have suggested, the psychologist may recommend strategies to patients to aid in their preoperative preparation and postoperative adherence and adjustment (LeMont, Moorehead, Parish, Reto, & Ritz, 2004; Sogg & Mori, 2009). Furthermore, the psychologist can recommend ways in which the surgical team can structure its interactions with specific patients, based on observed personality characteristics and cognitive styles and abilities.

Approaches to the Preoperative Psychological Consultation

At least three surveys have attempted to characterize common practices that constitute the preoperative psychological consultation (described as an "evaluation" in those papers; Bauchowitz et al., 2005; Fabricatore, Crerand, Wadden, Sarwer, & Krasucki, 2006; Walfish, Vance, & Fabricatore, 2007). Perhaps the strongest conclusion from these surveys is that no practice is universal. Nearly all respondents, however, reported use of a clinical interview. The majority of these also use psychological testing instruments, which may include paper-and-pencil symptom checklists, personality instruments, or tests of cognitive function. Several specific instruments are listed in Table 9.3, along with the frequency of use reported in three surveys. The list, however, is by no means exhaustive; the surveys found reference to over 50 specific tests!

Table 9.3. Percentage of respondents reporting use of formal tests as part of the preoperative psychological evaluation: findings from three surveys

Instrument	Survey		
	Bauchowitz et al., 2005*	Fabricatore et al., 2006**	Walfish et al., 2007***
Symptom Inventories			
Beck Depression Inventory	33.3	48.5	36
Beck Anxiety Inventory	7.4	15.5	13
Symptom Checklist-90	7.4	6.7	< 5%
Eating Disorders Inventory	3.7	7.2	17
Personality Tests			
Minnesota Multiphasic Personality Inventory	22.2	42.8	69
Personality Assessment Inventory	14.8	9.3	18
Millon Clinical Multiaxial Inventory	7.4	6.7	14
Behavioral Health Inventories			
Millon Behavioral Health Inventory	7.4	12.9	5
Millon Behavioral Medicine Diagnostic	3.7	16	25
Tests of Cognitive Function			
Mini Mental Status Examination	3.7	29.9	5
Shipley Institute of Living Scale	—	2.1	5

* Based on the 27 participants (total n = 81) who listed assessment instruments used in their evaluations.

** Based on the total sample (n = 194).

*** Based on the 77 participants (total n = 103) who reported using at least one test.

— Use not reported in this survey.

The tests and procedures selected for the evaluation depend on the domains the consultant believes are important to assess. Fabricatore and colleagues (2006) surveyed mental health professionals to whom ASMBS members (i.e., surgeons) referred patients for evaluations. Respondents were asked to list the "five most important things you assess for during your preoperative evaluations." Responses were open-ended and coded for content. Not surprisingly, psychiatric issues were mentioned by nearly all participants (92.3%). Many responses, however, were vague (e.g., "stability"), and no specific diagnostic class was mentioned by a majority of respondents. The most commonly cited classes of disorders were eating disorders (38%), mood disorders (31%), and substance use disorders (25%). Several non-psychiatric issues also were cited, including informed consent (i.e., capacity and knowledge; 60%), family/social support (53%), and issues related to adherence (47%).

The domains reported in the above-cited survey research are evident in two models for conducting preoperative psychological consultations. We review Wadden and Sarwer's (2006) "patient-oriented approach" to the behavioral assessment of bariatric surgery candidates, which is practiced at the University of Pennsylvania, and Sogg and Mori's (2008) approach, based on the Boston Interview for Bariatric Surgery.

Wadden and Sarwer's Patient-oriented Approach

This approach begins with a mental health professional who has expertise in obesity. The clinician's knowledge of the etiology, complications, and treatment of obesity helps focus the evaluation and inform recommendations. The evaluation consists of a clinical interview and completion of the Beck Depression Inventory (BDI; Beck, Steer, & Brown, 1996) and Weight and Lifestyle Inventory (WALI; Wadden & Foster, 2006). The WALI responses generally guide the interview, which addresses five primary domains.

One area of interest is the patient's knowledge of bariatric surgery. Informed consent requires an understanding of the procedure, as well as its benefits, risks, and behavioral and dietary requirements. Patients' expectations of weight loss and other changes should be assessed. Frequently, patients expect to lose considerably more weight than the procedure, on average, can offer (Bauchowitz, Azarbad, Day, & Gonder-Frederick, 2007). The clinical significance of unrealistic weight loss expectations with bariatric surgery is unknown. However, assessment of expected weight loss allows an opportunity for educating the patient and encouraging attention to changes in health and quality of life as important outcomes.

A second domain is the patient's weight and dieting history. Patients who appear to have a genetic predisposition to obesity (crudely estimated based on early age of onset and prominent family history) may be relieved of some of the guilt that they may harbor in relation to their condition. Exploration of additional biological factors or life events that were associated with weight gain may be useful for conceptualizing the problem and offering strategies for coping with similar situations in the future. Surveying the patient's history of weight loss attempts will determine whether more conservative options have been exhausted. Furthermore, details about the nature (e.g., active vs. passive), duration, and outcomes of the patient's efforts will provide insight into his or her history of making and sustaining behavioral change.

Eating and activity habits comprise the third area of focus, intended to identify behaviors that will require significant change postoperatively. Details about the number, composition, and timing of patients' meals and snacks may reveal that a dietary "overhaul" is necessary. Conversely, review of typical eating habits may show that large portions are the primary culprit behind weight gain. These scenarios have different implications for preparatory and postoperative dietary recommendations. (For example, a patient who typically forgoes breakfast, consumes a light lunch, and then eats a large dinner and snacks on high-calorie items before going to bed might be coached to eat more frequent meals, spaced evenly throughout the day)

Evaluation of eating behaviors should also include assessment for the presence of eating disorders. Bulimia nervosa is uncommon (Allison et al., 2006), but is considered by many experts to be a contraindication to surgery. Binge eating disorder is more frequently encountered in bariatric surgery candidates, but its prognostic significance is unclear. As described above, some studies show significantly less weight loss—though not necessarily greater risk of treatment failure—among patients with binge eating disorder, compared with non-binging controls. In preparation for surgery, practitioners may attempt to reduce binge frequency, which can be accomplished with behavioral weight control or cognitive-behavioral therapy of binge eating disorder with equivalent efficacy (Munsch, et al., 2007). Finally, clinicians should assess patients' current levels of physical activity, attitudes toward exercise, and barriers to increased activity to inform recommendations for initiating or expanding an exercise plan.

The fourth domain in Wadden and Sarwer's (2006) model is social/psychological status. This includes an informal mental status examination and a review of the patient's histories of mental health disorders and treatment. When patients are currently under the care of a psychologist, psychiatrist, or other mental health professional, the clinician seeks consent to contact the other provider, who can provide a more detailed assessment of the patient's status than what can be obtained in the brief (~1 hour) preoperative psychological consultation. A short telephone call typically reveals the patient's history of treatment adherence, engagement and progress in therapy, and likelihood of continuing treatment postoperatively. Importantly, the consultant should attend to areas of consistency and contrast with his/her own impressions of the patient. In some cases, the contact yields discrepant information from the patient's report, which may require additional evaluation. Evidence of untreated or undertreated disorders or distress prompts the recommendation that the patient seek targeted therapy preoperatively. In some cases, concerns (rather than disorders) trigger a recommendation for psychotherapy to be initiated either prior to or shortly after surgery. These issues may include body image disturbance or expectations of family discord.

The fifth area of assessment includes the timing of surgery and the patient's plan for postoperative care. Ideally, patients will be free of significant acute stressors and will not be planning major life changes in the months following surgery. These stressors, as well as the accumulation of minor hassles, are a concern insofar as they may overwhelm the patient's resources for coping, thereby compromising his/her adjustment and adherence to the postoperative lifestyle. Depending on the type of surgery and the scheduled progression from clear liquids to solid foods, patients may be advised to take more than a month to return to their jobs.

Wadden and Sarwer's (2006) patient-oriented approach concludes with a review of the findings with the patient, who leaves with a list of specific recommendations. The findings and recommendations are summarized in a brief report to the surgeon. The consultant provides an opinion about the patient's readiness and areas of concern, but the ultimate decision regarding a patient's candidacy is left to the surgeon.

Sogg and Mori's Boston Interview for Bariatric Surgery.

Sogg and Mori (2004) developed the Boston Interview for Gastric Bypass to guide the preoperative psychological evaluation of patients seeking gastric bypass surgery. The burgeoning popularity of adjustable gastric banding, as well as the increases in knowledge and data pertinent to bariatric surgery, led the authors to revise the instrument as the Boston Interview for Bariatric Surgery (BIBS; Sogg & Mori, 2008). The interview assesses the following seven domains: 1) weight, diet, and nutrition history; 2) eating pathology; 3) medical history; 4) understanding of surgical procedures, risks, and the postoperative regimen; 5) motivation and outcome expectations; 6) relationships and support system; and 7) psychiatric functioning. As this list demonstrates, the BIBS shares several points of focus with the Wadden and Sarwer (2006) approach. Thus, the details of each domain will not be reviewed here. The BIBS, however, has the advantage of being a structured protocol, which provides suggested language for guiding the interview.

Like the Wadden and Sarwer (2006) approach, the BIBS is ideally implemented by a professional with expertise in obesity, in general, and bariatric surgery, in particular. A deep knowledge of the condition and its treatment enhances not only the gathering of information, but also the incorporation of assessment data into treatment recommendations. For a thorough discussion of how the BIBS (or other preoperative psychological evaluation methods) can be used to inform interventions, the reader is referred to Sogg & Mori (2009).

Outcomes of the Preoperative Psychological Consultation

Preoperative evaluations typically yield one of three primary recommendations: 1) to proceed unconditionally with bariatric surgery; 2) to defer surgery until areas of concern have been addressed; and 3) outright denial of surgery. The available data suggest that unconditional approval is the most common recommendation. Chart reviews conducted by two independent research/clinical groups suggested that ~65%-70% of patients were "approved" for surgery without stipulation (Sarwer et al., 2004; Pawlow, O'Neil, White, & Byrne, 2005). Similarly, in one national survey of mental health providers who conduct preoperative psychological evaluations, respondents estimated, on average, that they unconditionally recommended surgery for 70% of candidates (Fabricatore et al., 2006). In these studies (Sarwer et al., 2004; Pawlow et al., 2005; Fabricatore et al., 2006), ~25%-30% of patients received a recommendation to defer surgery, pending resolution or improvement of specific issues (typically the recommended course of action was psychotherapy and/or dietary counseling). Outright denial appeared, in these studies, to be rare (i.e., < 5%). A more recent survey of psychologists who evaluate bariatric surgery candidates did not distinguish between deferral and denial, but found that the average respondent recommended deferral *or* denial for < 15% of candidates (Walfish et al., 2007). Whether the greater approval rate found in the more recent study is merely a function of sampling or reflective of a trend is unknown. Clinicians' reasons for recommending deferral or denial of surgery, and perceived contraindications, vary (Bauchowitz et al., 2005; Fabricatore et al., 2006; Walfish et al., 2007). There are, however, many commonalities, which are summarized in Table 4. We note that the disorders and issues cited therein are not evidence-based. Instead, they represent the opinions and practices of providers and bariatric surgery program representatives who responded to surveys. As stated previously, no psychological or behavioral factors have been demonstrated to be reliable predictors of treatment failure or complications.

Table 9.4. Issues and disorders commonly perceived and treated as contraindications to bariatric surgery

Substance Use Disorders
Severe Mental Illness (Active Psychosis, Bipolar Disorder)
Depressive Disorder/Symptoms (Especially Untreated)
Suicidal Ideation, Suicide Attempts
Eating Disorders
Questionable Informed Consent (Cognitive Impairment, Poor Understanding, Unrealistic Expectations)
Demonstrated Nonadherence

(Adapted from Bauchowitz et al., 2005; Fabricatore et al., 2006; Walfish et al. 2007).

Clinicians who withhold the recommendation to proceed with surgery must have a firm rationale for doing so. We recommend asking several questions. One is "what is the theoretical or empirically-demonstrated mechanism by which this patient's presentation may negatively affect their outcome?" The clinician should be able to articulate to the patient (and the rest of the surgical team) *why* the presentation is a concern, *how* the issue increases the risk of an unfavorable outcome, and *what* the patient (in concert with their support system and treatment team) can do to reduce that risk. A second important question is "how do the benefits and risks of undergoing surgery compare to those of forgoing surgery?" Consultations with surgeons and physicians about the patient's specific health risks may be necessary. Also necessary is an understanding of the literature about the surgical and nonsurgical treatment of obesity. The SOS study suggested that the average patient treated with gastric bypass can be expected to lose ~32% of their body weight in one year and maintain a loss of ~25% at 10 years (Sjöström et al., 2007). Matched controls treated with diet and exercise, by contrast, remained with 2% of their initial weight. Other studies show that intensive lifestyle modification, with or without pharmacotherapy, typically induces losses of 5-15% of initial weight at 1 year; the average patient regains most or all of their lost weight within 5 years of discontinuing treatment (Wadden et al., 2005; Look AHEAD Research Group, 2007; Dansinger, Tatsioni, Wong, Chung, & Balk, 2007). Clinicians should discuss with patients ways in which their health and quality of life may change (for better or worse) with each of their weight loss options.

Beyond Approval, Deferral, Or Denial

Ideally, a clinician's preoperative psychological consultation yields more than a simple "yea" or "nay" regarding the patient's readiness or appropriateness for bariatric surgery. Based on a detailed assessment of the patient's eating habits, lifestyle, environment, resources, psychosocial status, stress level, and concerns, the clinician may offer specific recommendations intended to enhance success and avoid problematic outcomes. In many cases, these will rely on the same behavioral and cognitive principles that are taught in lifestyle modification (e.g., self-monitoring, stimulus control, problem-solving; see Chapter X). They also may entail teaching patients strategies for effectively communicating with significant others who may be unsupportive or undermining of the patient's efforts. The universe of possibilities is too large to consider here. Specific recommendations will depend not only on the patient's unique circumstances, but also on the knowledge, experience, and creativity of the clinician.

Similarly, the psychological consultant may provide recommendations to the surgical team. As noted above, consultants often recommend that the team delay surgery for some patients until they have completed (or at least initiated) dietary counseling and/or treatment of psychiatric disorder. (Consultants also may recommend such courses of action postoperatively, as adjuncts to the surgical therapy.) Assessment of personality or cognitive abilities may inform recommendations regarding how the treatment team may adjust communication or typical instructions to optimize the likelihood that the patient will understand and comply.

Conclusion

Bariatric surgery is the most effective tool for the treatment of extreme obesity. In addition to producing large, durable weight losses for most patients, bariatric surgery often results in resolution or improvement of weight-related comorbidities. Surgery, however, is not fail-safe and numerous investigations have attempted to identify behavioral, psychological, or psychiatric factors that predict poor weight loss or other untoward outcomes of bariatric surgery. Despite inconsistent findings from these endeavors, the process of selecting and preparing patients for bariatric surgery typically includes a psychological evaluation. There is no consensus on how those evaluations should be conducted, what their focus should be, and what findings constitute contraindications to surgery. Until prospective studies identify behavioral factors that reliably predict outcomes, or randomized controlled trials conclude that patients who receive a preoperative psychological consultation have better outcomes than those who do not, the value of the mental health professional in the preoperative selection process will remain open to debate.

We suggest that mental health professionals should explicitly inform the surgical team of the potential benefits and limitations of their contributions. In the same way that cardiologists cannot predict which patients will suffer a myocardial infarction and endocrinologists cannot predict which diabetic patients will achieve normoglycemia postoperatively, mental health professionals cannot definitively say which patients will fail and which will succeed in their efforts to lose weight and improve their health and quality of life.

Despite our inability to predict the future, we contend that the preoperative psychological evaluation can be valuable for the patient as well as for the surgical team. At the very least, patients suffering from a mental disorder can be identified and referred for appropriate treatment. However, we encourage mental health providers to approach the preoperative encounter more as a consultation than as strictly an evaluation. Clinicians also have an opportunity to counsel patients on potential barriers to success or sources of distress.

Furthermore, they may use their expertise in cognition, emotion, and behavior to recommend strategies to assist patients in preventing or overcoming expected obstacles. Providers can also help patients to identify and use their intrapersonal, interpersonal, and environmental resources to maximize their likelihood of a successful outcome. Because bariatric surgery represents the "last chance" at weight loss and risk reduction for many extremely obese individuals, well-intentioned contributions from all relevant specialists are likely to be appreciated.

Acknowledgments

This work was supported, in part, by NIH grant K23 DK 070777 to Dr. Fabricatore. The authors wish to thank Drs. Stephanie Sogg and Thomas Wadden for their thoughtful review and valuable recommendations.

References

Adams, K. F., Schatzkin A., Harris, T. B., Kipnis, V., Mouw, T., Ballard-Barbash, R., Hollenbeck, A., & Leitzmann, M. F. (2006). Overweight, obesity, and mortality in a large prospective cohort of persons 50 to 71 years old. *New England Journal of Medicine, 355*(8), 763-778.

Adams, T. D., Gress, R. E., Smith, S. C., Halverson, R. C., Simper, S. C., Rosamond, W. D., Lamonte, M. J., Stroup, A. M., & Hunt, S. C. (2007). Long-term mortality after gastric bypass surgery. *New England Journal of Medicine, 357*(8), 753-761.

Allison, K. C., Wadden, T. A., Sarwer, D. B., Fabricatore, A. N., Crerand, C. E., Gibbons, L. M., Stack, R. M., Stunkard, A. J., & Williams, N. N. (2006). Night eating syndrome and binge eating disorder among persons seeking bariatric surgery: prevalence and related features. *Obesity, 14*(Suppl. 2), 77S-82S.

Ashton, D., Favretti, F., & Segato, G. (2008). Preoperative psychological testing—another form of prejudice. *Obesity Surgery, 18*(10), 1330-1337.

Barry, D., Pietrzak, R. H., & Petry, N. M. (2008). Gender differences in associations between body mass index and DSM-IV mood and anxiety disorders: results from the National Epidemiologic Survey on Alcohol and Related Conditions. *Annals of Epidemiology, 18*(6), 458–466.

Bauchowitz, A., Azarbad, L., Day, K., & Gonder-Frederick, L. (2007). Evaluation of expectations and knowledge in bariatric surgery patients. *Surgery for Obesity and Related Diseases, 3*(5), 554-558.

Bauchowitz, A. U., Gonder-Frederick, L. A., Olbrisch, M. E., Azarbad, L., Ryee, M. Y., Woodson, M., Miller, A., & Schirmer, B. (2005). Psychosocial evaluation of bariatric surgery candidates: A survey of present practices. *Psychosomatic Medicine, 67*(5), 825-832.

Beck, A. T., Steer, R. A., & Brown, G. K. (1996). *Beck Depression Inventory-II (BDI-II)*. San Antonio, TX: Psychological Corporation.

Berkowitz, R. I., & Fabricatore, A. N. (2005). Obesity, psychiatric status, and psychiatric medications. *Psychiatric Clinics of North America, 28*(1), 39-54.

Bocchieri, L. E., Meana, M., & Fisher, B. L. (2002). A review of psychosocial outcomes of surgery for morbid obesity. *Journal of Psychosomatic Research, 52*(3), 155–165.

Buchwald, H., & Consensus Conference Panel. (2005). Bariatric surgery for morbid obesity: health implications for patients, health professionals, and third-party payers. *Journal of the American College of Surgeons, 200*(4), 593-604.

Buchwald, H., & Williams, S. E. (2004). Bariatric surgery worldwide, 2003. *Obesity Surgery, 14*(9), 1157-1164.

Buchwald, H., Avidor, Y., Braunwald, E., Jensen, M. D., Pories, W., Fahrbach, K., & Schoelles, K. (2004). Bariatric surgery: a systematic review and meta-analysis. *Journal of the American Medical Association, 292*(14), 1724 –1737.

Buchwald, H., Estok, R., Fahrbach, K., Banel, D., & Sledge, I. (2007). Trends in mortality in bariatric surgery: a systematic review and meta-analysis. *Surgery, 142*(4), 621-632.

Carr, D., Jaffe, K. J., & Friedman, M. A. (2008). Perceived interpersonal mistreatment among obese Americans: do race, class, and gender matter? *Obesity, 16*(Supp. 2), S60-S68.

Dansinger, M. L., Tatsioni, A., Wong, J. B., Chung, M., Balk, E. M. (2007). Meta-analysis: the effect of dietary counseling for weight loss. *Annals of Internal Medicine, 147*(1), 41-50.

Fabricatore, A. N., Crerand, C. E., Wadden, T. A., Sarwer, D. B., & Krasucki, J. L. (2006). How do mental health professionals evaluate candidates for bariatric surgery? Survey results. *Obesity Surgery, 16*(5), 567-573.

First, M. B., Gibbon, M., Spitzer, R. L., Williams, J. B. W., & Benjamin, L. S. (1997). Structured Clinical Interview for DSM-IV Axis II Personality Disorder, (SCID-II). Washington, D.C.: American Psychiatric Press, Inc.

First, M. B., Spitzer, R. L., Gibbon, M., & Williams, J. B.W. (2002). Structured Clinical Interview for DSM-IV-TR Axis I Disorders, Research Version, Non-patient Edition (SCID-I/NP). New York: Biometrics Research, New York State Psychiatric Institute.

Fitzgibbon, M. L., Stolley, M. R., Kirschenbaum, D. S. (1993). Obese people who seek treatment have different characteristics than those who do not seek treatment. *Health Psychology, 12*(5), 342-345.

Flegal, K. M., Carroll, M. D., Ogden, C. L., & Johnson, C. L. (2002). Prevalence and trends in obesity among U.S. adults, 1999-2000. *Journal of the American Medical Association, 288*(14), 1723-1727.

Friedman, M. A., & Brownell, K. D. (1995). Psychological correlates of obesity: moving to the next research generation. *Psychological Bulletin, 117*(1), 3–20.

Greenberg, I., Sogg, S., & Perna, F. M. (2009). Behavioral and psychological care in weight loss surgery: best practice update. *Obesity, 17*(5), 880-884.

Herpertz S., Kielmann, R., Wolf, A. M., Langkafel, M., Senf, W., & Hebebrand J. (2003). Does obesity surgery improve psychosocial functioning? A systematic review. *International Journal of Obesity, 27*(11), 1300-1314.

Herpertz, S., Kielmann, R., Wolf, A. M., Hebebrand, J., Senf, W. (2004). Do psychosocial variables predict weight loss or mental health after obesity surgery? A systematic review. *Obesity Research, 12*(10), 1554-1569.

Kakoulidis, T. P., Karringer, A., Gloaguen, T., & Arvidsson, D. (In press). Initial results with sleeve gastrectomy for patients with class I obesity (BMI 30-35 kg/m^2). *Surgery for Obesity and Related Diseases.*

Kalarchian, M. A., Marcus, M. D., Levine, M., Courcoulas, A. P., Pilkonis, P. A., Ringham, R. M., Soulakova, J. N., Weissfeld, L. A., & Rofey, D. L. (2007). Psychiatric disorders among bariatric surgery candidates: relationship to obesity and functional health status. *American Journal of Psychiatry, 164*(2), 328-334.

Kalarchian, M. A., Marcus, M. D., Levine, M. D., Soulakova, J. N., Courcoulas, A. P., & Wisinski, M. S. (2008). Relationship of psychiatric disorders to 6-month outcomes after gastric bypass. *Surgery for Obesity and Related Diseases, 4*(4), 544-549.

Kolotkin, R. L., Crosby, R. D., & Williams, G. R. (2002). Health-related quality of life varies among obese subgroups. *Obesity Research, 10*(8), 748-756.

Kolotikin, R. L., Meter, K., & Williams, G. R. (2001). Quality of life and obesity. *Obesity Reviews, 2*(4), 219-229.

LeMont, D., Moorehead, M. K., Parish, M. S., Reto, C. S., & Ritz, S. J. (2004). Suggestions for the pre-surgical psychological assessment of bariatric surgery candidates. Retrieved June 10, 2009, from American Society for Metabolic and Bariatric Surgery Web site: http://www.asbs.org/html/pdf/PsychPreSurgicalAssessment.pdf.

Look AHEAD Research Group (2007). Reduction in weight and cardiovascular disease risk factors in individuals with type 2 diabetes: one-year results of the Look AHEAD trial. *Diabetes Care, 30*(6), 1374-1383.

Maggard, M. A., Shugarman, L. R., Suttorp, M., Maglione, M., Sugerman, H. J., Livingston, E. H., Nguyen, N. T., Li, Z., Mojica, W. A., Hilton, L., Rhodes, S., Morton, S. C., & Shekelle, P. G. (2005). Meta-analysis: surgical treatment of obesity. *Annals of Internal Medicine, 142*(7), 547-559.

Mather, A. A., Cox, B. J., Enn, M. W., & Sareen, J. (2009). Associations of obesity with psychiatric disorders and suicidal behaviors in a nationally representative sample. *Journal of Psychosomatic Research, 66*(4), 277–285.

Mauri, M., Rucci, P., Calderone, A., Santini, F., Oppo, A., Romano, A., Rinaldi, S., Armani, A., Polini, M., Pincheram, A., & Cassano, G. B. (2008). Axis I and II disorders and quality of life in bariatric surgery candidates. *Journal of Clinical Psychiatry, 69*(2), 295-301.

Munsch, S., Biedert, E., Meyer, A., Michael, T., Schlup, B., Tuch, A., & Margraf, J. (2007). A randomized comparison of cognitive behavioral therapy and behavioral weight loss treatment for overweight individuals with binge eating disorder. *International Journal of Eating Disorders, 40*(2), 102-113.

National Heart Lung and Blood Institute & North American Association for the Study of Obesity. (2000). *The Practical Guide: Identification, Evaluation, and Treatment of Overweight and Obesity in Adults*. Bethesda, MD: National Institutes of Health.

National Institutes of Health Consensus Development Conference Panel. (1991). Gastrointestinal surgery for severe obesity. *Annals of Internal Medicine, 115*(12), 956-61.

National Institutes of Health/National Heart, Lung, and Blood Institute (1998). *Clinical guidelines on the identification, evaluation, and treatment of overweight and obesity in adults: The evidence report*. Bethesda, MD: National Institutes of Health.

O'Brien, P. E., Dixon, J. B., Laurie, C., Skinner, S., Proietto, J., McNeil, J., Strauss, B., Marks, S., Schachter, L., Chapman, L., & Anderson, M. (2006). Treatment of mild to moderate obesity with laparoscopic adjustable gastric banding or an intensive medical program. *Annals of Internal Medicine, 144*(9), 625-633.

Ogden, C. L., Carroll, M. D., Curtin, L. R., McDowell, M. A., Tabak, C. J., & Flegal, K. M. (2006). Prevalence of overweight and obesity in the United States, 1999-2004. *Journal of the American Medical Association, 295*(13), 1549-1555.

Onyike, C. U., Crum, R. M., Lee, H. B., Lyketsos, C. G., & Eaton, W. W. (2003). Is obesity associated with major depression? Results from the third National Health and Nutrition Examination Survey. *American Journal of Epidemiology, 158*(12), 1139-1147.

Pawlow, L. A., O'Neil, P. M., White, M. A., & Byrne, T. K. (2005). Findings and outcomes of psychological evaluations of gastric bypass applicants. *Surgery for Obesity and Related Diseases, 1*(6), 523-527.

Peeters, A., O'Brien, P. E., Laurie, C., Anderson, M., Wolfe, R., Flum, D., MacInnis, R. J., English, D. R., & Dixon, J. (2007). Substantial intentional weight loss and mortality in the severely obese. *Annals of Surgery, 246(*6), 1028-1033.

Petry, N. M., Barry, D., Pietrzak, R. H., & Wagner, J. A. (2008). Overweight and obesity are associated with psychiatric disorders: results from the National Epidemiologic Survey on Alcohol and Related Conditions. *Psychosomatic Medicine, 70*(3), 288–297.

Puhl, R., & Brownell, K. D. (2001). Bias, discrimination, and obesity. *Obesity Research, 9*(12), 788-805.

Sarwer, D. B., Cohn, N. I., Gibbons, L. M., Magee, L., Crerand, C. E., Raper, S. E., Rosato, E. F., Williams, N. N., & Wadden, T. A. (2004). Psychiatric diagnoses and psychiatric treatment among bariatric surgery candidates. *Obesity Surgery, 14*(9), 1148-1156.

Sarwer, D. B., Wadden, T. A., & Fabricatore, A. N. (2005). Psychosocial and behavioral aspects of bariatric surgery. *Obesity Research,13*(4), 639–648.

Sarwer, D.B., Thompson J. K., & Cash, T. F. (2005). Body image and obesity in adulthood. *Psychiatric Clinics of North America, 28*(1), 69-87.

Simon, G. E., Von Korff, M., Saunders, K., Miglioretti, D. L., Crane, P. K., van Belle, G., & Kessler, R. C. (2006). Association between obesity and psychiatric disorders in the U.S. adult population. *Archives of General Psychiatry, 63*(7), 824-830.

Sjöström, L., Lindroos, A. K., Peltonen, M., Torgerson, J., Bouchard, C., Carlsson, B., Dahlgren, S., Larsson, B., Narbro, K., Sjöström, C. D., Sullivan, M., Wedel, H., & Swedish Obese Subjects Study Scientific Group. (2004). Lifestyle, diabetes, and cardiovascular risk factors 10 years after bariatric surgery. *New England Journal of Medicine, 351*(26), 2683-2693.

Sjöström, L., Narbro, K., Sjöström, C. D., Karason, K., Larsson, B., Wedel, H., Lystig, T., Sullivan, M., Bouchard, C., Carlsson, B., Bengtsson, C., Dahlgren, S., Gummesson, A., Jacobson, P., Karlsson, J., Lindroos, A. K., Lönroth, H., Näslund, I., Olbers, T., Stenlöf, K., Torgerson, J., Ågren, G., Carlsson, L. M., & Swedish Obese Subjects Study. (2007). Effects of bariatric surgery on mortality in Swedish obese subjects. *New England Journal of Medicine, 357*(8), 741-752.

Sogg S. (2007). Alcohol misuse after bariatric surgery: epiphenomenon or "Oprah" phenomenon? *Surgery for Obesity and Related Diseases, 3*(3), 366-368.

Sogg, S., & Mori, D. L. (2004). The Boston interview for gastric bypass: determining the psychological suitability of surgical candidates. *Obesity Surgery, 14*(3), 1-11.

Sogg, S., & Mori, D. L. (2008). Revising the Boston Interview: incorporating new knowledge and experience. *Surgery for Obesity & Related Diseases, 4*(3), 455-463.

Sogg, S., & Mori, D. L. (2009). Psychosocial evaluation for bariatric surgery: the Boston interview and opportunities for intervention. *Obesity Surgery, 19*(3), 369-377.

Sturm, R. (2003). Increases in clinically severe obesity in the United States, 1986-2000. *Archives of Internal Medicine, 163*(18), 2146-2148.

Tice, J. A., Karliner, L., Walsh, J., Petersen, A. J., & Feldman, M. D. (2008). Gastric banding or bypass? A systematic review comparing the two most popular bariatric procedures. *American Journal of Medicine, 121*(10), 885-893.

van Hout, G. C., Boekestein, P., Fortuin, F. A., Pelle, A. J., & van Heck, G. L. (2006). Psychosocial functioning following bariatric surgery. *Obesity Surgery. 16*(6), 787-794.

van Hout, G. C., Verschure, S. K., & van Heck, G. L. (2005). Psychosocial predictors of success following bariatric surgery. *Obesity Surgery, 15*(4), 552–560.

Wadden, T. A., & Foster, G. D. (2006). Weight and lifestyle inventory (WALI). *Obesity, 14*(Suppl. 2), 99S-118S.

Wadden, T. A., & Sarwer, D. B. (2006). Behavioral assessment of candidates for bariatric surgery: A patient-oriented approach. *Obesity, 14*(Suppl. 2), 53S-62S.

Wadden, T. A., & Stunkard, A. J. (1985). Social and psychological consequences of obesity. *Annals of Internal Medicine, 103*(6), 1062–1067.

Wadden, T. A., Berkowitz, R. I., Womble, L. G., Sarwer, D. B., Phelan, S., Cato, R. K., Hesson, L. A., Osei, S. Y., Kaplan, R., & Stunkard, A. J. (2005). Randomized trial of lifestyle modification and pharmacotherapy for obesity. *New England Journal of Medicine, 353*(20), 2111-2120.

Wadden, T. A., Sarwer, D. B., Fabricatore, A. N., Jones, L., Stack, R., & Williams, N. S. (2007). Psychosocial and behavioral status of patients undergoing bariatric surgery: what to expect before and after surgery. *Medical Clinics of North America, 91*(3), 451-469.

Walfish, S., Vance, D., & Fabricatore, A. N. (2007). Psychological evaluation of bariatric surgery applicants: Procedures and reasons for delay or denial of surgery. *Obesity Surgery, 17*(12), 1578-1583.

World Health Organization (n.d.). Global database on body mass index: an interactive surveillance tool for monitoring nutrition transition. Retrieved June 10, 2009, from World Health Organization Website: http://www.who.int/bmi/index.jsp.

World Health Organization. (1998). *Obesity: preventing and managing the global epidemic*. Geneva, Switzerland: Author.

In: Pathways to Obesity and Main Roads to Recovery
Editor: Piergiuseppe Vinai
ISBN: 978-1-61122-740-6

Chapter X

Psychosocial Contribution and Prevention of Childhood Obesity

***Yael Latzer*[1] *and Daniel Stein*[2]**
[1]Eating Disorders Clinic, Psychiatric Division, Rambam Medical Center, Haifa, Israel, affiliated with The Faculty of Social Welfare & Health Sciences, Haifa University, Haifa, Israel
[2]Pediatric Psychosomatic Department, the Edmond and Lily Safra Children's Hospital, The Chaim Sheba Medical Center, Tel Hashomer, affiliated with The Sackler Faculty of Medicine, Tel Aviv University, Tel Aviv, Israel

Abstract

The current review focuses on an updated critical analysis of the most relevant socio-cultural issues in childhood overweight issues. It is rooted on a comprehensive systematic literature search of the PUBMED, PSYCHLIT, PSYCHINFO, and ERIC between 1991 and 2010.

A dramatic rise in childhood overweight issues has been shown in many countries around the globe, both Western industrialized and Third World non-industrialized countries, in the past two to three decades. From the different environmental dimensions potentially associated with childhood overweight issues, this review highlights the role of gender, socio-economic status, cultural and familial background, social isolation, and a host of factors associated with the influence of modernization, particularly the influence of the media, changes in the food consumed, and reduction in physical activity.

These findings highlight the need for promoting health-generated strategies to reduce the risk of child and adolescent obesity. The findings of prevention studies, although not definite, emphasize two important points. Firstly, prevention programs should be multidisciplinary, combining the knowledge of experts from different professions, taking into consideration the important role of the family, and relevant influential social organizations, primarily the school. Secondly, no change can be induced without planned large-scale programs carried out on a public policy level.

Introduction

The investigation of the psychosocial aspects of childhood obesity has been the focus of long-standing theoretical and empirical endeavors (Renman et al., 1999; Strauss, 2000). In this review, we will relate to the classical definitions of obesity and being overweight. We will review first the socio-cultural factors including exposure to media contributing to childhood obesity and then present the psychsocial intervention for the prevention of childhood obesity. The review is based on a comprehensive systematic literature search of the PUBMED, PSYCHLIT, PSYCHINFO, and ERIC between 1991 and 2010.

Socio-Cultural Factors Contributing to Childhood Obesity

An inverse correlation has been repeatedly shown between being overweight and socio-economic status and education among adults, whereas among children and adolescents this relationship is less clear (Sweeting et al., 2008), particularly in industrialized countries. Accordingly, some studies have shown that the risk of childhood overweight issues is greater in children of higher socio-economic status (Hawkins et al., 2008; Strauss & Knight 1999). This has been associated with the absence of mothers because of long working hours, likely impeding young children's access to healthy foods and physical activity (Hawkins et al., 2008). Still, other studies in affluent societies have associated being overweight in children with lower socio-economic status, (Gray et al., 2007; McCullough et al., 2009; O'Dea & Wilson, 2006; Salanave et al., 2009), or have found no association between childhood obesity and socio-economic status (Sweeting et al., 2008).

By contrast, in most studies performed in Third World non-Western countries (Jiang et al., 2006; Jingxiong et al., 2009; Strauss & Knight, 1999), the elevated risk of being overweight in children of lower socio-economic status mirrors adult findings. A similar trend has been reported in minority groups (Crawford, 2001; Moreno et al., 2004; Novaes et al., 2008; Ogden et al., 2002; Speiser et al., 2005; Strauss & Knight, 1999) and in many (Casey et al., 2006; O'Dea & Wilson, 2006; Spinks et al., 2007) although not all (Kelly et al., 2006) studies assessing other less affluent populations in industrialized countries. Several factors have been suggested to account for this finding. First and foremost, the rise in the rate of childhood obesity is most prevalent in cultures considered to be in transition, i.e., experiencing considerable changes within a relatively brief period of time, as is the case with many other physical and emotional disorders (Speiser et al., 2005). Non-Western countries and minority groups have likely experienced such changes in recent decades. Specifically, elevated rates of childhood obesity have been found in environments with an inclination toward overfeeding of children, above-average levels of dietary intake of low nutritional-quality, high-fat, high-calorie foods and beverages, inadequate physical activity, and a greater amount of time spent in sedentary behaviors (Casey et al., 2006; O'Dea & Wilson, 2006; Spinks et al., 2007). Impoverished environments with limited availability of healthful foods and higher-than-average availability of fast food restaurants, along with exposure to ethnically targeted food marketing, may further contribute to reliance on high-calorie foods and beverages, these foods being also valued socially and culturally (Casey et al., 2006; Kumanyika, 2008). Another study suggests that that low-income mothers of overweight preschool children may use food to cope with the stresses of their economic situation, have difficulty setting limits for their children related to food, and are less committed to sustained behavioral change than high-income mothers (Chamberlin et al., 2002). Alternatively, experiences of poverty-associated food deprivation during childhood may super-motivate some women to actively avoid food insecurity in adulthood, both with respect to themselves and their children (Olson et al., 2007). As a result, food may be used in impoverished surroundings to meet emotional needs in childhood, directing overeating to become a generalized response to negative emotional states in later years (Olson et al., 2007). The association between childhood food insecurity and increased risk for being overweight remains significant after controlling for ethnicity, gender, age, and family poverty level (Casey et al., 2006).

Aside from the socio-economic domain, age, gender and cultural background are considered as particularly influential in the recent dramatic rise in childhood overweight issues. This increase has been shown to be particularly prominent in very young children [including in two years old; See Adair, (2008)], and to be greater in female than in male youngsters (Spinks et al., 2007) and in minority groups (Adair, 2008; Ogden et al., 2002). Specifically, African-American female adolescents are at greater risk to become overweight and obese in comparison to African-American male adolescents (Robinson et al., 2009) and other minority and non-minority populations (Adair, 2008; Crawford, 2001; Ogden et al., 2002). This female/male disparity in obesity prevalence in young black individuals has been related to parental education, as it is found primarily in families with low parental education (Robinson et al., 2009). Moreover, the influence of childhood psychosocial factors in general to predict obesity in later life is greater in females than in males (Kestilä et al., 2009).

Still, other socio-environment factors may also be of relevance in increasing the recent rise in childhood overweight and obesity. These include lack of social networks, social isolation and marginalization, single-parent families, parental lack of education and unemployment, child neglect, parental violence, and early sexual harassment and abuse (D'Argenio et al., 2009; Fuemmeler et al., 2009; Gilbert et al., 2008; Greenfield & Marks, 2009; Irish et al., 2009; Israel & Ivanova, 2002; Kestilä et al., 2009; Lissau & Sorenson, 1994; Noll et al., 2007; Puhl & Latner, 2007). Several processes may mediate in the association between early-life trauma and being overweight. These include greater rates of skipping meals to lose weight, problematic eating, and the use of food in response to stress, reduced physical activity (Fuemmeler et al., 2009; Gray et al., 2008; Greenfield & Marks, 2009), greater depression and other psychological squeals of the trauma (Gunstad et al., 2006; Noll et al., 2007), and hypothalamic-pituitary-adrenal axis dysregulation (Noll et al., 2007) found in girls with childhood abuse in comparison to controls. Interestingly, severity of early childhood trauma remains a significant predictor of later obesity even when the influence of minority (Noll et al., 2007) and of trauma-related psychiatric morbidity (D'Argenio et al., 2009) are taken into account.

Factors associated with the influence of modernization, primarily the decrease in physical activity and increase in sedentary behaviors in younger populations, the rise in the accessibility to low-quality snacks, high-fat products, high-energy drink consumption and fast food, the increase in the portion sizes in restaurants, and the decreased consumption of vegetables have also been found to increase the risk of childhood obesity (Bisset et al., 2007;

Campbell et al., 2006c; Colapinto et al., 2007; Forman et al., 2009; Israel & Ivanova, 2002; Kaiser Family Foundation, 2004; Novaes et al., 2008; Olstad and McCargar, 2009; Spinks et al., 2007).

According to the study of the Institute of Medicine from 2006 (McGinnis et al., 2006), at least 30 percent of the calories in the average American children's diet derives from sweets, soft drinks, salty snacks, and fast food. Soft drinks account for more than ten percent of the caloric intake, representing a doubling since 1980. One large-scale study in Canada has thus found that children report preference for portions of French fries, meats, and potato chips that are larger, and for vegetable portions that are smaller than what is recommended. Children from socio-economically disadvantaged families or who frequently eat while watching television and in fast-food restaurants prefer larger portions of French fries and potato chips. Consequences of consuming large portions of these foods have been found to include poor diet quality and increased energy intake, whereas the opposite findings are shown when consuming large portions of vegetables (Colapinto et al., 2007). Although most of these findings have been documented in Western countries, similar trends have been observed also in less industrialized countries (Moreno et al., 2004; Novaes et al., 2008).

Exposure to the Media

Children in the U.S. and other Western industrialized countries are exposed to the media for an average of three to five hours daily, which is greater than any other daily activity, except for sleeping (Center for Disease Control, 2004; Leatherdale & Wong, 2008; Manios et al., 2009; Van Zutphen et al., 2007), and exceeds the television-viewing recommendations of ≤2 hours/day (Davison et al., 2005; Spinks et al., 2007). Moreover, the prevalence (Manios et al., 2009; van Zutphen et al., 2007), and severity of being overweight (Leatherdale & Wong, 2008) have been found to be positively correlated with the amount of time spent in television watching (Spinks et al., 2007). The television-viewing habits of children are significantly correlated with those of their parents and siblings (Davison et al., 2005). Exposure to the media in youngsters contributes to around 60% of their overweight incidence via several mechanisms (CDC, 2004; Leatherdale & Wong, 2008; Maffeis et al., 2008; Manios et al., 2009); exposure time displacing time spent on physical activity [lower levels of physical activity have been found to be inversely correlated in children with weight status (Gray et al., 2008)], exposure to advertisements encouraging unhealthy food choices, use of popular characters to promote high-calorie foods, excessive eating while viewing television (primarily of energy-dense snacks that may promote fat gain) and exposure to distorted messages regarding the way to achieve an ideal weight. Interestingly, some studies have shown that the effect of television-viewing time on childhood obesity may be independent of the physical activity status of the child, attributed only to the increased total energy intake during television watching (Manios et al., 2009). This maladaptive influence of television on childhood overweight issues has been demonstrated in both cross-sectional and longitudinal studies of large cohorts (Dietz & Gortmaer, 1993), with females' weight being influenced by it to a greater extent than that of males.

Another topic of great concern relates to the great exposure of youngsters to unhealthy food via marketing and advertisements (Kelly et al., 2008). Food marketing to children is massive in many countries around the globe, expanding in a number of venues such as the television, placements in toys, games, educational materials, songs, movies, celebrity endorsements, cellular-telephone text and messages, and the Internet (Harris et al., 2009; McGinnis et al., 2006) A recent research performed by the Institute of Medicine in the USA in 2006 (McGinnis et al., 2006), which analyzed the results of 123 studies that addressed the issue of food marking and childhood obesity, supported the likelihood of a link between food marketing, children's food preferences, children's food consumption, and adiposity. According to this study, since 1994, U.S. companies have introduced about 600 new children's food products; half of them have been candies or chewing gums, and another fourth are other types of sweets or salty snacks. Only one-fourth is of healthier items, such as baby foods, bread products, and bottled waters.

More than a quarter of advertisements directed to young populations in recent years are for food, with quick-serve restaurants, non-core foods such as candy, cereal, and snacks, and soft drinks being the food products most commonly advertised in popular children's websites and in television (Alvy & Calvert, 2008; Harris et al., 2009; Powell et al., 2007) and around primary schools (Kelly et al., 2008). Many food-related advertisements have been found to use the term "super-charged" or a similar adjective to describe the powerful taste or other physical properties of unhealthy high-calorie dense food products. By contrast, statements or depictions that a food product is healthy or nutritious are quite rare among commercials (Page & Brewster, 2007). This condition is highly harmful, because food marketing and food-related media may influence food preferences, purchase and consumption in all youngsters (Alvy & Calvert, 2008; Dalmeny, 2003; Halford et al., 2008), but particularly in younger children (Swinburn et al., 2008), and in overweight children vs. normal-weight children (Halford et al., 2008; Kelly et al., 2009). For example, overweight children may show greater responsiveness to food branding, being, therefore, at risk in environments that are highly inundated with messages about food (Forman et al., 2009). Moreover, although exposure to food advertisements may produce a substantial increase in energy intake in all children, particularly of high-fat and/or sweet energy-dense snacks, this increase is the largest in obese children. This is evident by the positive associations found between the amount of food intake (in particular intake of high-fat snacks) following exposure to food-related commercials, and BMI (Halford et al., 2008). Lastly, the mean energy density of foods consumed in general is found to be significantly higher in obese and overweight children in comparison to normal-weight children (Maffeis et al., 2008). This, when bearing in mind that the taste of food preferred, for example, children's inclination to savory snacks, has been associated with overweight in prepubertal children (Maffeis et al., 2008).

It should be noted that although many studies highlight the detrimental influence of advertisements on food habits of children, this is not the case for all studies. Kopelman et al., (2007), for example, have found that although 9- to 11-year-old children demonstrate high-brand logo recognition abilities, no association is shown between higher brand logo recognition ability and poorer eating behaviors, food knowledge and food preferences.

Familial and Social Interventions for the Prevention of Childhood Obesity

The recent increase in childhood overweight issues places a significant burden on physical, psychological, and social health. It is, therefore, essential to alter those environmental and behavioral factors that may potentially increase the risk of childhood overweight issues (Hill & Peters, 1998). The premise underlying primary prevention programs for childhood obesity is that lifestyle behaviors such as dietary habits and physical activity, considered of paramount importance in reducing the risk of childhood obesity, although difficult to achieve (Maximova et al., 2008), can be modifiable (Cole et al., 2006). Nevertheless, targeted interventions that have involved only children, but not their families or social surroundings, have been for the most part ineffective in reducing the rate of pediatric overweight issues (Olstad and McCargar, 2009; Story, 1999). Another drawback of programs involving overweight children is their often sole focus on weight reduction, but not on reducing the influence of psychosocial risk factors such as media influence or peer pressure (Campbell et al., 2001), or how overweight children perceive their own weight. While on the one hand an accurate awareness of weight may lower the overweight youngster's self-esteem, accurately perceiving oneself as overweight/obese has nevertheless, been linked to greater motivation to change lifestyle behaviors (Maximova et al., 2008). It is interesting in this respect to note that overweight and obese youth may be more likely to misperceive their weight compared with non-overweight youth. Targeting this misperception may facilitate the adoption of healthy lifestyle behaviors among overweight/obese children, potentially improving the effectiveness of obesity prevention interventions (Maximova et al., 2008).

The Role of the Family

Involving Parents and Other Social Agencies

Involving parents and other social agencies in the attempt to prevent or reduce childhood overweight issues emerges, therefore, of vital importance (Sonneville et al., 2009). This is not surprising, as parents have primary influence over their children's food and activity environments (Olstad and McCargar, 2009), and the manner in which parents feel and act with respect to eating behaviors, food consumption and physical activity may have an important role in shaping their children's eating- weight- and physical activity-related perceptions and behaviors (Kröller & Warschburger, 2008: Larios et al., 2009; Neumark-Sztainer, 2009). Obese children often feel that initiation of a behavioral change requires the active intervention of a role model, in younger ages primarily a parent, whereas delayed parental recognition is recognized by them as an important barrier to take action (Murtagh et al., 2006). Parents may influence children's developing preferences and eating behaviors by promoting some food varieties and some patterns of food intake available and others may not (Savage et al., 2007). For example, an association may be found between parents' obesity and their children's energy-dense food intake at snack time (Maffeis et al., 2008). Several parameters have been found to mediate in the influence of parental feeding strategies on their children's food intake, including the child's weight, and family income and educational level (Kröller & Warschburger, 2008).

Moreover, parental (primarily maternal) obesity/overweight is the single most important predicator of obesity/overweight among children, both in industrialized (Novaes et al., 2008; Olstad and McCargar, 2009) and non-industrialized (Jiang et al., 2006; Jingxiong et al., 2009; Oliveira et al., 2007) countries. In addition, elevated parental psychopathology and distress may also considerably increase the risk for the development of overweight and obesity in their children (Davis et al., 2008; Gray et al., 2008; Kestilä et al., 2009; Koch et al., 2008; Moens et al., 2009; Novaes et al., 2008).

The Role of the Family in Promoting Healthy Eating and Weight Related Behavior

The entire family should be included in interventions attempting to promote healthy and reduce unhealthy eating and weight-related behaviors and to increase physical activity and decrease sedentary activities in younger individuals. This can be done either with focus groups that include only parents, or in groups including parents/children dyads (Sonneville et al., 2009). Drawing definite conclusions with respect to the effectiveness of such primary prevention interventions, as well as the factors improving and reducing their utility, is currently still limited. This is because most studies are open, include a relatively small number of families, and have no long-term follow up evaluations (Sonneville et al., 2009). Still, Bautista-Castano et al., (2004), analyzing the effectiveness of prevention strategies carried out during the 1990s, have concluded that despite a great variability in the design, duration and outcome assessments, these programs do have the potential to reduce the rate of overweight issues in some children. The findings of more recent programs are less optimistic (McGarvey et al., 2004) and have, thus, found that whereas the combination of psychoeducation with behaviorally targeted changes may affect the attitudes and behaviors of the parents, the effect of these parental changes on the overweight child is limited.

The role of the entire family food environment in changing eating behaviors and the amount and type of food consumed is of paramount importance (Campbell et al., 2006c). Neumark-Sztainer (2009) emphasizes the conflicts and confusion that parents often have with respect to the types of messages they should give, or not give, to their children regarding eating and weight. She outlines several strategies for parents to deal with potentially harmful eating-related societal pressures and to decrease their child's risk for becoming overweight. The first strategy, "model healthy behaviors for your children," emphasizes that parents should model behaviors they wish their children to emulate, particularly engaging in healthy eating of a variety of foods and exercising at an appropriate level. On the other hand, parents should refrain from behaviors and comments encouraging unhealthy eating and weight-related behaviors (e.g., dieting or excessive exercising). The second strategy, "provide an environment that makes it easy for your child to make healthy choices" proposes that instead of trying to restrict and control their children's dietary intake, parents should provide a home environment that includes an abundance of fruits and vegetables and a minimal number of televisions, and that encourages family meals [some have suggested also to increase the child's water consumption as a part of a healthy eating environment (see Sharma at el, 2005)]. The third strategy, "focus on adaptive attitudes and behaviors rather than on weight," encourages parents to assist their children in developing an identity that goes beyond physical appearance to non-appearance-related traits and accomplishments, moderating their children's interest and preoccupation with weight and dieting. The fourth strategy, "provide a supportive environment," encourages parents to support their children when teased outside home in relation to their weight.

Some randomized controlled studies (RCTs) have attempted to test these propositions. Fulkerson et al., (2010), for example, have recently examined the feasibility of a pilot parent/child obesity prevention intervention, including five sessions consisting of interactive nutrition education, taste testing, cooking skill building, parent discussion groups, and hands-on meal preparation. While significant favorable differences have been shown in research compared to control families at post-intervention with respect to healthy food choice, many of these changes have not held at six months follow-up, and changes in weight have not deferred according to group condition. Interestingly, in another study, frequency of meals, but not consumption of breakfast, has been found inversely associated with childhood overweight, even after controlling for socio-demographic and constitutional confounders (Toschke et al., 2009). Accordingly, eating three meals or less may increase the risk for overweight 4.5 more than eating five meals or more.

Parental Feeding Strategies and Styles

From another perspective, the inclination of parents to control and restrict food from their overweight children, while being highly prevalent, is particularly harmful in increasing the risk for the development of later obesity (Clark et al., 2008; Faith et al., 2004; Hughes et al., 2008; Novaes et al., 2008). This because focusing on restrictive approaches to feeding interferes with satiety cues and regulation of eating and increases opportunistic snacking and preferences towards unhealthy food. Restriction also interferes with children's natural ability to control and regulate their food intake and unfavorably affects their capacity to consume moderate amounts of food when restriction is no longer present (Anzman and Birch, 2009; Clark et al., 2008; Hughes et al., 2005). The subsequent eating behavior that may emerge during childhood, described in terms of eating in the absence of hunger, has been found, in turn, to predict weight gain and increase the risk for the development of being overweight in later years (Francis & Birch, 2005; Tanofsky-Kraff et al., 2009). Indeed, highly directive restrictive strategies have been consistently associated with higher weight status among children (Jaramillo et al., 2007; Silveira et al., 2006). Despite challenges to unraveling causal pathways, the most current data suggest that restrictive feeding practices are elicited by child characteristics (e.g., weight status or obesity risk) and depend on parent characteristics as well. Restriction, in turn, may maintain or exacerbate the child's overweight issues (Faith & Kern, 2005).

Another similar, although not identical, control-related feeding strategy found in some studies to be associated with eating problematic food with high-fat intake, and hence with a greater risk to develop overweight issues, relates to parental pressure to eat (Campbell et al., 2006b; Kröller & Warschburger, 2008; Moore et al., 2007). One possible reason for the inclination of some parents pressure their normal-weight children to overeat relates to the risk of them to misclassify their children as eating too little for their measured weight status, when, in fact, they are eating the right portions (up to 30% of parents, see Hirschler et al., 2006). From a different, although still risky, perspective, mothers may voice an inability to say no if a child claims to be hungry. Providing ample nourishment to their children may be, accordingly conceived an important and emotionally rewarding part of parenting that mothers seem unwilling and/or unable to relinquish (Hirschler et al., 2006).

On the other hand, several prospective longitudinal studies have shown that an authoritative parenting style that is both highly demanding and highly responsive may have the most beneficial effect on children's eating behaviors and weight (Hearn et al., 1998; Hughes et al., 2005; Rhee et al., 2006). In the feeding domain, authoritative parents encourage eating by using predominantly non-directive and supportive behaviors, including reasoning and complimenting. Most importantly, authoritative parenting style allows children to have control over their food choices. It nevertheless implies that although parents tend not to restrict available food, they do control the availability of food at home. This strategy has been found to maximize the consumption of healthy food and to minimize the consumption of unhealthy food in a non-restricting family atmosphere (Hughes et al., 2008; Kröller & Warschburger, 2008). Interestingly, feeding styles among parents may be associated with their educational level. For example, mothers with higher education may exert significantly greater control over their children's feeding and significantly lower emotional feeding than mothers with lower education (Hupkens et al., 1998; Saxton et al., 2009).

Parental Role in Promoting Adaptive Media Consuming Habits

Parents should have a role in reducing their children's media viewing habits and, in turn, their sedentary-related behaviors. Some cross-sectional (van Zutphen et al., 2007) and prospective longitudinal studies (Escobar-Chaves et al., 2010) have shown that parents of young children have the ability to psycho-educate their children to reduce snacking while watching television, to close the television while no one is watching, and to take the television out of the child's room, although actual television consumption time may not be significantly reduced. Even so, while these findings may seem promising, most of these studies are short-termed, and their effect on actual behavioral weight reduction in overweight children is highly difficult to analyze.

From a different angle, although parents may be concerned about overweight issues among children and adolescents in general, they are reluctant to take a health-promoting action when it comes to their own children (Booth et al., 2009). Studies have shown that between 30 to 50% of parents of overweight and obese children do nothing about their children's eating habits and weight (Hackie & Bowles, 2007; Nazario Rodriguez et al., 2008). This lack of activity is greater in the case of older children and in parents who feel incompetent about their ability to influence their children and to serve as role models (Nsiah-Kumi et al., 2009). Indeed, parents of 4- to 11-year-old obese children have been found to present themselves with lower levels of parenting self-efficacy in comparison to parents of normal-weight children (West & Sanders, 2009).

Promotion of Healthy Physical Activity

Promotion of healthy physical activity programs to reduce the risk of childhood obesity (Floriani & Kennedy, 2008) is also of great importance in the complex balance of reducing energy consumption while simultaneously increasing energy expenditure. Research has repeatedly shown that being inactive or minimally active during childhood and adolescence, as opposed to performing adequate activity during these critical developmental periods, may considerably increase the risk of developing obesity in childhood as well as in later life.

Greater frequency of physical activity also appears to be related to improved mental health status in overweight/obese children (Floriani & Kennedy, 2008). The findings of studies assessing the influence of physical activity on overweight in children are not definite. Some studies have, thus, shown that increasing children's activity can reduce weight gain (LeMura & Maziekas, 2002). By contrast, a rigorously designed RCT has shown no change in BMI following a physical activity intervention in Scottish preschool children at six and 12 months follow-up despite increasing the children's physical activity levels (Reilly et al., 2006). Methodological considerations such as the outcome measures used, the amount and quality of the physical activity introduced, and/or the selection and training of staff, may account for these inconsistencies (Yancey, 2006).

Yet, child and adolescent physical activity levels have been found to be positively associated with family support and modeling behavior (Pugliese & Tinsley, 2007). Indeed, an RCT involving parents and children in a two-hour weekly joint fun physical activities for a period as brief as two months has found both at post-intervention and at 12 months follow-up a significant improvement in the children's waist circumference, BMI, body composition, physical activity level, sedentary activities, cardiovascular fitness, and self-esteem in comparison to a control waiting-list group (Sacher et al., 2010). Similarly, sibling (Timperio et al., 2008) and peer (Salvy et al., 2007) engagement in physical activity, as well as environmental stimuli related to both physical activity and sedentary behaviors, may have a significant impact on overweight children's physical activity levels and hence their BMI.

School-based Prevention Programs

The School as a Health Promoting Agency

The social soundings of the overweight child outside home present another putative focus for preventive interventions. The findings concerning the efficacy of school-related programs remain debatable. Some interventions have been found useful in improving the food environment at school. For example, by removing whole milk and switching from low-fat to fat-free chocolate milk, New York City public school milk-drinking students have been served an estimated 5,960 fewer calories and 619 fewer grams of fat in 2009, than in 2004 (Center for Disease Control and Prevention, 2010). One means to achieve this change is with school programs delivering frequent and systemized positive messages about eating healthful food and modeling fruit and vegetable consumption (Folta et al., 2006). Indeed, several RCTs incorporating recommendations for healthy eating (Austin et al., 2005; Folta et al., 2006; Foster et al., 2008; Jan et al., 2009; Slavin, 2003; Veugelers & Fitzgerald, 2005), for example, changing of foods sold and served at school according to accepted guidelines (Foster et al., 2008), reducing the amount of consumption of carbonated drinks (James et al., 2004), as well as promoting healthy physical activity at school (Floriani & Kennedy, 2008; Veugelers & Fitzgerald, 2005), have shown a positive impact not only on children's knowledge and attitudes toward exercise and healthy eating and on their weight status, but also on their eating behaviors, overall lifestyle, and mental health. Other interventions considered effective included nutrition and physical activity education provided to the students, and in some in some cases also to the parents (e.g., Foster et al., 2008) Recently, a specific intervention for the prevention of overweight—edutainment—combining the active participation of youngsters and popular celebrities in a musical (active entertainment) with a lifestyle change workshop (education) initiated in Israel, has shown promising changes in the participants' physical activity, eating patterns and attitudes towards dieting (Levin-Zamir et al., 2004). The findings of this program are, however, still only preliminary, so that no definite conclusions can be drawn at this stage.

Promotion of Healthy Nutrition and Physical Activity at School

Conversely, other studies have shown that school-based obesity prevention programs have not altered school nutrition and physical activity (Dämon et al., 2005; Hawley et al., 2006; Nanney et al., 2008; Spinks et al., 2007; Yancey, 2006). One explanation for these unfavorable results has been that more impoverished schools are less likely to follow the programs' recommendations and to offer the intramural interventions required (Nanney et al., 2008). Alternatively, a recent critical review has concluded that although childhood obesity prevention programs have not been associated with unintended psychological harm, the negative findings of many of them may be accounted for by the inadequacy of the measurements used to assess efficacy (Carter & Bulik, 2008). Still, although children have been found to participate in less than the desired activity outside of school (Naughton et al., 2006), access to neighborhood parks may have the potential to increase physical activity and reduce the time spent in sedentary behaviors (Floriani & Kennedy, 2008).

Cole et al., (2006) have attempted to investigate the factors potentially increasing the efficacy of school-based intervention programs. Accordingly, they have reviewed all ten school-based interventions found effective in reducing the BMI of 4- to 14-year-old children. Nine out of these ten studies have used an experimental research design. The length of these studies has ranged from ten weeks to 24 months, and only two have reported follow-up outcomes. Healthy lifestyle education, focusing on teaching appropriate nutrition and physical activity behaviors, has been implemented in nine studies, a direct manipulation of dietary habits in four studies, and direct physical activity interventions in another four. Four of the ten studies have used a combination of all three intervention approaches. The authors conclude that effective school-based interventions should use a combination of multiple treatment modalities to address childhood overweight issues. These interventions would be most beneficial if including elements based on social cognitive and motivational perspectives (applied in eight of the ten studies), such as focusing on readiness for change, self-evaluation and self-monitoring, peer support, observational learning, appropriate social setting (the class), and appropriate modeling (teachers, school nurses and other facilitators familiar with the students).

From the all-important social surroundings perspective of the obese/overweight child, recent school prevention programs have failed to reduce the extent of weight-related teasing (Krukowski et al., 2008; Puhl & Latner, 2007). According to Puhl & Latner (2007), although providing external explanation for obesity at school can change children's cognitions about obesity, it is less likely to improve their overall negative attitudes. Still, as only a relatively brief period of time has elapsed since the implementation of these programs, it is too early to reach definite conclusions with respect to their efficiency or inefficiency.

One school-based strategy recently used in the attempts to reduce the rates of childhood obesity in several states in the USA relates to weight (and height) screening performed at school during the early school years. The assumption underneath this strategy is that sharing weight status information could increase family awareness of the child's weight, hence motivating the family to take appropriate actions to address a child's potential weight problem (Kalich et al., 2008). Whereas the usefulness of such programs is still not evident, perhaps because only a brief amount of time has elapsed since their implementation, they have caused a serious ongoing debate over their potential hazards. Eating disorders experts have been particularly concerned about the potential of such screenings to induce disordered eating- and weight-related attitudes and behaviors. Another focus of concern relates to their possible unfavorable influence on the well-being of the overweight/obese child at school. There are still no definite conclusions relating to any of these concerns. It has been found that whereas parents in general are usually supportive of school-based weight screening (Kubik et al., 2006), although even that is not always the case (Murnan et al., 2006), parents of children who are overweight or at risk for being overweight are significantly less likely to give active consent *to school-based survey researches on healthy eating and physical activity* (Mellor et al., 2008). Similarly, although the majority of the middle school students do not report discomfort with school-based weight screening more than a third of overweight students are uncomfortable with this intervention (compared to 8% of normal-weight youngsters; Kalich et al., 2008).

Intervention at the Public Policy Level

These interventions all suggest that programs aiming to prevent, or at least reduce, the ongoing rise in childhood obesity should be multi-faceted and focus on both the familial and social surroundings of the overweight child (Olstad and McCargar, 2009). However, this is not enough, as the influence of such interventions is at best transient and local. Levine and Smolak (2008) and others (Harris et al., 2009; Sallis et al., 2009; Swinburn et al., 2008), recommend that planned large-scale universal programs should be carried out also on a public policy level, focusing on important psychosocial factors such as the influence of the media on the child and the family, the reduction in physical activity and increase in sedentary activities in the society at large, the rise in accessibility to snacks in school and at home, the change in portion sizes in restaurants, and the increase in marketing of food products with a high-fat content on the market.

Along these lines, Schwartz and Brownell (2007) recommend that public policy prevention program should relate to pediatric obesity as a consequence of a "toxic environment" rather than a result of the population failing to take enough "personal responsibility." In order to make progress in decreasing the prevalence of obesity, policymakers should shift the view of obesity away from the medical model (which focuses on the individual) to a public health model (which focuses on the population at large).

Levine and Smolak (2008) and others (Wofford, 2008) further suggest that the combination of universal programs (aimed to influence government policies) and selective interventions (geared for non-symptomatic youngsters considered at risk to develop future overweight because of some broad factors, e.g., overweight issues in the family) are particularly relevant to children under the age of 11 and early adolescents. In these age groups, adequate interventions have a good chance to intervene with precursors for the development of overweight, both personal precursors, e.g., decreased physical activity, and socio-cultural precursors, for example peer teasing or food advertisements. Such programs can additionally alter the actual environments (home, school) in which children may develop problematic eating, and promote eating-related protective factors, for example healthy nutrition and exercising.

To increase their potential efficacy, prevention programs in overweight children and adolescents should take into consideration the developmental stage of the child and his/her capacity for change, his/her personality structure and psychopathology, the socio-economic status and the functioning of the family system, as well as issues related to ethnicity and socio-cultural background acceptability. Preventive interventions should be developed and piloted in consultation with the target community, in particular with respect to ethnic minorities, to improve acceptability and hence compliance (Kestilä et al., 2009; Levine and Smolak, 2008; Maynard et al., 2009). This because it has increasingly been acknowledged that individual behaviors and lifestyles, e.g., food choices or child-feeding practices, are responsive to the socio-cultural and ecological contexts in which they are practiced (Kumanyika, 2008). For that purpose, programs utilize appropriate settings such as home, post-natal clinics, day care centers, school, community centers, and places of worship to provide an opportunity for the involvement of family members and significant others in the program (Maynard et al., 2009). They should promote and implement changes in lifestyle, eating behavior, physical activity, reduction of sedentary behaviors, and media literacy. Specifically, multidisciplinary programs combining experts of different professions, advocating health promotion approaches, and communicating research findings to policymakers, may be a promising population-based initiative to prevent, or at least reduce, the risk of childhood overweight issues (Levine and Smolak, 2008; Maynard et al., 2009; Sallis et al., 2009; van Gerwen et al., 2009).

The American Academy of Pediatrics initiated in 2003, the following recommendations for action on a policy level, based on prospective longitudinal exploratory research: regulation of food advertisements targeted at children; expanding public education campaigns to promote healthy eating and exercise; introducing healthy food at school meals; incorporating messages about healthy lifestyles into television programming scripts; reducing the time children spend with media while promoting children's media literacy; implementing multiple treatment modalities in school-based interventions addressing childhood overweight issues; encouraging pediatricians and other health professionals to include a "media intake" when treating children and families; and including health promotion and media literacy in the curriculum of primary and secondary schools (American Academy of Pediatrics, 2003). It is further recommended that children should participate in a minimum of 30 to 90 (mean 60) minutes of physical activity daily and spend no more than two hours a day using electronic media for entertainment (Davidson et al., 2005; Irwin et al., 2005; Spinks et al., 2007). Currently, more than 50 countries around the globe have implemented laws that regulate television food advertising aimed at children (Nestle, 2006).

The regulation of food marketing has become another issue of specifically great importance in the global fight against the rise in childhood obesity (Nestle, 2006; Swinburn et al., 2008). This because research does show that restrictions at the public policy level may be effective for this purpose (Haby et al., 2006). Indeed, marketing-related regulatory codes have been advanced in recent years by the World Health Organization (2006), International Obesity Task Force (2007) and the United Nations (2007). Actions to reduce food marketing to children have been recommended to be statutory in nature, take a wide definition of commercial promotions, guarantee commercial-free childhood settings, and include cross-border media (Nestle, 2006; Swinburn et al., 2008). These actions should further be evaluated on a routine basis, monitored and enforced (Swinburn et al., 2008). The effect of these changes on the consummatory patterns of children and families and hence on the rate of childhood overweight issues in the next years, in the case of enforcing these regulations eventually, would be a main focus of future research.

Another drawback in the implementation of adequate prevention interventions relates to the lack of adequate knowledge and/or the presence of derogatory view points and prejudice about pediatric obesity among primary health care professionals in many (Khanna et al., 2009; Serrano et al., 2006; Spivack et al., 2009; Vaidya, 2006), although not on all surveys (Franc et al., 2009). For example, general practitioners and practice nurses may feel that obesity in children is a familial or social but not a medical problem (Walker et al., 2007). Additionally, trained personnel often feel a lack of comfort, practice, and confidence in addressing and/or preventing childhood overweight issues (Serrano et al., 2006) It is thus unfortunate, although not surprising, to find that primary caretakers may refrain from assessing vital obesity-related issues, particularly the child's activity level or television-viewing habits (O'Brien et al., 2004), but in many cases even the child's BMI is not routinely measured (Dorsey et al., 2005; Khanna et al., 2009). In other studies, over 35% of primary care providers have never discussed fast food, television, or candy use in parents of young overweight children, and 55% never discussed exercise (Spivack et al., 2009). In addition, health care professionals are more likely to obtain activity histories, note obesity in the physical examination, refer the patient to a nutritionist, obtain screening laboratory studies, and recommend follow-up monitoring in the case of overweight adolescents (76%) in comparison to preschool children (31%) (O'Brien et al., 2004).

Still in other studies, primary care providers have been found to have a fair knowledge about factors influencing the risk of overweight and obesity in children, but they have nevertheless often felt that many barriers exist that preclude adequate preventive interventions (King et al., 2007). Accordingly, in the opinion of many caretakers, providing diet and exercise advice do not show adequate impact upon a child's weight (Walker et al., 2007) because parents and patients may often fell negative about, and hence would not comply with, their advice (King et al., 2007; Serrano et al., 2006). Accordingly, their efforts toward reducing the risk of pediatric obesity are bound to fail (Franc et al., 2009; Spivack et al., 2009; van Gerwen et al., 2009). Another reason for the unfavorable viewpoints of caretakers about obesity prevention relates to the limited literature offered to them about the proper way to communicate and discuss a child's overweight issues with his or her parents (Mikhailovich & Morrison, 2007; Walker et al., 2007). Other likely barriers for adequate interventions include cultural issues, time constraint, lack of training and lack of resources (Serrano et al., 2006; Walker et al., 2007).

It is thus of immediate relevance to initiate programs designed to improve the knowledge, attitudes, sense of self-efficacy, and commitment of primary caretakers treating overweight youngsters (Crawford et al., 2004; Khanna et al., 2009; Serrano et al., 2006; Spivack et al., 2009). Accordingly, practitioners receiving a vocational training dedicated to childhood obesity and/or are familiar with national recommendations about its management have been found to improve their knowledge (Freedman & Alvarez, 2010) and feel more competent in their obesity-related preventive endeavors (Franc et al., 2009). Moreover, in a recent small study, a greater reduction in the child's BMI has been found in overweight children whose parents and primary caretakers have received training in motivational interviewing techniques in comparison to control participants of both sectors (Schwartz et al., 2007). Still, in another study, additional years of pediatric training have not improved overweight identification abilities of primary health caretakers (O'Brien et al., 2006).

Interestingly, school and kindergarten staffs have been found to possess more positive attitudes toward childhood obesity than primary medical caretakers. For example, in one study, kindergarten teachers were both aware of and concerned about overweight issues among children and felt that encouraging healthy eating and active play were part of their core responsibilities. They worked closely in partnership with parents, had several programs and policies in place, and identified a range of educational resources and professional development opportunities that they would find helpful, including how to discourage parents from sending unhealthy foods with their child and whether/how to raise their concerns about a child's weight with the parents (Pagnini et al., 2007b). This discrepancy might be perhaps associated with the fact that school and kindergarten staff, unlike primary caretakers, do not have to feel responsible, and hence inadequate, in their efforts to deal with the endless problems associated with managing obesity in children.

Conclusion

A dramatic rise in childhood overweight issues has been shown in many countries around the globe, both Western industrialized and Third World non-industrialized countries, in the past two to three decades. As the gene pool has likely not changed during this time period, environmental, social and psychological factors are largely thought to account for this rise. For and foremost, it is most prevalent in cultures in transition. From the different environmental dimensions potentially associated with childhood overweight, this review highlights the role of gender, socio-economic status, cultural and familial background, social isolation, and a host of factors associated with the influence of modernization, particularly the influence of the media, changes in the food consumed, and reduction in physical activity.

These findings highlight, from a psychosocial point of reference, the need to prevent, or at least reduce, the rate of overweight in children and adolescents. The findings of prevention studies, although not definite, emphasize two important points. Firstly, prevention programs should be multidisciplinary, combining the knowledge of experts from different professions, taking into consideration the important role of the family and relevant influential social organizations, primarily the school. Secondly, no change can be induced without planned large-scale programs carried out on a public policy level.

In line with the findings emphasized in this review, the following are our main suggestions at the policy level. Not surprisingly, they are in line and/or add to recommendations of previous researchers. 1. Education of primary health care professionals about childhood and adolescent overweight issues and obesity, to increase uniformity of assessment and to improve caretakers' knowledge, awareness, overall attitudes, and sense of self-efficacy in managing these disturbances 2. Regulation of the use of television-viewing and sedentary video games by youngsters, and the inclusion of health promotion and media literacy programs in schools' curricula. 3. Regulation of food/physical activity advertisements targeted at children. 4. Expanding public education and environmental changes to promote healthy eating and adequately increased physical activity and to reduce sedentary activities. 5. Promotion at the public policy level of legal, legislative, and industry-based activities in the attempt to regulate, even if to some extent, the type of food administered to young individuals and their families. 6. Prevention programs should always take into consideration the developmental stage of the obese child and socio-economic and socio-cultural background of his or her family. 7. Preventive interventions at the public policy level should coordinate all parties involved, including the obese children, their families, schools, primary care professionals, government, industry and media.

Limitation and Directions for Future Research

The limitations of the present status of the research in pediatric and adolescent overweight issues, reflected also in the present review, should be outlined. There is a paucity of well-designed studies that would encourage primary health care professionals to integrate the relevant psychosocial issues described in this review and others in their evaluation procedures and intervention strategies. Similarly, there is a paucity of well-designed studies that would enable policy level planning to integrate psychosocial parameters in nationwide recommendations.

Future research requires the design of prospective and longitudinal studies with appropriate sample sizes, inclusion of the families and social organizations in the interventions, and adequate long-term follow-up.

References

Adair, L.S. (2008). Child and adolescent obesity: epidemiology and developmental perspectives. *Physiology and Behavior, 94*, 8-16.

Alvy, L.M. & Calvert, S.L. (2008). Food marketing on popular children's web sites: a content analysis. *Journal of the American Dietetic Association, 108*, 710-713.

American Academy of Pediatrics Policy Statement (2003). Prevention of pediatric overweight and obesity. *Pediatrics, 112*, 424-430.

Anzman, S.L. & Birch, L.L. (2009). Low inhibitory control and restrictive feeding practices predict weight outcomes. *Journal of Pediatrics, 155*, 651-656.

Austin, S.B., Field, A.E., Wiecha, J., Peterson, K.E. & Gortmaker, S.L. (2005). The impact of a school-based obesity prevention trial on disordered weight-control behavior in early adolescent girls. *Archives of Pediatrics and Adolescent Medicine, 159*, 225–230.

Bautista-Castano, I., Doreste, J. & Serra-Majem, L. (2004). The effectiveness of interventions in childhood obesity. *European Journal of Epidemiology, 19*, 617-622.

Bellizzi, M.C. & Dietz, W.H. (1999). Workshop on childhood obesity: summary of the discussion. *American Journal of Clinical Nutrition, 70*, 173S-175S.

Bisset, S., Gauvin, L., Potvin, L. & Paradis, G. (2007). Association of body mass index and dietary restraint with changes in eating behavior throughout late childhood and early adolescence: a 5-year study. *Public Health Nutrition, 10*, 780-789.

Booth, M.L., King, L.A., Pagnini, D.L., Wilkenfeld, R.L. & Booth, S.L. (2009). Parents of school students on childhood overweight: the Weight of Opinion Study. *Journal of Paediatrics and Child Health, 45*, 194-198.

Campbell, K., Waters, E., O'Meara. S. & Summerbell, C. (2001). Interventions for preventing obesity in children. *The Cochrane Database of Systematic Reviews*. The Cochrane Library, Issue 1. Wiley J & Sons, Ltd. Chichester, UK.

Campbell, K.J., Crawford, D.A. & Ball, K. (2006b). Family environment and dietary behaviors likely to promote fatness in 5–6-year-old children. *International Journal of Obesity, 30*, 1272–1280.

Campbell, K.J., Crawford, D.A. & Ball, K. (2006c). Family food environment and dietary behaviors likely to promote fatness in 5-6 year-old children. *International Journal of Obesity, 30*, 1272-1280.

Carter, F. & Bulik, C.M. (2008). Childhood obesity prevention programs: how do they affect eating pathology and other psychological measures? *Psychosomatic medicine, 70(3)*, 363-371.

Casey, P.H., Simpson, P.M., Gossett, J.M., Bogle, M.L., Champagne, C.M., Connell, C., Harsha, D., McCabe-Sellers, B., Robbins, J.M., Stuff, J.E. & Weber J. (2006). The association of child and household food insecurity with childhood overweight status. *Pediatrics, 118*, e1406-1413.

Center for Disease Control and Prevention (2004). Overweight among U.S. Children and adolescents. *National Health and Nutrition Examination Survey*. January.

Center for Disease Control and Prevention. (2010). Effects of switching from whole to low-fat/fat-free milk in public schools—New York City, 2004-2009. *MMWR Morbidity and Mortality Weekly Report*, 59, 70-73.

Chamberlin, L.A., Sherman, S.N., Jain, A., Powers, S.W., Whitaker, R.C. (2002). The challenge of preventing and treating obesity in low-income, preschool children: perceptions of WIC health care professionals. *Archives of Pediatrics and Adolescent Medicine, 156*, 662–668

Clark, H.R., Goyder, E., Bissell, P., Blank, L., Walters, S.J. & Peters. J. (2008). A pilot survey of socio-economic differences in child-feeding behaviors among parents of primary-school children. *Public Health Nutrition, 11*, 1030-1036.

Colapinto, C.K., Fitzgerald, A., Taper, L.J. & Veugelers, P.J. (2007). Children's preference for large portions: prevalence, determinants, and consequences. *Journal of American Dietetic Association, 107*, 1183-1190.

Cole, T.J., Bellizzi, M.C., Flegal, K.M. & Dietz, W.H. (2000). Establishing a standard definition for child overweight and obesity worldwide: international survey. *British Medical Journal, 320*, 1240-1243.

Cole, K., Waldrop, J., D'Auria, J. & Garner, H. (2006). An integrative research review: effective school-based childhood overweight interventions. *Journal for Specialists in Pediatric Nursing, 11*, 166-177.

Crawford, P.B. (2001). Ethnic Issues in the epidemiology of childhood obesity. *Pediatric Clinics of North America, 48*, 855-878.

Crawford, P.B., Gosliner, W., Strode, P., Samuels, S.E., Burnett, C. & Craypo, L. (2004). Walking the talk Fit WIC wellness programs improve self-efficacy in pediatric obesity prevention counseling. *American Journal of Public Health, 94*, 1480-1485.

Dalmeny, K. (2003). Food marketing: the role of advertising in child health. *Consumer Policy review, 13*, 2-7

Dämon, S., Dietrich, S. & Widhalm, K. (2005). PRESTO—Prevention Study of Obesity: a project to prevent obesity during childhood and adolescence. *Acta Paediatrica, 94S*, 47-48.

D'Argenio, A., Mazzi, C., Pecchioli, L., Di Lorenzo, G., Siracusano, A. & Troisi, A. (2009). Early trauma and adult obesity: is psychological dysfunction the mediating mechanism? *Physiology and Behavior, 98*, 543-546.

Davis, M., Young, L., Davis, S.P. & Moll, G. (2008). Parental depression, family functioning and obesity among African American children. *Journal of Cultural Diversity, 15*, 61-65.

Davison, K.K., Francis, L.A. & Birch, L.L. (2005). Links between parents' and girls' television viewing behaviors: a longitudinal examination. *Journal of Pediatrics, 147*, 436-442.

Dietz, W. & Gortmaer, S. (1993). Do we fatten our children at the TV set? Obesity and television viewing in children and adolescents. *Pediatrics, 91*, 499-500.

Dorsey, K.B., Wells, C., Krumholz, H.M. & Concato, J.C. (2005). Diagnosis, evaluation, and treatment of childhood obesity in pediatric practice. *Archives of Pediatrics and Adolescent Medicine, 159*, 632-638.

Escobar-Chaves, S.L., Markham, C.M., Addy, R.C., Greisinger, A., Murray, N.G. & Brehm, B. (2010). The Fun Families Study: intervention to reduce children's television viewing. *Obesity, 18S*:S99-101.

Faith, M.S., Scanlon, K.S., Birch, L.L., Francis, L.A. & Sherry, B. (2004). Parent-child feeding strategies and their relationships to child eating and weight status. *Pediatrics, 114*, e429-436.

Faith, M.S. & Kerns, J. (2005). Infant and child feeding practices and childhood overweight: the role of restriction. *Maternal and Child Nutrition, 1*, 164-168.

Floriani, V. & Kennedy, C. (2008). Promotion of physical activity in children. *Current Opinion in Pediatrics, 20*, 90-95.

Folta, S.C., Goldberg, J.P., Economos, C., Bell, R., Landers, S. & Hyatt, R. (2006). Assessing the use of school public address systems to deliver nutrition messages to children: Shape up Somerville—audio adventures. *Journal of School Health, 76*, 459-464.

Forman, J., Halford, J.C., Summe, H., MacDougall, M. & Keller, K.L. (2009). Food branding influences ad libitum intake differently in children depending on weight status. Results of a pilot study. *Appetite, 53*, 76-83.

Foster, G.D., Sherman, S., Borradaile, K.E, Grundy, K.M., Vander Veur, S.S., Nachmani, J., Karpyn, A., Kumanyika, S. & Shults, J. (2008). A policy-based school intervention to prevent overweight and obesity. *Pediatrics, 121*, e794-802.

Franc, C., Van Gerwen, M., Le Vaillant, M., Rosman, S. & Pelletier-Fleury, N. (2009). French pediatricians' knowledge, attitudes, beliefs towards and practices in the management of weight problems in children. *Health Policy, 91*, 195-203

Francis, L.A. & Birch, L.L. (2005). Maternal weight status modulates the effects of restriction on daughters' eating and weight. *International Journal of Obesity, 29*, 942-949.

Freedman, M.R. & Alvarez, K.P. (2010). Early childhood feeding: assessing knowledge, attitude, and practices of multi-ethnic child-care providers. *Journal of the American Dietetic Association, 110*, 447-451.

Fuemmeler, B.F., Dedert, E., McClernon, F.J. & Beckham, J.C. (2009). Adverse childhood events are associated with obesity and disordered eating: results from a U.S. population-based survey of young adults. *Journal of Traumatic Stress, 22*, 329-333.

Fulkerson, J.A., Rydell, S., Kubik, M.Y., Lytle, L., Boutelle, K., Story, M., Neumark-Sztainer, D., Dudovitz, B. & Garwick, A. (2010). Healthy Home Offerings via the Mealtime Environment (HOME): feasibility, acceptability, and outcomes of a pilot study. *Obesity, 18S*, S69-74.

Gilbert, R., Widom, C.S., Browne, K., Fergusson, D., Webb, E. & Janson, S. (2009). Burden and consequences of child maltreatment in high-income countries. *Lancet, 373*, 68-81.

Gray, V.B., Byrd, S.H., Cossman, J.S., Chromiak, J., Cheek, W.K. & Jackson, G.B. (2007). Family characteristics have limited ability to predict weight status of young children. *Journal of the American Dietetic Association, 107*, 1204-1209.

Gray, W.N., Janicke, D.M., Ingerski, L.M. & Silverstein, J.H. (2008). The impact of peer victimization, parent distress and child depression on barrier formation and physical activity in overweight youth. *Journal of Developmental and Behavioral Pediatrics, 29*, 26-33.

Greenfield EA, Marks NF. (2009). Violence from parents in childhood and obesity in adulthood: using food in response to stress as a mediator of risk. *Social Science and Medicine, 68*, 791-798.

Gunstad, J., Paul, R.H., Spitznagel, M.B., Cohen, R.A., Williams, L.M., Kohn, M. & Gordon, E. (2006). Exposure to early life trauma is associated with adult obesity. *Psychiatry Research, 142*, 31-37.

Haby, M.M., Vos, T., Carter, R., Moodie, M., Markwick, A., Magnus, A., Tay-Teo, K.S. & Swinburn B. (2006). A new approach to assessing the health benefit from obesity interventions in children and adolescents: the assessing cost-effectiveness in obesity project. *International Journal of Obesity, 30*, 1463-1475.

Hackie, M. & Bowles, C.L. (2007). Maternal perception of their overweight children. *Public Health Nursing, 24*, 538-546.

Halford, J.C., Boyland, E.J., Hughes, G.M., Stacey, L., McKean, S. & Dovey, T.M. (2008). Beyond-brand effect of television food advertisements on food choice in children: the effects of weight status. *Public Health Nutrition, 11*, 897-904.

Harris, J.L., Pomeranz, J.L., Lobstein, T. & Brownell, K.D. (2009). A crisis in the marketplace: how food marketing contributes to childhood obesity and what can be done. A crisis in the marketplace: how food marketing contributes to childhood obesity and what can be done. *Annual Reviews of Public Health, 30*, 211-225.

Hawkins, S.S., Cole, T.J. & Law, C. (2008). Maternal employment and early childhood overweight: findings from the UK Millennium Cohort Study. *Internation Journal of Obesity, 32*, 30-38.

Hawley, S.R., Beckman, H. & Bishop, T. (2006). Development of an obesity prevention and management program for children and adolescents in a rural setting. *Journal of Community Health Nursing, 23*, 69-80.

Hearn, M., Baranowski, T., Baranowski, J., Doyle, C., Smith, M., Lin, L.S. & Resnicow, K. (1998). Environmental influences on dietary behavior among children: Availability and accessibility of fruit and vegetables enable consumption. *Journal of Health Education, 29*, 26-32.

Hill, J.O. & Peters, J.C. (1998). Environmental contributions to the obesity epidemic. *Science, 280*, 1371–1377.

Hirschler, V., Gonzalez, C., Talgham, S. & Jadzinsky, M. (2006). Do mothers of overweight Argentinean preschool children perceive them as such? *Pediatric Diabetes, 7*, 201-204.

Hughes, S.O., Power, T.G., Fisher, J.O., Mueller, S. & Nicklas, T.A. (2005). Revisiting a neglected construct: Parenting styles in a child-feeding context. *Appetite, 44*, 83-92.

Hughes, S.O., O'Connor, T.M. & Power, T.G. (2008). Parenting and children's eating patterns: Examining control in a broader context. *International Journal of Child and Adolescent Health, 1*, 323-330.

Hupkens, C.L., Knibbe, R.A., Van Otterloo, A.H. & Drop, M.J. (1998). Class differences in the food rules mothers impose on their children: a cross-national study. *Social Science and Medicine, 47*, 1331-1339.

International Obesity Taskforce Sidney Principles, 2007 www.iotf.org/sydneyprinciples (accessed December 2007).

Irish, L., Kobayashi, I. & Delahanty, D.L. (2010). Long-term Physical Health Consequences of Childhood Sexual Abuse: A Meta-Analytic Review. *Journal of Pediatric Psychology, 35*, 450–461.

Irwin, J.D., He, M., Bouck, L.M., Tucker, P. & Pollett, G.L. (2005). Preschoolers' physical activity behaviors: parents' perspectives. *Canadian Journal of Public Health, 96*, 299-303.

Israel, A.C. & Ivanova, M.Y. (2002). Global and dimensional self-esteem in preadolescent and early adolescent children who are overweight: age and gender differences. *International Journal of Eating Disorders, 3*, 424-429.

James, J., Thomas, P., Cavan, D. & Kerr, D. (2004). Preventing childhood obesity by reducing consumption of carbonated drinks: Cluster randomized controlled trial. *British Medical Journal. 328*, 1237-1242.

Jan, S., Bellman, C., Barone, J., Jessen, L. & Arnold, M. (2009). Shape it up: a school-based education program to promote healthy eating and exercise developed by a health plan in collaboration with a college of pharmacy. *Journal of Managed Care Pharmacy, 15*, 403-413.

Jaramillo, S., Tsuei, E., Owens, B., Hughes, S., Nicklas, T., Shewchuk, R. & Franklin, F. (2007). Feeding styles and overweight status in preschool. *Annals of Behavioral Medicine, 33*, S083.

Jiang, J., Rosenqvist, U., Wang, H., Greiner, T., Ma, Y. & Toschke, A.M. (2006). Risk factors for overweight in 2- to 6-year-old children in Beijing, China. *International Journal of Pediatric Obesity, 1*, 103-108.

Jingxiong, J., Rosenqvist, U., Huishan, W., Koletzko, B., Guangli, L., Jing, H. & Greiner, T. (2009). Relationship of parental characteristics and feeding practices to overweight in infants and young children in Beijing, China. *Public Health Nutrition, 12*, 973-978.

Kaiser Family Foundation. (2004). The role of media in childhood obesity, February 2004, pp. 12.

Kalich, K.A., Chomitz, V., Peterson, K.E., McGowan, R., Houser, R.F. & Must, A. (2008). Ort and utility of school-based weight screening: the student perspective. *BMC Pediatrics, 8*, 9.

Kelly, L.A., Reilly, J.J., Fisher, A., Montgomery, C., Williamson, A., McColl, J.H., Paton, J.Y. & Grant, S. (2006). Effect of socio-economic status on objectively measured physical activity. *Archives of Disease in Childhood, 91*, 35-38.

Kelly, B., Cretikos, M., Rogers, K. & King, L. (2008). The commercial food landscape: outdoor food advertising around primary schools in Australia. *Australian and New Zealand Journal of Public Health, 32*, 522-528.

Kelly, B., Hughes, C., Chapman, K., Chun-Yu L. J., Dixon, H., Crawford, J., King, L., Daube, M. & Slevin, T. (2009). Consumer testing of the acceptability and effectiveness of front-of-pack food labeling systems for the Australian grocery market. *Health Promotion International, 24(2)*, 120-129.

Kestilä, L., Rahkonen, O., Martelin, T., Lahti-Koski, M. & Koskinen, S. (2009). Do childhood social circumstances affect overweight and obesity in early adulthood? *Scandinavian Journal of Public Health, 37*, 206-219.

Khanna, R., Kavookjian, J., Scott, V.G., Kamal, K.M., Miller, L.A. & Neal, W.A. (2009). Using the theory of reasoned action to determine physicians' intention to measure body mass index in children and adolescents. *Research in Social and Administrative Pharmacy, 5*, 170-181.

King, L.A., Loss, J.H., Wilkenfeld, R.L., Pagnini, D.L., Booth, M.L. & Booth, S.L. (2007). Australian GPs' perceptions about child and adolescent overweight and obesity: the Weight of Opinion study. *British Journal of General Practice, 57*, 124-129.

Koch, F.S., Sepa, A. & Ludvigsson, J. (2008). Psychological stress and obesity. *Journal of Pediatrics, 153*, 839-844.

Kopelman, C.A., Roberts, L.M. & Adab, P. (2007). Advertising of food to children: is brand logo recognition related to their food knowledge, eating behaviors and food preferences? *Journal of Public Health, 29*, 358-367.

Kröller, K. & Warschburger, P. (2008). Associations between maternal feeding style and food intake of children with a higher risk for overweight. *Appetite, 51*, 166-172.

Krukowski, R.A., West, D.S., Siddiqui, N.J., Bursac, Z., Phillips, M.M. & Raczynski, J.M. (2008). No change in weight-based teasing when school-based obesity policies are implemented. *Archives of Pediatrics and Adolescent Medicine, 162*, 936-942.

Kubik, M.Y., Fulkerson, J.A., Story, M. & Rieland, G. (2006). Parents of elementary school students weigh in on height, weight and body mass screening at school. *Journal of School Health, 76*, 496-501.

Kumanyika, S.K. (2008). Environmental influences on childhood obesity: ethnic and cultural influences in context. *Physiology and Behavior, 94*, 61-70.

Larios, S.E., Ayala, G.X., Arredondo, E.M., Baquero, B. & Elder, J.P. (2009). Development and validation of a scale to measure Latino parenting strategies related to children's obesigenic behaviors. The parenting strategies for eating and activity scale (PEAS). *Appetite, 52*, 166-172.

Leatherdale, S.T. & Wong, S.L. (2008). Modifiable characteristics associated with sedentary behaviors among youth. *International Journal of Pediatric Obesity, 3*, 93-101.

LeMura, L.M. & Maziekas, M.T. (2002). Factors that alter body fat, body mass, and fat-free mass in pediatric obesity. *Medicine and Science in Sports and Exercise, 34*, 487-496.

Levin-Zamir, D., Friedman, A. & Neumark-Sztainer, D. (2004). *"The Matter of Measure"* Program Evaluation Report. Department of Health Education and Promotion, Clalit Health Services.

Levine, M.P. & Smolak, L. (2008). "What exactly are we waiting for?" The case for universal-selective eating disorders prevention programs. *International Journal of Child and Adolescent Health, 1*, 295-304.

Lissau, I. & Sorenson, T.I.A. (1994). Parental neglect during childhood and increased risk of obesity in young adulthood. *Lancet, 343,* 324-327.

Maffeis, C., Grezzani, A., Perrone, L., Del Giudice, E.M., Saggese, G. & Tatò, L. (2008). Could the savory taste of snacks be a further risk factor for overweight in children? *Journal of Pediatric Gastroenterology Nutrition, 46*, 429-437.

Manios, Y., Kourlaba, G., Kondaki, K., Grammatikaki, E., Anastasiadou, A. & Roma-Giannikou, E. (2009). Obesity and television watching in preschoolers in Greece: the GENESIS study. *Obesity, 17*, 2047-2053.

Maximova, K., McGrath, J.J., Barnett, T., O'Loughlin, J., Paradis, G. & Lambert, M. (2008). Do you see what I see? Weight status misperception and exposure to obesity among children and adolescents. *International Journal of Obesity, 32*, 1008-1015.

Maynard, M.J., Baker, G., Rawlins, E., Anderson, A. & Harding, S. (2009). Developing obesity prevention interventions among minority ethnic children in schools and places of worship: The DEAL (DiEt and Active Living) study. *BMC Public Health, 9*, 480.

McCullough, N., Muldoon, O. & Dempster, M. (2009). Self-perception in overweight and obese children: a cross-sectional study. *Child Care Health and Development, 35*, 357-364.

McGarvey, E., Keller, A., Forrester, M., Williams, E., Seward, D. & Suttle, D.E. (2004). Feasibility and benefits of a parent-focused preschool child obesity intervention. *American Journal of Public Health*, *94*, 1490-1495.

McGinnis, J.M., Gootman, J.A. & Kraak, V.I., (Eds.) (2006). *Food Marketing to Children and Youth: Threat or Opportunity?* Washington, DC.: National Academies Press.

Mellor, J.M., Rapoport, R.B. & Maliniak, D. (2008). The impact of child obesity on active parental consent in school-based survey research on healthy eating and physical activity. *Evaluation Review, 32*, 298-312.

Mikhailovich, K. & Morrison, P. (2007). Discussing childhood overweight and obesity with parents: a health communication dilemma. *Journal of Child Health Care, 11*, 311-322.

Moens, E., Braet, C., Bosmans, G. & Rosseel, Y. (2009). Unfavorable family characteristics and their associations with childhood obesity: a cross-sectional study. *European Eating Disorders Review, 17*, 315-323.

Moore, S.N., Tapper, K. & Murphy, S. (2007). Feeding strategics used by mothers of 3-5-year-old children. *Appetite, 49*, 704-707.

Moreno, L.A., Thomas, C., Gonzales-Gross, M., Bueno, G., Perez-Gonzalez, J.M. & Bueno, M. (2004). Micro-environmental and socio-demographic determinants of childhood obesity. *International Journal of Obesity and Related Metabolic Disorders, 28,* S16-S20.

Murnan, J., Price, J.H., Telljohann, S.K., Dake, J.A. & Boardley, D. (2006). Parents' perceptions of curricular issues affecting children's weight in elementary schools. *Journal School Health, 76*, 502-511.

Murtagh, J., Dixey, R. & Rudolf, M. (2006). A qualitative investigation into the levers and barriers to weight loss in children: opinions of obese children. *Archives of Disease in Childhood*, 91, 920-923.

Nanney, M.S., Bohner, C. & Friedrichs, M. (2008). Poverty-related factors associated with obesity prevention policies in Utah secondary schools. *Journal of the American Dietetic Association, 108*, 1210-1215.

Naughton, G.A., Carlson, J.S. & Greene, D.A. (2006). A challenge to fitness testing in primary schools. *Journal of Science and Medicine in Sport, 9,* 40-45.

Nazario Rodriguez, I.J., Figueroa, W.I., Rosado, J. & Parrilla Idel C. (2008). Perception of parents regarding their children's weight. *Boletin- Asociacion Medica de Puerto Rico, 100*, 33-38.

Nestle, M. (2006). Food marketing and childhood obesity—a matter of policy. *New England Journal of Medicine, 354*, 2527-2529.

Neumark-Sztainer D. (2009). Preventing obesity and eating disorders in adolescents: what can health care providers do? *The Journal of adolescent health: official publication of the Society for Adolescent Medicine, 44(3)*, 206-13.

Noll, J.G., Zeller, M.H., Trickett, P.K. & Putnam, F.W. (2007). Obesity risk for female victims of childhood sexual abuse: a prospective study. *Pediatrics, 120*, e61-67.

Novaes, J.F., Franceschini Sdo, C. & Priore, S.E. (2008). Mother's overweight, parents' constant limitation on the foods and frequent snack as risk factors for obesity among children in Brazil. *Archives of Latinoamerican Nutrition, 58*, 256-264.

Nsiah-Kumi, P.A., Ariza, A.J., Mikhail, L.M., Feinglass, J. & Binns, H.J. (2009). Pediatric Practice Research Group. Family history and parents' beliefs about consequences of childhood overweight and their influence on children's health behaviors. *Academic Pediatric, 9*, 53-59.

O'Brien, S.H., Holubkov, R. &, Reis, E.C. (2004). Identification, evaluation, and management of obesity in an academic primary care center. *Pediatrics, 114*, e154-159.

O'Dea, J.A. & Wilson, R. (2006). Cognitive and nutritional factors associated with body mass index in children and adolescents: possibilities for childhood obesity prevention. *Health Education Research, 21*, 796-805.

Ogden, C.L., Flegal, K.M., Carroll, M.D. & Johnson, C.L. (2002). Prevalence and trends in overweight among U.S. children and adolescents, 1999-2000. *JAMA, 288*, 1728-1732.

Ogden, C.L., Carroll, M.D., Curtin, L.R., McDowell, M.A., Tabak, C.J. & Flegal, K.M. (2006). Prevalence of overweight and obesity in the United States, 1999–2004. *JAMA, 295*, 1549–1555.

Oliveira, A.M., Oliveira, A.C., Almeida, M.S., Oliveira, N. & Adan, L. (2007). Influence of the family nucleus on obesity in children from northeastern Brazil: a cross-sectional study. *BMC Public Health, 7*, 235.

Olson, C.M., Bove, C.F. & Miller, E.O. (2007). Growing up poor: long-term implications for eating patterns and body weight. *Appetite, 49*, 198-207.

Olstad, D.L. & McCargar, L. (2009). Prevention of overweight and obesity in children under the age of 6 years. *Applied Physiology Nutrition and Metabolism, 34*, 551-570

Page, R.M. & Brewster, A. (2007). Emotional and rational product appeals in televised food advertisements for children: analysis of commercials shown on U.S. broadcast networks. *Journal of Child Health Care, 11*, 323-340.

Pagnini, D., Wilkenfeld, R., King, L., Booth, M. & Booth, S. (2007b). Early childhood sector staff perceptions of child overweight and obesity: the Weight of Opinion Study. *Health Promotion Journal of Australia, 18*, 149-154.

Powell, L.M., Szczypka, G. & Chaloupka, F.J. (2007). Exposure to food advertising on television among U.S. children. *Archives of Pediatric and Adolescent Medicine, 161*, 553-560.

Pugliese, J. & Tinsley, B. (2007). Parental socialization of child and adolescent physical activity: a meta-analysis. *Journal of Family Psychology, 21*, 331-343

Puhl, R.M. & Latner, J.D. (2007). Stigma, obesity, and the health of the nation's children. *Psychological Bulletin, 133*, 557-580.

Reilly, J.J., Kelly, L., Montgomery, C., Williamson, A., Fisher, A. & McColl, J.H. (2006). Physical activity to prevent obesity in young children: cluster randomized controlled trial. *British Medical Journal, 333*, 1041.

Renman, C., Engstrom, I., Silverdal, S.A. & Aman, J. (1999). Mental health and psychosocial characteristics in adolescent obesity: a population based case-control study. *Acta Paediatrica, 88*, 998-1003.

Rhee, K., Appugliese, D., Kaciroti, N. & Bradley, R. (2006). Parenting styles and overweight in first grade. *Pediatrics, 117*, 2047-2054.

Robinson, W.R., Gordon-Larsen, P., Kaufman, J.S., Suchindran, C.M. & Stevens, J. (2009). The female-male disparity in obesity prevalence among black American young adults: contributions of socio-demographic characteristics of the childhood family. *American Journal of Clinical Nutrition, 89*, 1204-1212.

Sacher, P.M., Kolotourou, M., Chadwick, P.M., Cole, T.J., Lawson, M.S., Lucas, A. & Singhal, A. (2010). Randomized controlled trial of the MEND program: a family-based community intervention for childhood obesity. *Obesity, 18S*, S62-68.

Salanave, B., Peneau, S., Rolland-Cachera, M.F., Hercberg, S. & Castetbon, K. (2009). Stabilization of overweight prevalence in French children between 2000 and 2007. *International Journal of Pediatric Obesity, 4*, 66-72.

Sallis, J.F., Linton, L.S., Kraft, M.K., Cutter, C.L., Kerr, J., Weitzel, J., Wilson, A., Spoon, C., Harrison, I.D., Cervero, R., Patrick, K., Schmid, T.L. & Pratt, M. (2009). The Active Living Research program: six years of grant making. *American Journal of Preventive Medicine, 36S*, S10-21.

Salvy, S.J., Bowker, J.W., Roemmich, J.N., Romero, N., Kieffer, E., Paluch, R. & Epstein, L.H. (2007). Peer influence on children's physical activity: an experience sampling study. *Journal of Paediatrics and Child Health, 43*, 458-463.

Savage, J.S., Fisher, J.O. & Birch, L.L. (2007). Parental influence on eating behavior: conception to adolescence. *Journal of Law Medicine and Ethics, 35*, 22-34.

Saxton, J., Carnell, S., van Jaarsveld, C.H. & Wardle, J. (2009). Maternal education is associated with feeding style. *Journal of the American Dietetic Association, 109*, 894-898.

Schwartz, M.B. & Brownell, K.D. (2007). Actions necessary to prevent childhood obesity: creating the climate for change. *Journal of Law Medicine and Ethics, 35*, 78-89.

Serrano, E., Gresock, E., Suttle, D., Keller, A. & McGarvey, E. (2006). Fit WIC: attitudes, perceptions and practices of WIC staff toward addressing childhood overweight. *Journal of Nutrition Education and Behavior, 38*, 151-156.

Sharma, M., Wagner, D.I. & Wilkerson, J. (2005). Predicting childhood obesity prevention behaviors using social cognitive theory. *International Quarterly of Community Health Education, 24*, 191-203.

Silveira, D., Taddei, J.A., Escrivão, M.A., Oliveira, F.L. & Ancona-Lopez, F. (2006) Risk factors for overweight among Brazilian adolescents of low-income families: a case-control study. *Public Health Nutrition, 9*, 421-428.

Slavin, J. (2003). Why whole grains are protective: Biological mechanisms. *The Proceedings of the Nutrition Society, 62*, 129–134.

Sonneville, K.R., La Pelle, N., Taveras, E.M., Gillman, M.W. & Prosser, L.A. (2009). Economic and other barriers to adopting recommendations to prevent childhood obesity: results of a focus group study with parents. *BMC Pediatrics, 9*, 81.

Speiser, P.W., Rudolf, M.C.J., Anhalt, H., Camacho-Hubner, C., Chiarelli, F., Eliakim, A., Freemark, M., Gruters, A., Hershkovitz, E., Iughetti, L., Krude, H., Latzer, Y., Lustig, R.H., Hirsch Pescovitz, O., Pinhas-Hamiel, O., Rogol, A.D., Shalitin, S., Sultan, C., Stein, D., Vardi, P., Werther, G.A., Zadik, Z., Zuckerman-Levin, N. & Hochberg, Z. (2005). CONSENSUS STATEMENT: Childhood Obesity. *The Journal of Clinical Endocrinology & Metabolism, 90,* 1871–1887.

Spinks, A.B., Macpherson, A.K., Bain, C. & McClure, R.J. (2007). Compliance with the Australian national physical activity guidelines for children: relationship to overweight status. *Journal of Science and Medicine in Sport, 10*, 156-163.

Spivack, J.G., Swietlik, M., Alessandrini, E. & Faith, M.S. (2009). Primary Care Providers' Knowledge, Practices, and Perceived Barriers to the Treatment and Prevention of Childhood Obesity. *Obesity*, Nov 12. [Epub ahead of print]

Story, M. (1999). School-based approaches for preventing and treating obesity. *International Journal of Obesity and Related Metabolic Disorders, 23,* S43-S51.

Strauss, R.S. & Knight, J. (1999). Influence of the home environment on the development of obesity in children. *Pediatrics, 103,* e85.

Strauss, R.S. (2000). Childhood obesity and self-esteem. *Pediatrics, 105*, 1-5.

Sweeting, H., West, P. & Young, R. (2008). Obesity among Scottish 15 year olds 1987-2006: prevalence and associations with socio-economic status, well-being and worries about weight. *BMC Public Health, 8*, 404-410.

Swinburn, B., Sacks, G., Lobstein, T., Rigby, N., Baur, L.A., Brownell, K.D., Gill, T., Seidell, J. & Kumanyika, S. (2008). International Obesity Taskforce Working Group on Marketing to Children. 'Sydney Principles' for reducing the commercial promotion of foods and beverages to children. *Public Health Nutrition*, 11, 881-886.

Tanofsky-Kraff, M., Yanovski, S.Z., Schvey, N.A., Olsen, C.H., Gustafson, J. & Yanovski, J.A. (2009). A prospective study of loss of control eating for body weight gain in children at high risk for adult obesity. *International Journal of Eating Disorders, 42*, 26-30.

Timperio, A., Salmon, J., Ball, K., Baur, L.A., Telford, A., Jackson, M., Salmon, L. & Crawford, D. (2008). Family physical activity and sedentary environments and weight change in children. *International Journal of Pediatric Obesity,3,* 160-167.

Toschke, A.M., Thorsteinsdottir, K.H., von Kries, R. (2009). GME Study Group. Meal frequency, breakfast consumption and childhood obesity. *International Journal of Pediatric Obesity, 4*, 242-248.

United Nations System Standing Committee on Nutrition (2007). *Issued by the Working Groups on Nutrition throughout the Life Cycle and Nutrition, Ethics and Human Rights.* Rome, Italy, 26 February—5 March.

Vaidya, V. (2006). Psychosocial aspects of obesity. *Advances in Psychosomatic Medicine, 27*, 73-85.

van Gerwen, M., Franc, C., Rosman, S., Le Vaillant, M., Pelletier-Fleury, N. (2009). Primary care physicians' knowledge, attitudes, beliefs and practices regarding childhood obesity: a systematic review. *Obesity Reviews, 1,* 227-236.

van Zutphen, M., Bell, A.C., Kremer, P.J. & Swinburn, B.A. (2007). Association between the family environment and television viewing in Australian children. *Journal of Pediatric and Child Health, 43*, 458-463.

Veugelers, P.J. & Fitzgerald, A.L. (2005). Effectiveness of school programs in preventing childhood obesity: a multilevel comparison. *American Journal of Public Health*, *95*, 432-435.

Walker, O., Strong, M., Atchinson, R., Saunders, J. & Abbott, J. (2007). A qualitative study of primary care clinicians' views of treating childhood obesity. *BMC Family Practice, 8*, 50.

West, F. & Sanders, M. R. (2009). The Lifestyle Behavior Checklist: a measure of weight-related problem behavior in obese children. *International Journal of Pediatric Obesity, 4(4)*, 266-273.

Wofford, L.G. (2008). Systematic review of childhood obesity prevention. *Journal of Pediatric Nursing, 23*, 5-19.

World Health Organization. (2006). Marketing of food and non-alcoholic beverages to children: report of a WHO forum and technical meeting. Oslo, Norway, 2-5 May.

Yancey, A. (2006). Tackling childhood obesity requires a shift in social norms, not just an exercise program. *British Medical Journal, 333*, 1031-1032.

In: Pathways to Obesity and Main Roads to Recovery
Editor: Piergiuseppe Vinai
ISBN: 978-1-61122-740-6

Chapter XI

Improving Healthy Eating Habits and Daily Physical Activity

Sabrina Guidi
Ville Turina e Amione clinic, San Maurizio Canavese, Turin, Italy

Abstract

Metabolic syndrome (MS) is a combination of medical disorders that increase the risk of developing cardiovascular disease, insulin resistance, glucose intolerance, abdominal obesity, hypertension and dyslipidemia. This pathology has both clinical and economic impact; a low physical activity and being overweight are predictors of MS. There is great interest in identifying the best therapeutic approach to the MS. In this chapter are reviewed the available data regarding influence of changing lifestyles on metabolic syndrome.

Introduction

Ageing is associated with increase in body weight and worsening in glucose tolerance; therefore, prevalence of metabolic syndrome is in constant growth (Ford et al., 2004; Hillier et al., 2006). There is great interest in identifying the best therapeutic approach to patients affected by obesity and metabolic disorders, both for the clinical and economic impact they have. BMI (Pan et al., 1997), bad alimentary habits, low physical activity and low cardio breathing fitness (Laaksonen et al., 2002) have assessed a predictive role for metabolic syndrome. Changes in way of life have demonstrated a reduction of metabolic syndrome (MS) from 40% to 80% in the group of subjects under observation (Bo et al., 2005; Matthews et al., 1982).

An Apple a Day ... Influence of Dieting on Metabolic Syndrome

Metabolic syndrome is a combination of medical disorders increasing the risk of cardiovascular disease, insulin resistance, glucose intolerance, abdominal obesity, hypertension and dyslipidemia. There are no well-accepted diagnostic criteria for MS; currently recommended and widely used, with minor modifications, are those proposed by the National Cholesterol Education Program (NCEP) Adult Treatment Panel III (ATP III) (2001). The presence of three or more of the following symptoms allow diagnosis of the MS:

- Elevated waist circumference: men equal to or greater than 40 inches (102 cm), women equal to or greater than 45 inches (88 cm)
- Elevated triglycerides: equal to or greater than 150 mg/dl
- Reduced HDL cholesterol: men less than 40 mg/dl, women less than 50 mg/dl
- Elevated blood pressure: equal to or greater than 130/85 mmHg
- Elevated fasting glucose: equal to or greater than 110 mg/dl

This group of metabolic disorders concurs to increase the risk for type 2 diabetes, coronary heart disease and all mortality causes (Salmeron et al., 2001; American Diabetes Association 2002). Obesity is the key factor of the syndrome. There is a well-known strong correlation between insulin resistance and obesity: abdominal obesity (Bogardus, 1985) is positively correlated to insulin resistance and influences the synthesis of lipoproteins, glucose utilization and hemodynamic disorders. (Desprès, 1989). Much more than subcutaneous peripheral fat, the abdominal fat is well responsive to reduction in caloric supply and animal fats. Normalization of body weight and in particular loss of abdominal fat represents the primary goal of the clinical management of MS. A hypo-caloric diet improves glucose utilization and reduces hepatic glucose production as well as VLDL proteins in overweight diabetic patients (Wiest-Kent et al., 1986). Weight loss due to a hypo-caloric diet in patients affected by visceral obesity significantly contributes to reduce glycemic rates, insulin, cholesterol and triglycerides levels, and to normalize systolic and diastolic blood pressure rates. (Desprès, 1991).

A diet study conducted on a group of Norwegian patients affected by "insulin resistance syndrome" (The Oslo Diet and Exercise Study) found that loss of weight is strictly related to reduction of insulin-resistance (Torjesen, 1997). Glycemic reaction to food depends on carbohydrate quota, type of sugar (glucose, fructose, sucrose, and lactose), type of amides (amylase, amylopectin), food preparation and other components of food such as fats or other substances that may slow down digestion. There is evidence that consuming low glycemic rate food improves insulin sensitivity, therefore reducing type 2 diabetes risks and increasing HDL cholesterol level. (Wolever, 2000).

Fiber Intake

Epidemiological studies correlated fiber intake to a low risk of type 2 diabetes and cardiovascular diseases (Marlett et al., 2002). Pharmacological doses of soluble fibers and low glycemic level diet have shown positive effects on insulin sensitivity, HDL cholesterol levels and inflammatory markers (Jenkins et al., 2000).

On the contrary, non-soluble fibers of flours seem not to have impact on risk factors. Soluble fibers delay the glucose absorption, increase the hepatic extraction and the sensitivity to insulin of the tissues. (Tabatabai, 2000). A meal rich in fibers usually has a low caloric and fat content and is consumed more slowly, therefore giving a bigger sense of satiety; it is useful in the treatment and prevention of obesity. (Marlett, 2002). In patients with type 2 diabetes a diet rich in fibers improves post-meal glycemia, insulin level range and plasma lipids. (Tabatabai, 2000).

Twenty-five grammes per day fiber consumption, 50% of which being soluble, has produced positive effects on glucose homeostasis and on hyperlipidemia in patients with type 2 diabetes (Mc Intosh & Miller, 2001). Fasting insulin and LDL cholesterol levels are highly influenced by fibers contained in whole meal food, especially in overweight patients, more than by fibers of complex carbohydrates (Mc Keown, 2002). High-fiber foods have also a high-protein/carbohydrate ratio: the great quantity of vegetable proteins seems to support the protective effect of fibers; in fact, they could have positive effects in LDL cholesterol reduction (Jenkins et al., 2000).

It is, therefore, recommended a norm caloric diet in patients affected by metabolic syndrome, with intake > 50 % of complex carbohydrates with at least 30 g of fiber and drastic reduction of simple sugars. A protein intake of about 20% of the whole daily caloric consumption (vegetable proteins are preferred), and fat intake of about the 30 %, mainly represented by poly and mono-unsaturated fatty acids (olive oil), are recommended.

A reverse correlation between intracellular magnesium and insulin-resistance has been reported; (Paolisso et al., 1989) so magnesium supplements may improve insulin sensitivity in men.

It is also necessary to reduce alcohol consumption, but not to abolish it because low quantities of alcohol, in particular in red wine, seem to have a protective action against cardiovascular diseases due to its antioxidant action. (Hjartaker A, Langiou, 2002).

Fat Intake

An excessive intake of saturated animal fats seems to be the most important factor contributing to onset of obesity, type 2 diabetes and insulin-resistance. In the Saint Luis Valley Diabetes Study (1997), it was observed in a large sample of population from South Colorado that excessive intake of lipids and saturated fats was associated with hyperinsulinemia and insulin-resistance (Marshall et al., 1997). It has been demonstrated that a diet rich in saturated fats generates an increase of triglycerides and a change in tissue phospholipids composition that has negative effects on physical and chemical properties of the muscle fiber membrane and transmission of the insulin message (Storlien et al., 1991). There are discordant epidemiological evidences on the metabolic effect of specific fatty acids (Grundy, 1991). Several studies reported an association between the amount of lipids in diet and incidence of diabetes (Salmeron, 1997). The results are influenced by inadequate survey methods of nutritional data and of an incomplete control of confounding factors (Clandinin, 1993). Polyunsaturated fatty acids seem to play a protective role. An increase in the diet of 5% of the amount of polyunsaturated acids seems to reduce the relative risk of diabetes from 1.39 to 0.60 (32). Besides, supplements of polyunsaturated omega 3 fatty acids reduce levels of triglycerides (Borkman, 1993). One of the mechanisms proposed to explain the role of polyunsaturated fatty acids on insulin sensitivity could be the different composition in fatty acids of cellular membranes that modulates insulin action (Purnell & Brunzell, 1997); a greater amount of saturated fats in the phospholipidic membrane could increase resistance to insulin action (Meyer, 2000). There is an association between a high intake of trans fatty acids (e.g., margarine derived from hydrogenation of vegetable oils) and hyperglycemia. If fatty acids were consumed in their natural forms, incidence of diabetes would be reduced by 40% (Clandinin, 1993). Besides, as well as saturated fats, they increase LDL cholesterol levels and lower HDL cholesterol (Borkman et al., 1993). Some metabolic studies have demonstrated that by correcting the amount and caloric intake, diets poor in saturated fats and rich in carbohydrates are effective in lowering LDL cholesterol levels (Borkman et al., 1993). Substitution of saturated fats with unsaturated (arachidonic acid) and monounsaturated fatty acids (oleic and linoleic acid) normalizes insulin sensitivity (Purnell & Brunzell, 1997). In an iso-caloric diet, only 10% of saturated fats could be tolerated, which should be associated with 10% of polyunsaturated fats and with 10% of mono unsaturated fatty acids, easily found in olive oil.

Complex-Carbohydrate Intake

However, if a reduction in the consumption of fats is linked to an increase in carbohydrate intake, the diet does not generate a real metabolic benefit; in particular, it does not improve insulin sensitivity. In fact, a diet poor in fats and rich in carbohydrates can even lead to a worsening of the metabolic syndrome. On the other hand, other authors have emphasized the extremely positive role of diets rich in complex carbohydrates (Meyer et al., 2000). Carbohydrates influence glucose levels and insulin secretion, even if studies on it have contradictory evidence. Studies on healthy subjects and on subjects at risk of developing type 2 diabetes confirm the importance of including food rich in complex carbohydrates in a diet for diabetic subjects, especially cereals, fruit, vegetables and milk (Borkman et al., 1993). Lowering the extent of glycemic and insulin response after meals could be a way to interrupt wrong metabolic cycle where insulin resistance causes hyperinsulinemia, which makes insulin sensitivity even worse (Laaksonen, 2002).

Influence of Physical Activity on Metabolic Syndrome

Poor physical activity is an important risk factor. Given the widespread increase in obesity, type 2 diabetes and metabolic syndrome (Katzmarzyk et al., 2004, Mokdad et al., 2001, Zimmet et al., 2001, Zimmet et al., 2001), it is necessary to further understand as metabolic risk factors are influenced by the patient's way of life. It has been demonstrated that energy expenditure is inversely related to a cluster of metabolic risk factors in healthy subjects and that energy expenditure inversely predicts progression toward the metabolic syndrome independently from aerobic fitness and fatty tissue mass (Franks et al., 2004; O'Donovan et al., 2005). In a randomized controlled trial of 258 male and female healthy subjects at risk for type 2 diabetes, Ekelund & coll. (2005) demonstrate that total body fitness is inversely and independently associated with three out of six risk factors (triglycerides on an empty stomach, HDL cholesterol, insulin) and to all metabolic risk factors after adjustment by age, sex and obesity. Physical activity predicted progression toward the metabolic syndrome, independent of baseline metabolic syndrome, body fat and other confounding factors. In conclusion, physical activity is inversely associated with cardiovascular and metabolic risk factors and with metabolic risk cluster independently from type of activity and obesity.

Insulin resistance is typical of patients affected by type 2 diabetes. It is often present years before the onset of glucose intolerance or before overt diabetes. Insulin resistance mechanism leads to an increase of fatty acids (e.g., high calorie intake or obesity) and to altered conditions of degradation/oxidation balance of muscular fatty acids. Several studies found that an increase in physical activity could delay the onset of type 2 diabetes, while a poor physical activity is a risk factor for onset of this pathology. The mechanism responsible for insulin sensitivity increase after physical activity has been studied for a longtime, but it is not completely understood (Ekelund et al., 2007).

Some studies compared the benefits in sensitivity to insulin due to either a moderate or a vigorous physical activity The results suggest that vigorous long-term physical activity can generate durable effects on insulin action, if compared with moderate-vigorous fitness, which can only produce temporary effects (Ostergard et al., 2007).

Lee and colleagues (2005) assessed physical activity effects on reduction in visceral or total adipose tissue, muscular mass and corporal composition in thin men and in obese women with and without type 2 diabetes. Twenty-four men practiced supervised moderate-intensity aerobic activity five times a week for 60 minutes (approximately 60% of max VO2). Corporal composition of visceral and total body fat mass has been observed by means of Nuclear Magnetic Resonance Imaging (NMRI), while muscular mass composition by means of Computerized Axial Tomography (CAT) and cardio breathing capacity was assessed through gradual intensity test. Body weight did not change in any of the groups after exercise. A relevant reduction in total body fat, subcutaneous and visceral fat has been observed in every group but reduction in visceral fat was significantly greater among obese subjects as well as in those affected by type 2 diabetes. In conclusion, regular physical exercise, without weight decrease, is associated with a significant reduction in the total and visceral fat and in the muscle lipids, in both groups of obese and type 2 diabetes subjects (DiPietro et al., 2006).

Physical exercise reduces postprandial lypidemia, but this is generally described as a short-term result. The exact mechanism responsible for this reduction has not been completely identified yet, but at least two mechanisms seem to be involved: a reduction in secretion of triglycerides in the liver, and an increase in plasma triglycerides recovery from muscles. Changes in metabolism of other lipids, e.g., in HDL cholesterol, have been observed only when physical exercise is practiced in the hours before a meal rich in lipids. The most important factors determining a high reduction in postprandial lipidemia seem to be the reduction of energy intake during the meal and the intensity of physical activity. Therefore, healthy subjects can induce a positive change in postprandial lipidemia through aerobic physical exercise. This is effective if practiced between 16 hours before and one and a half hours after meals and if it induces an energy consumption of about 500 Kcal (Lee et al., 2005).

Obese subjects at risk of developing coronary disease should be treated with an appropriate weight loss program (Katsason, 2006), but to lose weight only through a diet therapy involves a reduction in free fat mass and a reduction in lipid oxidation after the end of the diet, which could contribute to gain weight again afterwards. To avoid this, it is highly recommended to treat obesity with a combination of physical activity and low caloric intake (Jansses & Ross, 1999). Walking is an aerobic exercise affordable by every social strata of the population, as it is cheap, easy, and suitable. Since intensity of activity during the march is under threshold value of lactic acid production, walking is considered a low-intensity exercise. Aerobic fitness, a common activity especially among women, represents a moderate-vigorous physical activity. For example, Okura & coll. (2003) report that low-intensity physical activity (walking) or moderate-vigorous one (aerobic fitness) associated with a slimming diet, have different effects on cardiovascular risk (Jakicic et al., 2002). Ninety obese women have been divided into different groups: the first only treated with a diet, the second with the same diet and walking, the third with diet and aerobic fitness. Blood pressure, lipoprotein and fasting glycemic levels have been used as cardiovascular risk indicators. These variables have been measured before and after a 14-week period. Results show that fat mass in excess in every layer is significantly reduced ($p<0.001$). Total weight loss and adipose tissue and non-bone masses reduction are significantly inferior in the group performing diet associated with aerobic fitness (respectively -1.5 Kg e -0.1 kg) if compared to the group on diet (respectively -2.1 kg e -0.4 kg) and to the diet + walking (respectively-2.5 Kg e-0.5 kg). Risk for developing a cardiovascular disease is greatly reduced in every group. Reduction in LDL cholesterol level and fasting glycemia are higher in the diet + aerobic fitness group. Different from what was expected, a high-intensity physical activity program associated to a slimming diet could not be protective but rather be a risk factor for cardiovascular disease, if compared with low-intensity activity.

Low physical activity levels, non-aerobic fitness and obesity are associated with a higher risk of developing type 2 diabetes (Okura et al., 2003; Williams et al., 2003; Church et al., 2005; Toledo et al., 2005, 2006). Both scarce physical activity, particularly aerobic activity, and being overweight are predictors of type 2 diabetes and of metabolic disease. (Stump et al., 2003; Mootha et al., 2003; Petersen et al., 2004; Morino et al., 2005; Menshinova et al., 2005). Lee et al., (2005) found that a regular exercise, also without weight loss, is associated with a substantial reduction in total and visceral fat and in skeletal muscle lipid in both obesity and T2D

Stallmann et al., (2007) hypothesized that among adolescents, fat intake, intense physical activity and their interaction can be predictive on percentage of total body fat mass and on adipose tissue, and that a sedentary way of life as well as intake of dairy products, fruit, vegetables and cereals could be related to the amount of adipose tissue. A group of 661 healthy white and black adolescents was studied. The results show that caloric intake and visceral adipose tissue are predictive factors on fat mass percentage. Time spent for watching TV and the percentage of protein in daily caloric intake are positive predictive factors for thin mass percentage. After adjustment for calorie intake, none of the independent variables were significantly predictive for fat mass percentage. Caloric intake is the only and unique predictive factor for adipose visceral tissue.

Pesactello and coll. (2000) examined the impact of habitual low-intensity physical activity on serum lipid values and other cardiovascular risk factors in older adults in an observational study on 155 old subjects (average age 74 years). After adjustment for age, sex, adiposity, medicines, a greater amount of physical activity was associated with a better lipid profile. Subjects practicing five or more hours of fitness had a higher HDL cholesterol level (0.23 mmol/l) and a lower total/HDL cholesterol level (-0.92). They also had a lower LDL cholesterol value (-0.39 mmol/l), as well as a lower ratio between triglycerides and HDL cholesterol (-1.31). Total cholesterol values were similar in both groups. Glycemia was 1.49 mmol/l lower in the group practicing more physical activity, independently from sex, age, adiposity, use of medicines and postprandial state.

Conclusion

The levels of physical exercise are inversely associated with the concentration of inflammatory markers, whereas fiber consumption is negatively related with fasting glucose values, regardless of changes in body weight. Both these conditions may play a role in predicting the metabolic syndrome in healthy subjects. Both low physical activity, in particular the one poor in aerobic activity, and overweight are predictors of type 2 diabetes and of metabolic disease. Changes in lifestyle may be an effective non-pharmacological strategy to reduce blood concentrations of inflammatory markers and prevent metabolic deterioration. In conclusion: physical activity, even of low-intensity, is a sufficient tool to improve glycemic levels and lipid profile in adult subjects, independently from visceral adiposity and body fat mass.

References

A.A.V.V. (2001). Executive summary of the third report of the national cholesterol education program (NCEP) expert panel on detection, evaluation and treatment of high blood cholesterol in adults (adult treatment panel III). *JAMA, 285,* 2846-2497.

A.A.V.V. (2002). American Diabetes Association: Evidence-Based nutrition principles and recommendations for the treatment and prevention of diabetes and related complications. *Diabetes Care, 25*, S50-60.

Bo, S., Gentile, L., Ciccone, G., Baldi, C., Benini, L., Dusio, F., Lucia, C., Forastiere, G., Nuti, C., Cassader, M., Pagano, G.F. (2005). The metabolic syndrome and high C-reactive protein: prevalence and difference by sex in a Southern-European population-based cohort. *Diab Metab Res Rev, 21*,515-24.

Bogardus, C., Lillioja, S., Mott, D.H., Hollenbeck, C., Reaven, G. (1985). Relationship between degree of obesity and in vivo insulin-action in man. *Am J Physiol., 248,* 286-290.

Borkman, M., Storlien, L.H., Pan, D.A., Jenkins, A.B., Chisholm, D.J., Campbell, S.V. (1993). The relationship between insulin sensitivity and the fatty acid composition of scheletal muscle phospholipids. *N Engl J Med, 328,* 238-244.

Carroll, S., Cooke, C.B., Butterly, R.J. (2000). Metabolic clustering, physical activity and fitness in non-smoking, middle-aged men. *Med Sci Sports Exerc, 32*, 2079-2086.

Church, T.S., La Monte, M.J., Barlow, C.E., Blair, S.N. (2005). Cardio respiratory fitness and body mass index as predictors of cardiovascular disease mortality among men with diabetes. *Arch Intern Med, 165,* 2114-2120.

Clandinin, M.T., Cheema, S., Field, C.J., Baracos, V.E. (1993). Dietary lipids influence insulin action. *Ann N Y Acad Sci, 683*,151-163.

Desprès, J.P., Pauliot, M.C., Moorjani, S. (1991). Loss of abdominal fat and metabolic response to exėrcise training in obese women. *Am J Physiol, 261,* E159-167.

Desprès, J.P., Nadeau, A., Tremblay, A., Ferland, M., Morjani, S., Lupien, P.J., Thierault, G., Pinault, S., Bouchard, C. (1989). Role of deep abdominal fat in the association between regional adipose tissue distribution and glucose tolerance in obese women. *Diabetes Care, 38,* 304-309.

Di Pietro L, Dziura J, Yeckel CW, Neufer PD. (2006). Exercise and improved insulin sensitività in older women: evidence of the enduring benefits of higher intensity training. *Journal of Applied Physiology, 100* (1), 142-149.

Eckel, R.H., Grundy, S.M., Zimmet, P.Z. (2005). The metabolic syndrome. *Lancet, 365,* 1415-1428.

Ekelund, U., Brage, S., Franks, P.W., Hennings, S., Emms, S., Wareham, N.J. (2005). Physical activity energy expenditure predicts progression toward the metabolic syndrome independently of aerobic fitness in middle-aged healthy Caucasians: The medical Research Council Ely Study. *Diabetes Care, 28,* 1195-2000.

Ekelund, U., Griffin, S.J., Wareham, N.J. (2007). Physical activity and metabolic risk in individuals with a family history of type 2 diabetes, *Diabetes Care, 30*, 337-342.

Ford, E.S., Giles, W.H., Mokdad, A.H. (2004). Increasing prevalence of the metabolic syndrome among U.S. adults. *Diabetes Care, 27,* 2444-2449.

Franks, P.W., Ekelund, U., Brage, S., Wong, M.J., Wareham, N.J. (2004). Does the association of habitual physical activity with the metabolic syndrome differ by level of fitness? *Diabetes Care, 27,* 1187-1193.

Fung, T.T., Hu, F.B., Yu, J., Chu, N.F., Spiegelman, D., Tofler, G.H., Willet, W.C., Rimm, E.B. (2000). Leisure time physical activity, television watching, and plasma biomarkers of obesity and cardiovascular disease risk. *Am J Epidemiol, 152,* 1171-1178.

Goodpaster, B.H., Katsiaras, A., Kelley, D.E. (2003). Enhanced fat oxidation trough physical activity is associated with improvements in insulin sensitivity in obesity. *Diabetes, 52,* 2191-2197.

Grundy, S.M. (1991). Dietary therapy in diabetes mellitus. Is there a single best diet? *Diabetes Care, 14*, 796-801.

Henry, R.R., Wiest-Kent, T.A., Schaeffer, L., Kolterman, O.G., Olefsky, J.M. (1986). Metabolic consequences of very-low-caloric diet therapy in obese noninsulin-dependent diabetic and non diabetic subjects. *Diabetes, 35,* 155-164.

Hillier, T.A., Fagot-Campagna, A., Eschwège, E., et al., (2006). Weight change and changes in the metabolic syndrome as the French population moves towards overweight: the DESIR Cohort. *Internat J Epidemiol.,35,* 190-196.

Hjartaker, A., Langiou, A., et al., (2002). Consumption of dairy products in the European Prospective Investigation into Cancer and Nutrition (EPIC) cohort: data from 35 955 24-

hour dietary recalls in 10 European countries. *Public Health Nutr, Dec, 5(6b),* 1259-1271.

Jakes, R.W., Day, N.E., Khaw, K.T., Luben, R., Oakes, S., Welch, A., Bingham, S., Wareham, N.J. (2003). Television viewing and low participation in vigorous recreation are independently associated with obesity and markers of cardiovascular disease risk: EPIC-Norfolk population-based study. *Eur J Clin Nutr, 57,* 1089-1096.

Jakicic, J.M., Clark, K., Coleman, E., et al., American. (2002). College of Sports Medicine position stand. Appropriate intervention strategies for weight loss and prevention of weight regain for adults. *Med Sci Sports Exerc,10,* 757-766.

Jansses, I., Ross, R., (1999). Effects of sex on the change in visceral, subcutaneous adipose tissue and skeletal muscle in response to weight loss. *Int J Obes Relat Metab Disord, 23,* 1035-1046.

Jenkins, D.J., Axelsen, M., Kendall, C.V., Augustin, L.S., Vuksan, V., Smith, U. (2000). Dietary fibre, lente carbohydrates and the insulin-resistant diseases. *British Journal of Nutrition, 83,* 157-163.

Katsason, C.S. (2006). Prescribing aerobic exercise for the regulation of postprandial lipid metabolism: current research and recommendations. *Sports Med, 36 (7),* 547-560.

Katzmarzyk, P., Church, T.S., Blair, S.N. (2004). Cardiorespiratory fitness attenuates the effects of the metabolic syndrome on all-cause and cardiovascular disease mortality in men, *Arch Intern Med, 164,* 1092-1097.

Laaksonen, D.E., Lakka, H.M., Niskanen, L.K., Kaplan, G.A., Salonen, J.T., Lakka, T.A. (2002). Metabolic syndrome and development of diabetes mellitus: application and validation of recently suggested definitions of the metabolic syndrome in a prospective cohort study, *Am J Epidemiol, 156,* 1070-1077.

Laaksonen, D.E., Lakka, H.M., Niskanen, L.K., Kaplan, G.A., Salonen, J.T., Lakka, T.A. (2002). Low levels of leisure-time physical activity and cardiorespiratory fitness predict development of the metabolic syndrome. *Diabetes Care, 25,* 1612-1618.

Lee, S., Kuk, J.1., Davidson, L.E., Hudson, R., Kilpatrick, K., Graham, T.E., Ross, R. (2005). Exercise without weight loss is an effective strategy for obesity reduction in obese individuals with or without. Type 2 diabetes. *Journal of Applied Physiology Sep, 99, (3),* 1120-1125.

Marlett, J.A., Mc Bumey, M.1., Slavin, J.L. (2002). Position of the American Dietetic Association: health implications of dietary fiber. *J Am Diet Assoc.,* 102 (7), 993-1000.

Marshall, J.A., Bessesen, D.H., Hamman, R.F. (1997). High saturated fat and low starch and fibre are associated with hyperinsulinemia in a non-diabetic population: The San Luis Valley Diabetes Study. *Diabetologia 40,* 430-438.

Matthews, D.R., Hosker, J.P., Rudenski, A.S., Naylor, B.A., Treacher, D.F., Turner, R.C. (1985). Homeostasis model assessment: insulin resistance and β-cell function from fasting plasma glucose and insulin concentrations in man. *Diabetologia, 28,* 412-419.

Mc Keown, N.M., Meigs, J.B., Wilson, P.W., Jacques, P.F. (2002).Whole grain intake is favourably associated with metabolic risk factors for type 2 diabetes and cardiovascular disease in the Framingham Offspring Study. *Am J Clin Nutr., 76 (2),* 390-398.

Mc lntosh, M., Miller, C. (2001). A diet containing food rich in soluble and insoluble fiber improves glycemic control and reduces hyperlipidemia among patients with type 2 diabetes mellitus. *Nutr Rev., 59 (2),* 52-55.

Menshinova, E.V., Ritov, V.B., Fairfull, L., Ferrel, R.E., Kelley, D.E., Goodpaster, B.H. (2006). Effects of exercise on mitochondrial content and function in aging human skeletal muscle, *J Gerontol A Biol Sci Med Sci, 61,* 534-540.

Menshinova, E.V., Ritov, V.B., Toledo, F.G., Ferrel, R.E., Goodpaster, B.H., Kelley, D.E. (2005). Effects of weight loss and physical activity on skeletal muscle mitochondrial function in obesity. *Am J Endocrinol Metab, 288,* E818-E825.

Meyer, K.A., Kushi, L.H., Jakobs, D.R. Jr., Slavin, J., Sellers, T.A., Folsom, A.R. (2000). Carbohydrates, dietary fiber and incident type 2 diabetes in older women. *American Journal of Clinical Nutrition, 71 (4),* 921-930.

Mokdad, A.H., Ford, E.S., Bowman, B.A., Dietz, W.H., Vinicor, F., Bales, V.S., Marks, J.S. (2001). Prevalence of obesity-related health risk factors, *JAMA, 289,*76-79.

Mootha, V., Lindgren, C.M. L, Eriksson, K.F., Subramanian, A., Sihag, S., Lehar, J., Puigserver, P., Carlsson, E., Ridderstrale, M., Laurila, E., Houstis, N., Daly, M., Patterson, N., Mesirow, J., Golub, T., Tamayo, P., Spiegelman, B., Lander, E., Hirschorn, J., Altshuler, D., Groop, L. (2003). PGC- 1alpha responsive genes involved in oxidative phosphorilation are coordinately down-regulated in human diabetes. *Nat Genet, 34,* 267-273.

Morino, K., Dufor, S., Befroy, D., Frattini, J., Shatzkes, N., Neschen, S., White, M., Bilz, S., Sono, S., Pypaert, M., Shulman, G.I. (2005). Reduced mitochondrial density and increased IRS-1 serine phosphorylation in muscle of insulin-resistant offspring of type 2 diabetes patients. *J Clin Invest, 115,* 3587-3593.

Nascetti, S., Linarello, S., Scurti, M., Grandi, E., Gaddoni, M., Noera, G., Gaddi, A. (2004). Assessment of the health status in the Massa Lombarda cohort: a preliminary description of the program evaluating cardio-cerebro-vascular disease risk factors and quality of life in an elderly population. *Arch Gerontol Geriatr, suppl (9),* 309-314.

O'Donovan, G., Owen, A., Kearney, E.M., Jones, D.W., Nevill, A.M., Woolf-May, K., Bird, S.R. (2005). Cardiovascular disease risk factors in habitual exercises, lean sedentary men and abdominally obese sedentary men. *Int J Obes Relat Metab Disord, 29*, 1063-1069.

Okura, T, Nakata, Y, Tanaka, K. (2003). Effects of exercise intensity on physical fitness and risk factors for coronary heart disease. *Obes Res Sep, 11 (9),* 1131-1139.

Ostergard, T., Jessen, N., Schimtz, O., Mandarino, L.J. (2007). The effect of exercise, training, and inactivity on insulin sensitivity in diabetics and their relatives: what is new? *Applied Physiology Nutrition Metabolism Jun,* 32, 541-548.

Pan, X.R., Li, G.W., Hu, Y.H., et al., (1997). Effects of diet and exercise in preventing NIDDM in people with impaired glucose tolerance. The Da Qing IGT and Diabetes Study. *Diabetes Care, 20,* 537-544.

Paolisso, G., Sgambato, S., Pizza, G., Passariello, N., Varricchio, M., D'Onofrio, F. (1989). Improved insulin response and action by chronic magnesium administration in aged NIDDM subjects. *Diabetes Care 12,* 265-269.

Pescatello LS, Murphy D, Costanzo D. (2000). Low intensity physical activity benefits blood lipids and lipoproteins in older adults living at home. *Age Ageing. Sep, 29 (5)*: 433-439.

Petersen, K.F., Dufor, S., Befroy, D., Garcia, R., Shulman, G.I. (2004). Impaired mitochondrial activity in the insulin- resistant offspring of patients with type 2 diabetes, *New England Journal of Medicine, 350,* 664-671.

Purnell, J.Q., Brunzell, J.D. (1997). The central role of dietary fat, not carbohydrate, in the insulin resistance syndrome. *Curr Opin Lipidol., 8,* 17-22.

Rainwater, D.L., Mitchell, B.D., Comuzzie, A.G., Vandeberg, J.L., Stern, M.P., MacCluer, J.W. (2000). Association among 5-year changes in weight, physical activity, and cardiovascular disease risk factors in Mexican Americans. *Am J Epidemiol, 152,* 974-982.

Salmeron, J., Ascherio, A., Rimm, E.B., Coldlitz, G.A., Spiegelman, D., Jenkins, D.J., Stampfer, M.J., Wing, A.L., Willett, W.C. (1997). Dietary fiber, glycemic load and risk of NIDDM in men. *Diabetes Care, 20 (4),* 545-550.

Salmeron, J., Hu, B.F., Manson, J.A., Stampfer, M.J., Graham, A.C., Rimm, E.B., Willett, W. Dietary fat intake and risk of type 2 diabetes in women. (2001). *Am J Cin Nutr, 73,* 1019-1026.

Stallmann-Jorgensen IS, Gutin B, Hatfield-Laube JL, Humphries MC, Johnson MH, Barbeau P. (2007). General and visceral adiposity in black and white adolescents and their relation with reported physical activity and diet. *International Journal of Obesity. (London) Apr, 31* (4): 622-629.

Storlien, L.H., Jenkins, A.B., Chisolm, D.J., Pascal, W.S., Kouri, S., Kraegen, E.W. (1991). Influence of dietary fat composition on development of insulin resistance in rats: relationship to muscle triglyceride and ω-3 fatty acids in muscle phospholipid. *Diabetes 40,* 280-289.

Stump, C., Short, K., Bigelow, M., Schimke, J., Nair, S. (2003). Effect of insulin on human skeletal muscle mitochondrial ATP production, protein synthesis and mRNA transcripts, *Proc Natl Acad Sci USA, 100,* 7996-8001.

Stumvoll, M., Goldstein, B.J., Van Haften, T.W. (2005). Type 2 diabetes: principles of pathogenesis and therapy. *Lancet, 365,* 1333-1346.

Tabatabai, A., Li, S. Dietary fiber and type 2 diabetes. (2000). *Clin Excell Nurse Pract., 4 (5),* 272-276.

Toledo, F.G., Watkins, S., Kelley, D.E. (2006). Changes induced by physical activity and weight loss in the morphology of intermyofibrillar mitochondria in obese men and women. *J Clin Endocrinol Metab, 91,* 3224-3227.

Toledo, F.G.S., Kelley, D.E. (2005). Mitochondrial dysfunction in the pathogenesis of insulin resistance associated with obesity, diabetes, and aging. *Current Opinions in Endocrinology and Metabolism, 12,* 157-162.

Torjesen, P.A., Birkeland, K.I., Anderssen, S.A., Hjermam, I., Holme, I., Urdal, P. (1997) Lifestyle changes may reverse development of the Insulin Resistance Syndrome. *Diabetes Care, 20,* 26-31.

Williams, K.V., Bertoldo, A., Kinahan, P., Cobelli, C., Kelley, D.E. (2003). Weight loss-induced plasticity of glucose transport and phosphorilation in the insulin resistance of obesity and type 2 diabetes. *Diabetes, 52,* 1619-1626.

Wing, R., Koeske, R., Epstein, L., Nowalk, M., Gooding, W., Becker, D. (1987). Long-term effects of modest weight loss in type 2 diabetic patients. *Arch Intern Med,147,* 1749-1753.

Wolever, T.M. (2000). Dietary carbohydrates and insulin action in humans. *British Journal of Nutrition, 83 (suppl 1),* S97-S102.

Zimmet, P., Alberti, K.G., Shaw, J. (2001). Global and societal implications of the diabetes epidemic, *Nature, 414,* 782-787.

In: Pathways to Obesity and Main Roads to Recovery
Editor: Piergiuseppe Vinai
ISBN: 978-1-61122-740-6

Chapter XII

Dieting

Anna Tagliabue
Department of Applied Health Sciences, Section of Human Nutrition and Dietetics, Faculty of Medicine, University of Pavia, Italy

Abstract

Dieting, defined as intentional caloric restriction to reduce body weight, is part of a multi-factorial approach and not the only strategy for weight loss. A correct diet requires a caloric deficit of 500 to 1000 kcal/day, usually inducing a weight loss at the rate of 1 to 2 lb/ week. It has to be prescribed by a clinical nutritionist or registered dietitian in order to ensure an adequate nutrient composition. The short-term efficacy of low-calorie diets has been consistently demonstrated independent of the macronutrient composition of the diets, but has to be integrated with other approaches (exercise, psychological support) as needed by each patient, to improve long-term treatment outcome.

Introduction

The excessive fat accumulation, which defines obesity and determines health threats, is determined by a positive energy balance; i.e., the energy intake has been relatively abundant compared to the subject's physical activity. This can easily be the case in our society characterized by a "sedentary lifestyle" and an abundant food supply. A balanced and medically supervised low-caloric diet can induce a reasonable weight loss of about 5 to 10 %, which significantly reduces the medical risks associated with obesity (National Institute of Health Clinical Guidelines, 1998). The diet alone is not sufficient to obtain long-term weight maintenance and has to be integrated with exercise, behavior modification, nutritional education and psychological support, but this does not undermine its significance.

Indications, Contraindications, Caveat

According to the National Institute of Health Clinical Guidelines (1998), dieting is recommended, in combination with increased physical activity and behavior therapy, for adult patients with a Body Mass Index of 30 or more, before considering a pharmacological or surgical approach. It should also be considered for overweight subjects (i.e., with a BMI between 25 and 29.9) or subjects with a high-risk waist circumference and two or more risk factors (hypertension, dyslipidemia, etc.). The slimming regimen should be prescribed by a clinical nutritionist or registered dietitian in order to ensure that the diet is adequate in its nutrient composition and is part of a multi-factorial approach and not the only strategy for weight loss. To follow a self-prescribed, uncontrolled very low-caloric diet for many months can induce side effects due to an inadequate intake of micronutrients and fibers. The clinical manifestations vary according to the diet and may comprise dehydration, hypotension, anemia or constipation.

The desire to lose weight and the subsequent dieting attitude is not only restricted to overweight people. It also extends to include normal or underweight people who may wish to lose weight for cultural, social, or psychological reasons. In a national telephone survey in the United States, Biener and Heaton (1995) reported that almost half of the White women and one quarter of the Black women who were trying to lose weight at any particular time were not overweight. Notably, the majority of normal-weight dieters reported that their primary motivation was to improve their health, and they thus appeared to be heeding public health messages. Dieting is unadvisable in subjects who do not need to lose weight for medical reasons, their request to lose weight being due to a psychological distress have to be properly assessed and treated. Aim of the NIH guidelines was to provide a guide to health care professionals to deal with these patients.

Healthy and Unhealthy Diets

Diets used in the treatment of obesity are by definition low-calorie diets in order to induce a negative energy balance and weight loss. The initial target of a weight loss program should be to decrease body weight by 5 to 10 %, at which point a new target or a weight management program can be set. Even a 5 % weight reduction alleviates risk factors and risk of co-morbidities. Final weight goals should be individualized and chosen realistically with reduction of body fat as the focus.

To calculate a definite energy deficit, it is necessary to estimate the actual energy requirements of the subject. The Food and Nutrition Board of the Institute of Medicine (2004) has established a new approach for this calculation that is based on the direct measurement of total energy expenditure by doubly labeled water (see Table 12.1)

The Guidelines issued by the National Institute of Health (1998) suggest losing weight at the rate of 1 to 2 lb/ week; this requires a calorie deficit of 500 to 1000 kcal/day. Therefore, the energy level of a diet results from the energy requirement of the patient minus the desired energy deficit.

Table 12.1. Estimated Energy Requirements modified from Food and Nutrition Board Institute of Medicine, National Academies

Height in meters	Physical Activity Level (PAL)	Men Estimated Energy Requirements (kcal/day)		Women Estimated Energy Requirements (kcal/day)	
		BMI 18.50	BMI 24.99	BMI 18.50	BMI 24.99
1.5	Sedentary	1.848	2.080	1.652	1.762
	Low Active	2.009	2.267	1.803	1.956
	Active	2.215	2.506	2.025	2.198
	Very Active	2.554	2.898	2.291	2.489
1.65	Sedentary	2.068	2.349	1.816	1.982
	Low Active	2.254	2.566	2.016	2.202
	Active	2.490	2.842	2.267	2.477
	Very Active	2.880	3.296	2.567	2.807
1.8	Sedentary	2.301	2.635	2.015	2.211
	Low Active	2.513	2.884	2.239	2.459
	Active	2.782	3.200	2.519	2.769
	Very Active	3.225	3.720	2.855	3.141

Estimated energy requirements for subject, 30 years old; for each year below 30, add 7 kcal/day for women and 10 kcal /day for men. For each year above 30, subtract 7 kcal /day for women and 10 kcal /day for men. Derived from the following regression equation based on doubly labeled water data:

Men EER= 662-9.53 x years of age + PA* x (15.91 x (kg of weight + 539.6 x height in meters).

Women EER = 354—6.91 x years of age + PA* x (9.36 x kg of weight + 726 x height in meters).

* PA refers to coefficient for Physical Activity Level:

Men Sedentary: PA = 1; Low Active: PA = 1.11; Active: PA – 1.25; Very Active: PA = 1.48.

Women Sedentary: PA = 1; Low Active: PA = 1.12; Active: PA = 1.27; Very Active: PA = 1.45.

Low-energy diets (LED), also called “traditional diets,” usually provide 1200 to 1800 kcal /day and consist of natural foods, but sometimes a higher energy level may be needed. The diet should meet requirements for essential nutrients other than energy and should be acceptable to the patient. Clearly a low-energy diet is not the preferred by an obese subject, so, as it is possible, it is important to consider matters of taste, social, economic and religious factors, to devise a diet as much as possible acceptable for the patient.

A traditional balanced low-calorie diet is made up of 50 to 55% of carbohydrates using sources such as vegetables, fruits, beans and whole grains, 15 to 25 % of protein and no more than 30 % of fat. An adequate intake of fiber is recommended to reduce caloric density, to promote satiety by delaying stomach-emptying time and to prevent constipation. LED introduces healthy eating habits early in the weight-reduction program to familiarize the patient with the dietary changes that are central elements in a weight-maintenance program. An example of such a diet is illustrated in Table 12.2.

Table 12.2. Sample Menu

Breakfast	Lunch	Dinner
cereal *3/4 cup* skim milk *1/2 cup* banana *1* whole wheat toast *1 slice* sliced almonds *1/2 oz*	lentil soup *1 cup* hard roll *1* olive oil *1/2 tbsp* spinach *1 cup* romaine lettuce *1 cup* chopped mushrooms *1/4 cup* radishes *2* balsamic vinegar *1/2 oz*	pasta *1 1/2 cup* tomatos *1/2 cup* broccoli *1/2 cup* squash/zucchini *1/2 cup* sweet peppers *1/4 cup* chopped mushrooms *1/4cup* olive oil *2 tbsp* parmesan cheese *1 tbsp* white beans *1.2 cup* red wine vinegar *1/2 oz* garlic *1 clove* whole wheat bread *1 slice* grapes *1/2 cup*

Snack

- plain yogurt *1 cup*
- blueberries *1/2 cup*

This diet provides the following

Calories	1800
Protein	15%
Carbohydrates	58%
Fat	27%
Fiber	34 gm

A correct dietary approach also provides suggestions to cut calories (Table 12.3).

Table 12.3. Ways to Shave Calories. (Modified from the American Dietetic Association)

When it comes to healthy weight management, small steps add up. In fact, little changes in eating and activity level have a more positive impact on health than drastic ones.
Lighten up your favorite coffee drink with non-fat milk and sugar-free syrup.
Trim all fat from beef, pork and chicken. Remove the skin from poultry.
Dish up slow-churned, reduced-calorie ice cream in place of regular.
Enjoy raw vegetables with salsa or fat-free ranch dip instead of chips.
Downsize Your Dishes. Our brains think we are getting more when the same amount of food is placed in a smaller dish. ***Savor Your Meals.*** Eating too quickly leads to overeating and feeling uncomfortably full afterwards.
Leave Some Food on Your Plate. Don't Eat Out of a Bag or Box, because you are likely to keep eating until it's all gone—no matter how many servings the package actually contains. Pour one serving into a small bowl.
Choose Your Glass Wisely. Use slender glasses for any beverage except water. People tend to fill short and wide glasses with more and to drink more.
Rethink Your Drinks. Whenever possible, replace caloric drinks with plenty of water.

Table 12.4. Macronutrient composition of popular diets compared with average intakes and recommendations

	Carbohydrate	Protein	Fat
Average U.S. intake	51—53	15	32—34
Recommendation	45-65	10-35	20-35
Low carb diets			
-Atkins	< 10	Unrestricted	unrestricted
-Zone diet	40	30	30
-Scarsdale	34	43	22

Vitamin and mineral supplements that meet age-related requirements are usually recommended with low-calorie diets, especially if they provide less than 1200 kcal for women or 1800 for men, because it is difficult to choose foods to maintain this calorie level and meet all nutritional requirements every day.

The macronutrient composition of LED has been debated, and low-carbohydrate diets have been suggested to produce a greater weight loss than the conventional balanced diet (Foster et al., 2003). A systematic review by Bravata et al., (2003) on 94 low-carb dietary interventions found insufficient evidence to conclude that lower-carbohydrate content is independently associated with greater weight loss compared with higher carbohydrate content. The authors did find a relationship between weight loss and decreased caloric intake or increased diet duration.

Table 12.5. Staying Away from Fad Diets, following the suggestion of the American Dietetic Association http://www.eatright.org/default.aspx

If a diet sounds too good to be true, it probably is false.

Steer clear of any diet claiming:

"Rapid Weight Loss!"

"Eat as much as you want of a single food"

"Eat only Specific Food Combinations!"

"Follow Rigid Menus!"

"No Need to Exercise!"

Slow, steady weight loss is more likely to last than dramatic weight changes and less likely to regain the pounds quickly afterwards.

Ditch diets that allow unlimited quantities of any food, such as grapefruit and cabbage soup, or eliminate or severely restricts entire food groups, such as carbohydrates.

There is no evidence that combining certain foods or eating foods at specific times of day will help with weight loss.

Limiting food choices or following rigid meal plans can be an overwhelming, distasteful task.

Regular physical activity (30 to 60 minutes a day) is essential for good health and healthy weight management.

A plethora of weight-reducing diets is available to the public, ranging from healthy diets to questionable, complex single-food regimen. Popular diets can be divided into categories based on their macronutrient content and varies from high fat, low-carbohydrate to low- and very low-fat diets. All of these unbalanced diets reduce caloric intake and therefore can result in short-term weight loss, but no controlled clinical trials are available on weight maintenance after weight loss or long-term health benefits and risks (Freedman M. et al., 2001). The macronutrient composition of popular diets compared with average intakes and recommendations is shown in Table 12.4.

Moreover, these diets emphasize fast results with minimal effort risking to encourage unrealistic expectations, setting the dieter up for failure, subsequent guilt and feelings of helplessness at ever overcoming their weight problem.

The American Dietetic Association http://www.eatright.org/default.aspx indicated claims to identify (and avoid) fad diets; they are summarized in Table 12.5.

Very low-energy diets provide 800 kcal/day or less. Their use without a medical supervision is not justified, and they should not be recommended, both for their questionable cardiac safety and because they do not facilitate the gradual modification of eating habits, nutritional knowledge and skills, which are required for long-term weight maintenance.

Efficacy and Limits

A correct dieting approach can help to improve dietary habits and maintaining a long-term healthy nutrition. Therefore, it should be included in every obesity treatment program.

Short-term Efficacy

The short-term efficacy of low-calorie diets has been consistently demonstrated independent of the macronutrient composition of the diets. A calorie deficit of 500 to 1000 kcal/day can determine a weight loss of about 1 to 2 lb/week and is therefore recommended in every obesity treatment (NHI, 1998).

Long-term Efficacy

The limit of this approach consists in the metabolic adaptation of the organism to a low-calorie intake. The restriction of energy intake and the subsequent weight loss are associated with compensatory changes in energy expenditure, which oppose the maintenance of a body weight that is different from the usual weight (Leibel, 1995). These compensatory changes may account for the poor long-term efficacy of dieting if not adequately integrated with physical exercise. The reduction of dieting-induced weight loss is one of the factors leading to treatment drop-out, which is rather high and reaches 30 to 50 % of patients at one year (Melin I et al., 2006; Dansinger ML et al., 2005; Dalle Grave, 2005). The reasons for dropping out are currently under investigation and comprise socio-demographic (age, gender, employment), anthropometric (initial body weight, number of dieting attempts) and psychological (lower quality of life, mental distress) factors.

Other "downfalls of dieting" are the lack of satisfaction and feelings of hunger that may lead some people to engage in binge eating once food is available. Restrictive eating may also promote preoccupation with food and eating and other psychopathological problems. A small but significant minority of young women, who diet in pursuit of an ever-thinner ideal, is at risk for anorexia nervosa and/or bulimia nervosa. Dieting has also been reported to be associated with depression, low self-esteem, and negative body image. Results of a classic study of average-weight male volunteers, who reduced their body weight to 24% below normal limits, revealed marked symptoms of depression, apathy, and food preoccupation, in addition to binge eating (Keys, 1950). According to the above-quoted observations, some investigators have suggested that dieting is associated with the development of eating disorders (Hsu, 1997; McFarlanc, 1999). Whereas aggressive dieting may clearly have these side effects in normal-weight people, the relevance of these findings to obese individuals who wish to lose weight through modest caloric restriction is negligible as demonstrated by Wadden et al., (2004). The authors conclude that concerns about the possible adverse behavioral consequences of dieting should not dissuade primary care providers from recommending energy restrictions to obese individuals.

Conclusion

A correct dieting approach should be part of any obesity treatment because an obese subject needs to modify his energy balance and dietary habits. It is important that the effects and limitations of the dieting approach be clear to obese subjects before the beginning of the treatment. Dieting should be integrated with other approaches (physical exercise, psychological support) as needed by the individual patient to improve treatment outcome.

References

American Dietetic Association http://www.eatright.org/default.aspx

Biener L. & Heaton A. (1995) Women dieters of normal weight: their motives, goals and risks. *Am J Public Health* 85, 714–717.

Bravata D.M., Sanders L., Huang J., Krumholz H.M., Olkin I., Gardner C.D., Bravata D.M. (2003). Efficacy and safety of low-carbohydrate diets: a systematic review. *JAMA, 289(14),* 1837-50.

Dalle Grave R., Calugi S., Molinari M., Petroni M.L., Bondi M., Compare A., Marchesini G. and the QUOVADIS Study Group. (2005). Weight Loss Expectations in Obese Patients and Treatment Attrition: An Observational Multicenter Study. *Obesity Res.*, 13 (11), 1961—69.

Dansinger, M.L., Gleason JA, Griffith J.L., Selker H.P., Schaefer E.J. *(2005)* Comparison of the Atkins, Ornish, Weight Watchers, and Zone Diets for Weight Loss and Heart Disease Risk Reduction A Randomized Trial. *JAMA, 293,*:43-53.

Freedman M., King J, and Kennedy E. (2001). Popular diets: a scientific review. *Obesity Research 9,* 1-40.

Food and Nutrition Board, Institute of Medicine (2004). Dietary Reference Intakes: The Essential Guide to Nutrient Requirements. Washington DC, National Academies Press (http://www.nap.edu).

Foster G.D., Wyatt H.R., Hill J.O., McGuckin B.G., Brill C., Mohammed B.S., Szapary P.O., Rader D.J., Edman J.S and Klein S. (2003) A randomized trial of a Low-Carbohydrate Diet for Obesity *N Engl J Med 348,* 2082-90.

Hsu L.K. (1997) Can dieting cause an eating disorder*? Psychological Medicine*, *27,* 509-513.

Keys A., Brozek J., Henschel A., Mickelsen F., Taylor H.L. (1950). *The biology of human starvation*. Minneapolis: University of Minneapolis Press,.

Leibel R.L., Rosenbaum M., Hirsch J. (1995). Changes in energy expenditure resulting from altered body weight. *N Engl J Med*, *332(10),* 621-8.

McFarlane T., Polivy J., McCabe R.E. (1999). Help, not harm: psychological foundation for a nondieting approach toward health. *J Soc Issues*, *55*, 261–76.

Melin. I, Reynisdottir S., Berglund L., Zamfir M., Karlström B. (2006). Conservative treatment of obesity in an academic obesity unit. Long-term outcome and drop-out. *Eat Weight Disord. 11*, 22-30.

National Institute of Health, National Health, Lung and Blood Institute (1998). Clinical Guidelines on the identification, evaluation and treatment of overweight and obesity in adults—the evidence report. NIH Publication, N° 98-4083.

Wadden T.A., Foster G.D., Sarwer D.B., Anderson D.A., Gladis M., Sanderson R.S., Letchak R.V., Berkowitz R.I., and Phelan S. (2004). Dieting and the development of eating disorders in obese women: results of a randomized controlled trial *Am J Clin Nutr 80*, 560–8.

In: Pathways to Obesity and Main Roads to Recovery
Editor: Piergiuseppe Vinai
ISBN: 978-1-61122-740-6

Chapter XIII

Self-help

Ilyse Dobrow DiMarco
American Institute for Cognitive Therapy, New York, USA

Abstract

This chapter reviews what is currently known about self-help weight loss treatment programs. These programs are classified into one of two groups: "traditional" self-help programs, which utilize written materials, and internet-based self help programs, which contain features accessible only via the internet. The specific features of the programs are described with a focus on the myriad differences among the programs. Extant evidence supporting the programs is reviewed. Limitations of the programs are highlighted, and suggestions for addressing these limitations are presented. Finally, recommendations are provided for clinicians who work with individuals pursuing self-help weight loss options.

Introduction

The most widely studied and empirically supported treatment for weight loss is group behavioral weight loss (BWL) treatment. Group BWL programs vary in terms of the specific dietary and exercise prescriptions they provide, but generally incorporate strategies such as self-monitoring of food intake, exercise, and weight; problem solving; cognitive restructuring; social support initiatives; education about nutrition and physical activities; and the use of stimulus control techniques and reinforcement (Wadden, Crerand, & Brock, 2005; West, Gore, & Leuders, 2007). Taken together, results from studies of group BWL suggest that individuals in such groups lose approximately 9 to 10% of their initial body weight (Wadden & Foster, 2000; Wing, 2002). This represents a clinically significant weight loss (NHLBI Obesity Education Initiative Expert Panel, 1998). However, weight maintenance has been more elusive. Long-term maintenance of weight loss among individuals in BWL groups has been found to be poor (Latner & Wilson, 2007a).

An alternative to group treatment for weight loss is self-help treatment, in which participants guide themselves through a weight-loss protocol. Self-help is significantly less costly and more easily disseminable than is group treatment and is thus a more feasible option for most overweight/obese individuals (Wadden & Osei, 2002). Self-help strategies may also be more empowering and less stigmatizing than other forms of treatment (Latner, 2001, 2008). In addition, studies of continuing-care self-help programs have indicated that self-help treatment might help facilitate weight-loss maintenance (Latner & Wilson, 2007a; see below for a more detailed discussion of these programs). In their studies of the National Weight Control Registry, a sample of thousands of successful weight losers, Wing and colleagues (i.e., Butryn, Phelan, & Wing, 2007) found that approximately 1/3 of registry participants lost weight using self-guided methods; 96% of these participants maintained their weight loss at two-year follow-up. This suggests that self-help is a popular and viable method for weight loss.

This chapter will describe extant research on self-help treatment programs, both in terms of the structure of these programs and the evidence for their efficacy. The limitations of this research and its applicability to clinical practice will be discussed.

"Traditional" Self-help Programs

Over the past 20 years, a number of studies have described and evaluated self-help programs for overweight/obesity. However, there is a great deal of variation among the programs that have been studied, as far as what types of materials are given to participants, how much clinician contact is provided, and the extent to which all of the elements of traditional BWL treatment are incorporated into the treatment. Below, the various types of self-help programs will be described. Then, the results of studies of these programs will be summarized, with a focus on common themes in the findings. These programs have been labeled "traditional" self-help programs, in order to distinguish them from the newer internet-based self-help programs.

Most traditional self-help programs provide some form of written materials that participants are expected to follow. The quality and quantity of the materials provided vary widely. Some programs' materials consist of basic information about nutrition and exercise (i.e., Ash et al., 2006; Byrne, Meerkin, Laukkanen, Ross, Fogelholm, & Hills, 2006; Christian et al., 2008; Goulis et al., 2004; Heshka et al., 2003). Others provide materials emphasizing certain crucial aspects of BWL programs, like self-monitoring of diet and exercise (i.e., Goulis et al., 2004; Miller, Eggert, Wallace, Lindeman, & Jastremski, 1993), or utilize texts based on popular diet plans, such as Zone (Sears, 1997; Sears & Lawren, 1995), Atkins (Atkins, 1998, 2002; Atkins & Gare, 1995), Weight Watchers (Weight Watchers Publishing Group, 1998), and Ornish (Ornish, 1997, 2001) (i.e., Dansinger, Gleason, Griffith, Selker, & Schaefer, 2005; Foster et al., 2003; Gardner et al., 2007). Still others provide comprehensive behavioral weight-loss texts, such as the LEARN program for weight management (Brownell, 2004) (i.e., Carels, Young, Coit, Clayton, Spencer & Hobbs, 2008a; Carels et al., 2008b; Foster et al., 2003; Gardner et al., 2007; Wing, Venditti, Jakicic, Polley, & Lang, 1998; Womble et al., 2004). A few programs even provide participants with personalized materials, in which behavioral goals are custom-tailored to the individual via a computer program (i.e.,

Adachi, Sato, Yamatsu, Ito, Adachi, & Yamagami, 2007; Byrne et al., 2006; Christian et al., 2008).

Traditional self-help programs have also differed as far as the amount and type of clinician contact they provide. Some of these programs can be considered "pure" self-help programs, because there is little to no clinician contact. In such programs, participants are essentially told to follow study materials and typically report to a study center only to complete assessments (i.e., Ash et al., 2006; Byrne et al., 2006; Carels et al., 2008a; Miller et al., 1993; Wing et al., 1998). Others are better characterized as "guided self-help" programs, because participants have regular (if minimal) contact with clinicians. In some programs, this contact occurs on an individual, face-to-face basis, during which clinicians review aspects of the written materials and monitor participant progress (Christian et al., 2008; Foster et al., 2003; Goulis et al., 2004; Heshka et al., 2003; Womble et al., 2004). Other programs have group meetings, during which study materials are reviewed (Dansinger et al., 2005; Gardner et al., 2007; Hellerstedt & Jeffery, 1997). Still others keep in contact with participants via regular phone sessions (Carels et al., 2008b; Hellerstedt & Jeffrey, 1997; Park, Perri, & Rodrigue, 2003) or letters (Adachi et al., 2007).

Another difference between the various traditional self-help programs concerns the aspects of BWL they emphasize. For example, some encourage (and even mandate) regular return of food and exercise self-monitoring records (i.e., Carels et al., 2008a, 2008b; Goulis et al., 2004; Miller et al., 1993; Park et al., 2003) while others do not (i.e., Diabetes Prevention Program [DPP] Research Group, 2002; Foster et al., 2003). Those programs utilizing a structured BWL manual, like LEARN (Brownell, 2004), impart the full package of BWL techniques (i.e., problem solving; cognitive restructuring; social support initiatives; psychoeducation; stimulus control), while other programs merely emphasize certain aspects of BWL, such as dietary change. Another difference concerns who provides the treatment; across different studies, medical doctors, psychologists, dieticians, and graduate students have been study clinicians.

As the types of self-help programs in the literature vary widely, so, too, do the results of these programs. Some studies report negligible post-treatment weight losses. For example, mean weight loss in Christian et al.'s (2008) intervention group, in which participants received individually tailored eating and exercise goals, was .081 kg after 12 months. However, other programs have yielded substantial weight reduction; for example, in Goulis et al.'s (2004) intervention group, in which participants were mandated to transmit self-monitoring data, mean weight loss was 12.4 kg after six months. Taken together, results of studies of traditional self-help programs indicate that such programs yield minimal to modest weight losses. Few of the studies followed participants after one year, and those that did invariably found that substantial weight regain had occurred (i.e., DPP Research Group, 2002; Heshka et al., 2003, Wing et al., 1998).

In examining the results of studies of traditional self-help programs, some general observations can be made. First, there is substantial evidence (i.e., Goulis et al., 2004; Miller et al., 1993; Park et al., 2003) that participants who have more contact with clinicians lose significantly more weight than those who are given a manual and left to their own devices. In their comprehensive review of minimal contact self-help studies, Butryn and colleagues (Butryn, Phelan, & Wing, 2007) hypothesized that regular contact with a professional may cause participants to feel "accountable" to someone for their behaviors, and, therefore, serves to increase their motivation to follow the prescribed program. It is worth noting, however, that the more clinician contact a program entails, the more labor-intensive the program becomes. This, in turn, makes the program less available and accessible to participants. In addition, several studies (i.e., Carels et al., 2008a, 2008b; Hellerstedt & Jeffery, 1997) did not find a correlation between more clinician contact and better therapeutic outcomes. In fact, Hellerstedt and Jeffery (1997) found that participants who received bibliotherapy and minimal clinician contact lost twice as much weight as participants who received weekly clinician check-in phone calls for 24 weeks.

Butryn and colleagues (2007) also conclude that in general, traditional self-help programs that are more structured appear to yield better results. One aspect of a program's structure that appears to be particularly important is the regular keeping of self-monitoring records, in which participants record both energy intake and exercise. A number traditional self-help studies found that when programs encouraged and/or mandated completion of self-monitoring records, participants lost more weight than when record keeping was not encouraged/mandated (i.e., Adachi et al., 2007; Goulis et al., 2004). Not surprisingly, several studies (i.e., Carels et al., 2008a; Park et al., 2003) found a significant association between the amount of weight participants lost and the amount of self-monitoring records they completed. Also not surprisingly, other markers of adherence to the weight loss program (i.e., number of guided self-help sessions attended, adherence to dietary and exercise recommendations) have been found to be significantly associated with amount of weight lost (i.e., Dansinger et al., 2005; Heshka et al., 2003; Womble et al., 2004).

The few studies examining self-help bibliotherapy using popular weight-loss books, including Zone, Atkins, Weight Watchers, and Ornish (i.e., Dansinger et al., 2005; Foster et al., 2003; Gardner et al., 2007), have reported mixed results. Dansinger and colleagues (Dansinger et al., 2005) found that followers of Zone, Atkins, Weight Watchers, and Ornish books lost similarly modest amounts of weight at one year (approximately 2 to 3 kg). Gardner et al., (2007) found that followers of the Atkins book lost significantly greater amounts of weight at one year (4.7 kg) than those following LEARN, Zone, and Ornish (each group lost approximately 2 kg). Foster and colleagues (2003) found no significant difference between weight losses of participants following LEARN versus Atkins. At one year, LEARN participants lost 2.5 % of body weight, while Atkins participants lost 4.4% of body weight. There is, therefore, no consistent evidence to suggest that any popular diet books are any more effective than a standard behavioral weight-loss protocol.

Finally, two studies (Adachi et al., 2007; Byrne et al., 2006) found that participants given individually tailored diet and exercise goals were more successful than those without personalized goals. A third study comparing a personalized program to a more generic one did not find any significant differences in weight loss between the two groups (and in fact, neither group lost significant amounts of weight; Christian et al., 2008). Results of studies of internet weight-loss programs, which will be discussed below, further support the idea that tailored weight-loss programs might be more effective than more generic programs.

Internet-based Self-help Programs

In recent years, researchers have been attempting to disseminate weight loss programs via the internet. The internet is in many ways an ideal medium for delivering self-help weight loss treatment—it is accessible to most, relatively inexpensive, and can put participants in touch with clinicians to whom they otherwise might not have access. Most of the internet programs that have been evaluated have been created by research teams at academic centers; very few commercial weight loss sites have been evaluated (there are, however, exceptions; see Gold, Burke, Pintauro, Buzzell, & Harvey-Berino, 2007, Tate, Jackvony, & Wing, 2006; Womble et al., 2004).

As with the traditional self-help programs, there is much variety in the specific features offered by the various internet self-help programs. For example, some of these programs are structured behavioral weight-loss programs, and include all elements of standard BWL, including lessons on key behavioral concepts and an emphasis on goal setting and self-monitoring (i.e., Gold et al., 2007; Micco, Gold, Buzzell, Leonard, Pintauro & Harvey-Berino, 2007; Tate, Jackvony, & Wing, 2003; Tate et al., 2006; Tate, Wing, & Winett, 2001; Webber, Tate, & Bowling, 2008). Others are less structured, encouraging a self-guided approach through the various website features and emphasizing certain weight-loss elements such as diet and exercise (i.e., Rothert et al., 2006; Womble et al., 2004).

Studies of internet programs have also varied the amount of clinician contact that is available to participants. On one extreme, some studies feature a treatment group(s) that was given no opportunity for interaction with a clinician (i.e., Digenio, Mancuso, Gerber, & Dvorak, 2009; Rothert et al., 2006; Tate et al., 2001; 2003, 2006; White et al., 2004; Wing, Pinto, Crane, Kumar, Weinberg, & Gorin, 2009). Other programs give feedback to participants in the form of automated messages, tailored to dietary and exercise information that participants provide (e.g., Rothert et al., 2006; Tate et al., 2006). Several programs include feedback from a "live" counselor who emails participants with suggestions and comments based on inputted diet/exercise data; in some of these studies, participants have the opportunity to communicate with the clinician and ask questions, via email or an online moderated group "chat" session (e.g., Digenio et al., 2009; Hunter et al., 2008; Morgan, Lubans, Collins, Warren, & Callister, 2009; Tate et al., 2001, 2003, 2006; White et al., 2004). Towards the other extreme, some programs offer weekly group BWL sessions online, led by a clinician who is available to chat with participants (e.g., Gold et al., 2007; Micco et al., 2007). Others enhance the internet program with regular telephone or face-to-face meetings with clinicians (e.g., Christian et al., 2008; Digenio et al., 2009; Micco et al., 2007; Williamson et al., 2006).

As with studies of traditional self-help, results of studies of internet programs vary. In the more efficacious internet programs (e.g., Gold et al., 2007; Micco et al., 2007; Tate et al., 2003), results are comparable to those of successful traditional self-help BWL programs and superior to the results of standard care, with 12-month weight losses averaging approximately 5 kg. In a recent review of internet weight loss treatments, Saperstein and colleagues (Saperstein, Atkinson, & Gold, 2007) maintain that a critical feature of a successful internet program is the provision of personalized feedback to participants. Several studies have shown that an internet BWL program yielded greater weight losses than a less-structured website (i.e., Gold et al., 2007; Rothert et al., 2006; Tate et al., 2001; Womble et al., 2004)

As with the traditional self-help studies, the majority of the evidence from internet studies suggests that participants who have more access to clinicians lose more weight than those with limited or no clinician contact (i.e., Digenio et al., 2009; Tate et al., 2003). However, this contact need not occur on a face-to-face basis. Interestingly, Tate and colleagues (Tate et al., 2006) found no significant differences in treatment outcome between participants receiving automated feedback and those receiving feedback from clinicians, suggesting that a "computerized clinician" can be effective. Further, Micco and colleagues (2007) found no differences in weight loss between participants meeting in-person for monthly group sessions and those who attended group meetings through an online chat forum, suggesting again that it is not necessarily "face time" with a clinician that matters. Rather, it might simply be that any form of personalized support can lead to better outcomes.

As discussed above, the more clinician contact a program entails, the more labor-intensive the program becomes; this, in turn, makes the program less accessible to participants. A program that involves regular clinician contact in addition to an internet site (i.e., one of the groups in Digenio and colleagues' [2009] study featured weekly face-to-face contact with a clinician for three months) cannot be offered to large numbers of people. Further, while many of the most effective internet programs appear to be those offered by academic research sites, such programs are not widely available for commercial use.

Finally, and not surprisingly, in many studies, adherence to the internet program (i.e., amount of log-ins to the program, amount of monitoring records completed) was correlated with weight loss; those who signed on to internet programs more often were likely to be more successful than those who signed on intermittently (i.e., Digenio et al., 2009; Gold et al., 2007; Tate et al., 2001, 2003; Webber et al., 2008). A challenge for creators of weight-loss websites is to somehow motivate users to continuously log-in. Recently, Webber and colleagues (Webber et al., 2008) attempted to address this issue by beginning their internet weight-loss program with a face-to-face clinician session utilizing motivational enhancement techniques; one of two treatment groups also received weekly calls from clinicians who utilized these same techniques. However, results indicated that these weekly calls conferred no additional benefit for participants.

Studies of internet programs are still relatively new, and follow-up data are lacking. Several studies suffer from methodological limitations (i.e., basing results on self-reported weights; Rothert et al., 2006, only presenting completer analyses; Booth, Nowson, & Matters, 2008). More methodologically rigorous research, with longer follow-up periods, is necessary. As there has been very little work examining popular commercial internet programs, evaluations of such programs would be particularly valuable.

Limitations and Caveats

Traditional and internet-based self-help weight loss programs share several limitations. As mentioned, few studies of these programs have followed participants over the long-term. Those studies that included longer-term follow-ups reported poor outcomes, with many participants re-gaining weight (i.e., DPP Research Group, 2002; Heshka et al., 2003, Wing et al., 1998). Another problem endemic to nearly all types of weight-loss programs is participant attrition. The attrition rate in behavioral weight-loss treatments is 32% on average (Davis & Addis, 1999). Even among those who continue to attend weight-loss programs, adherence to program components (i.e., for example, self-monitoring) is often poor.

Further, weight losses reported in most trials of self-help treatment are quite modest. Participants in these programs do not typically lose substantial amounts of weight, as they might with a severely restrictive diet or weight-loss surgery. Therefore, self-help treatments are not appropriate for morbidly obese individuals for whom substantial weight loss is a primary goal. Self-help weight-loss treatment is perhaps best viewed as the least intensive treatment option in a stepped-care treatment plan (Latner & Wilson, 2007b), to be tried initially by individuals looking to lose 5 to 10% of their body weight. If self-help treatment is not effective, more intensive interventions must be pursued.

Obesity treatment researchers have attempted to address several of the apparent limitations of self-help weight-loss programs. For example, some (i.e., Latner & Wilson, 2007a; Perri, Sears, & Clark, 1993; Wing, Tate, Gorin, Raynor, & Fava, 2006) have stressed the importance of continuing to provide support to participants who have completed the active phase of weight-loss treatment (be it self-help treatment or a more intensive treatment). This ongoing support can come in several forms: as regular in-person "check-in" meetings with a clinician; as continued group support meetings; or as internet-based contact. Internet contact can include regular videos of/emails from clinicians, posted behavioral lessons, online group chats/lessons, uploading of self-monitoring records, or simply access to a website geared towards weight-loss maintenance.

In general, studies have shown that participants in continuing-care programs experience significantly less weight regain than those who do not participate in such programs (see reviews by Latner, 2008; Latner & Wilson, 2007a; and Milsom, Perri, & Rejeski, 2007 for comprehensive discussions of continuing care programs). Results of recent studies comparing internet-based continued care with in-person continued care have been equivocal; some studies found both types of care to be basically equivalent (Harvey-Berino, Pintauro, Buzzell, & Gold, 2004; Wing et al., 2008), while others found in-person care to be superior (Harvey-Berino et al., 2002; Svetkey et al., 2008). The type of internet-based continued care that is offered varies from program to program; some simply offer access to a weight-maintenance website (i.e., Svetkey et al., 2008), while others provide regular contact with clinicians via internet chat or email contact (i.e., Harvey-Berino et al., 2002, 2004; Wing et al., 2008).

Ongoing support can clearly help participants in weight-loss programs maintain their treatment gains. However, not all participants who are offered ongoing support will avail themselves of this support, either because they cannot access it due to logistical or financial concerns or because they are not motivated to continue with treatment. Dropout rates from behavioral weight-loss programs rise steadily over time. To address this problem, some self-help weight-loss maintenance programs, like the Trevose Behavior Modification Program (see Latner & Wilson, 2007a), have made treatment adherence a necessary condition of program participation. Individuals in the Trevose program must follow specific rules throughout monthly maintenance meetings; these rules include attending every meeting, achieving specific weight-loss goals, and consistently completing and submitting food records. Anyone who does not meet these requirements is removed from the program. A number of individuals do not succeed in following the rules; however, those who do have excellent outcomes. In a study by Latner and colleagues (Latner, Wilson, Stunkard, & Jackson, 2002), 43.8% of individuals in the program remained after two years, and lost an average of 19% of their body weight.

Another potentially useful method for addressing attrition and adherence issues involves incorporating motivational interviewing techniques into self-help treatment. As described by Miller and Rollnick (2002), MI is as "a participant-centered, directive method for enhancing intrinsic motivation to change by exploring and resolving ambivalence" (Miller & Rollnick, 2002, p. 25; see Miller & Rollnick, 2002 for an in-depth description of MI principles and techniques). Several studies have examined MI as an adjunct to self-help/guided self-help BWL (Carels et al., 2008a, 2008b; Christian et al., 2008; Dobrow DiMarco, Klein, Clark, &

Wilson, 2009; Webber et al., 2008). Three of the studies directly compared a guided self-help treatment enhanced with MI techniques against one without enhancement. In their pilot study of the use of MI with the LEARN manual (Brownell, 2004), Dobrow DiMarco and colleagues (Dobrow DiMarco et al., 2009) found significant differences in the areas of eating concern and control over eating, favoring MI-enhanced guided self-help. Between-group effect size estimates indicated a small advantage for MI-enhanced guided self-help in weight loss. Carels et al., (2008a, 2008b) also studied the use of MI with the LEARN manual (Brownell, 2004). They, however, found no treatment differences between a manual-only group and a group receiving one face-to-face motivational enhancement session, one problem-solving session, and weekly phone check-ins. In the Webber et al., (2008) study, as mentioned above, participants receiving a one session face-to-face MI intervention as an adjunct to an internet program fared equally well as those receiving this introductory session plus weekly online chat sessions conducted in the MI style. As MI was utilized in both conditions, it is difficult to make conclusions about its efficacy; it is possible that MI was most useful as a stand-alone introductory treatment rather than as a supplement during active treatment. Further research must be conducted before firm conclusions can be reached concerning the role of MI in self-help weight-loss treatment.

Conclusion

As the above review of research attests, successful self-help programs can help participants achieve modest weight losses. What is also clear from past research, however, is that not all self-help/guided self-help programs are created equal. In working with individuals who wish to lose weight with minimal guidance, clinicians can make several key recommendations. First, participants should be encouraged to follow a structured behavioral weight-loss program, such as the program detailed in Brownell's LEARN (2004) manual. The few studies of popular weight-loss diet books (i.e., Atkins, Ornish, Weight Watchers, Zone) have not consistently found these books to be superior to behavioral manuals. Therefore, clients would be best served to utilize manuals based on the treatment (BWL) that has received the most consistent empirical support. If participants wish to utilize the internet in their weight-loss efforts, they should be educated about the various available internet options. Websites developed at academic research centers have thus far been found to be more effective than popular weight-loss websites, which have been understudied. Clients should be encouraged to seek out the former, if available (the VTrim program, the behavioral website utilized by Gold et al., 2007 and Micco et al., 2007, is now commercially available). If clients wish to use a popular or fad website, they should also be encouraged to use a structured BWL manual to accompany the site.

Self-guided dieters should be encouraged to self-monitor their weight, eating, and exercise while they are actively losing weight and should continue to monitor their weight while trying to maintain weight loss. Studies (i.e., Klem, Wing, McGuire, Seagle, & Hill, 1997; Linde, Jeffery, French, Pronk, & Boyle, 2005; Wing, Tate, Gorin, Raynor, Fava, & Machan, 2007) have indicated that daily weighing is associated with successful weight-loss maintenance. If daily weights begin trending upwards, clients can then resume utilizing essential BWL strategies (i.e., for example, monitoring of eating and exercise). Goal-setting is also a very important part of BWL programs, and clients should be encouraged to set both short- and long-term goals for diet and exercise as well as for other lifestyle changes (i.e., changing food shopping habits, seeking family support for weight loss efforts).

Clients may not be successful with self-guided weight-loss efforts. Clinicians can address motivational issues by utilizing a motivational interviewing-style intervention (Miller & Rollnick, 2002). Clinicians need not be formally trained in MI; rather, they can simply guide clients through a decisional balance exercise, in which the short- and long-term pros and cons of weight-loss efforts are articulated. If clients are seemingly motivated and adhering to a self-guided BWL program but are unable to lose weight, clinicians might recommend a more intensive form of treatment. As mentioned above, self-help weight-loss efforts are most appropriate as the first step in a stepped care model of weight loss. Later steps might include participation in a behavioral weight-loss group or individual treatment or, at the extreme end, weight-loss surgery. Further, self-help programs could be used as adjuncts to more intensive types of treatments, such as very low-calorie diets (VLCDs) or weight-loss medications (Latner, 2001).

It is also important to remember that weight regain is a potential problem for all individuals who have lost weight, whether via a self-help program or an intensive intervention. Clinicians should make their clients aware of this issue and discuss a maintenance plan that is appropriate for each individual client. As discussed above, ongoing support from a clinician and/or peer group has been shown to facilitate maintenance of weight loss. Clients could also be encouraged to seek out a peer support group in their community.

Acknowledgments

The author would like to acknowledge G. Terence Wilson, Ph.D. for his helpful review and comments on earlier drafts of this chapter.

References

Adachi, Y., Sato, C., Yamatsu, K., Ito, S., Adachi, K., & Yamagami, T. (2007). A randomized controlled trial on the long-term effects of a one-month behavioral weight control program assisted by computer tailored advice. *Behavior Research and Therapy. 45,* 459-470.

Ash, S., Reeves, M., Bauer, J., Dover, T., Vivanti, A., Leong, C., et al., (2006). A randomized control trial comparing lifestyle groups, individual counseling and written information in the management of weight and health outcomes over 12 months. *International Journal of Obesity, 30,* 1557-1564.

Atkins, R. (1998). *Dr. Atkins' new diet revolution.* New York: Harper Collins.

Atkins, R. (2002). *Dr. Atkins' new diet revolution, revised edition.* New York: Harper Collins.

Atkins, R, & Gare, F. (1995). *Dr. Atkins' new diet cookbook.* New York: M Evans and Co. Inc.

Booth, A.O., Nowson, C.A., & Matters, H. (2008). Evaluation of an interactive, internet-based weight loss program: A pilot study. *Health Education Research, 23,* 371-381.

Brownell, K.D. (2004). *The LEARN Program for Weight Management* (10th ed.). Dallas: American Health Publishing Company.

Butryn, M.L., Phelan, S., & Wing, R.R. (2007). Self-guided approaches to weight loss. In J.D. Latner & G.T. Wilson (Eds.), *Self-help approaches for obesity and eating disorders* (pp. 3-20). New York: Guilford Press.

Byrne, N.M., Meerkin, J.D., Laukkanen, R., Ross, R., Fogelholm, M., & Hills, A.P. (2006). Weight loss strategies for obese adults: personalized weight management program vs. standard care. *Obesity, 14,* 1777-1788.

Carels, R.A., Young, K.M., Coit, C, Clayton, A.M., Spencer, A., & Hobbs, M. (2008a). Can following the caloric restriction recommendations from the Dietary Guidelines for Americans help individuals lose weight? *Eating Behaviors, 9,* 328-335.

Carels, R.A, Young, K.M., Coit, C.B., Darby, L.A., Clayton, A.M., Spencer, A.C., et al., (2008b). The failure of therapist assistance and stepped-care to improve weight loss outcomes. *Obesity, 16,* 1460–1462.

Christian, J.G., Bessesen, D.H., Byers, T.E., Christian, K.K., Goldstein, M.G., & Bock, B.C. (2008). Clinic-based support to help overweight patients with type 2 diabetes increase physical activity and lose weight. *Archives of Internal Medicine, 168,* 141-146.

Dansinger, M.L., Gleason, J.A., Griffith, J.L., Selker, H.P., & Schaefer, E.J. (2005). Comparison of the Atkins, Ornish, Weight Watchers, and Zone diets for weight loss and heart disease risk reduction: A randomized trial. *Journal of the American Medical Association, 293,* 43-53.

Davis, M. J., & Addis, M. E. (1999). Predictors of attrition from behavioral medicine treatments. *Annals of Behavioral Medicine, 21*, 339-349.

Diabetes Prevention Program Research Group. (2002). Reduction in the incidence of type 2 diabetes with lifestyle intervention or metformin. *New England Journal of Medicine, 346,* 393-403.

Digenio, A.G., Mancuso, J.P., Gerber, R.A., & Dvorak, R.V. (2009). Comparison of methods for delivering a lifestyle modification program for obese patients: a randomized trial. *Annals of Internal Medicine, 150,* 255-262.

Dobrow DiMarco, I., Klein, D.A., Clark, V.L., & Wilson, G.T. (2009). The use of motivational interviewing techniques to enhance the efficacy of guided self-help behavioral weight loss treatment. *Eating Behaviors, 10,* 134–136.

Foster, G. D., Wyatt, H. R., Hill, J. O., McGuckin, B. G., Brill, C., Mohammed, B. S., et al., (2003). A randomized trial of a low-carbohydrate diet for obesity. *New England Journal of Medicine, 348*, 2082-2090.

Gardner, C.D., Kiazand, A., Alhassan, S., Kim, S., Stafford, R.S., Balise, R.R., et al., (2007). Comparison of the Atkins, Zone, Ornish, and LEARN diets for change in weight and related risk factors among overweight premenopausal women. The A to Z weight loss study: A randomized trial. *JAMA, 297,* 969-977.

Gold, B.C., Burke, S., Pintauro, S., Buzzell, P., & Harvey-Berino, J. (2007). Weight loss on the web: A pilot study comparing a structured behavioral intervention to a commercial program. *Obesity, 15,* 155-164.

Goulis, D.G., Gialis, G.D., Boren, S.A., Lekka, I., Bontis, E., Balas, E.A., et al., (2004). Effectiveness of home-centered care through telemedicine applications for overweight and obese patients: A randomized controlled trial. *International Journal of Obesity, 28,* 1391-1398.

Harvey-Berino, J., Pintauro, S.J., Buzzell, P., & Casey Gold, E. (2004). Effect of Internet support on the long-term maintenance of weight loss. *Obesity Research, 12,* 320-329.

Harvey-Berino, J., Pintauro, S.J., Buzzell, P., DiGiulio, M., Casey Gold, E., Moldovan, C., et al., (2002). Does using the Internet facilitate the maintenance of weight loss? *International Journal of Obesity, 26,* 1254-1260.

Hellerstedt, W.L., & Jeffery, R.W. (1997). The effects of a telephone-based intervention on weight loss. *American Journal of Health Promotion, 11,* 177-182.

Heshka, S., Anderson, J.W., Atkinson, R.L., Greenway, F.L., Hill, J.O., Phinney, S.D., et al., (2003). Weight loss with self-help compared with a structured commercial program: A randomized trial. *JAMA, 289,* 1792-1798.

Hunter, C.M., Peterson, A.L., Alvarez, L.M., Poston, W.C., Brundige, A.R., Haddock, K., et al., (2008). Weight management using the internet: A randomized controlled trial. *American Journal of Preventive Medicine, 34,* 119-126.

Klem, M.L., Wing, R.R., McGuire, M.T., Seagle, H.M., & Hill, J.O. (1997). A descriptive study of individuals successful at long-term maintenance of substantial weight loss. *American Journal of Clinical Nutrition, 66,* 239-246.

Latner, J.D. (2001). Self-help in the long-term treatment of obesity. *Obesity Reviews, 2,* 87-97.

Latner, J.D. (2008). Obesity and the challenge of long-term weight loss: The role of continuing care and self-help. *The Behavior Therapist, 31,* 112-113.

Latner, J.D., & Wilson, G.T. (2007a). Continuing care and self-help in the treatment of obesity. In J.D. Latner & G.T. Wilson (Eds.), *Self-help approaches for obesity and eating disorders* (pp. 223-239). New York: Guilford Press.

Latner, J.D., & Wilson, G.T. (2007b). Preface. In J.D. Latner & G.T. Wilson (Eds.), *Self-help approaches for obesity and eating disorders* (pp. xi-xiv). New York: Guilford Press.

Latner, J.D., Wilson, G.T., Stunkard, A.J., & Jackson, M.L. (2002). Self-help and long-term behavior therapy for obesity. *Behavior Research and Therapy, 40,* 805-812.

Linde, J.A., Jeffery, R.W., French, S.A., Pronk, N.P., & Boyle, R.G. (2005). Self-weighing in weight gain prevention and weight loss trials. *Annals of Behavioral Medicine, 30,* 210-216.

Micco, N., Gold, B., Buzzell, P., Leonard, H., Pintauro, S., & Harvey-Berino, J. (2007). Minimal in-person support as an adjunct to internet obesity treatment. *Annals of Behavioral Medicine, 33,* 49-56.

Miller, W.C., Eggert, K.E., Wallace, J.P., Lindeman, A.K., & Jastremski, C. (1993). Successful weight loss in a self-taught, self-administered program. *International Journal of Sports Medicine, 14,* 401-405.

Miller, W. R., & Rollnick, S. (2002). *Motivational interviewing: Preparing people for change* (2nd ed.). New York: Guilford Press.

Milsom, V.A., Perri, M.G., & Rejeski, W.J. (2007). Guided group support and the long-term management of obesity. In J.D. Latner & G.T. Wilson (Eds.), *Self-help approaches for obesity and eating disorders* (pp. 205-222). New York: Guilford Press.

Morgan, P.J., Lubans, D.R., Collins, C.E., Warren, J.M., & Callister, R. (2009). The SHED-IT randomized controlled trial: Evaluation of an internet-based weight-loss program for men. *Obesity* advance online publication, 2 April 2009 (DOI:10.1038/oby.2009.85).

National Heart, Lung, and Blood Institute Obesity Education Initiative Expert Panel (1998). *Clinical guidelines on the identification, evaluation, and treatment of overweight and obesity in adults: The evidence report* (NIH Publication No. 98-4083). Washington, DC: National Institutes of Health.

Ornish, D. (1997). *Every Day Cooking with Dean Ornish.* New York: Harper Collins.

Ornish, D. (2001). *Eat more, weigh less*. New York: Harper Collins.

Park, T.L., Perri, M.G., & Rodrigue, J.R. (2003). Minimal intervention programs for weight loss in heart transplant candidates: A preliminary examination. *Progress in Transplantation, 13,* 284-288.

Perri, M.G., Sears, S.F. Jr., & Clark, J.E. (1993). Strategies for improving maintenance of weight loss: Toward a continuous care model of obesity management. *Diabetes Care, 16,* 200-209.

Rothert, K., Strecher, V.J., Doyle, L.A., Caplan, W.M., Joyce, J.S., Jimison, H.B., et al., (2006). Web-based weight management programs in an integrated health care setting: A randomized, controlled trial. *Obesity, 14,* 266-272.

Saperstein, S.L., Atkinson, N.L., & Gold, R.S. (2007). The impact of internet use for weight loss. *Obesity Reviews, 8,* 459-465.

Sears, B. (1997). *Zone perfect meals in minutes.* New York: Harper Collins.

Sears, B., & Lawren, W. (1995). *Enter the zone*. New York: Harper Collins.

Svetkey, L.P., Stevens, V.J., Brantley, P.J., Appel, L.J., Hollis, J.F., Loria, C.M., et al., (2008). Comparison of strategies for sustaining weight loss: the weight loss maintenance randomized controlled trial. *JAMA, 299,* 1139-1148.

Tate, D.F., Jackvony, E.H., & Wing, R.R. (2003). Effects of internet behavioral counseling on weight loss in adults at risk for type 2 diabetes: A randomized trial. *JAMA, 289,* 1833-1836.

Tate, D.F., Jackvony, E.H., & Wing, R.R. (2006). A randomized trial comparing human e-mail counseling, computer-automated tailored counseling, and no counseling in an internet weight loss program. *Archives of Internal Medicine, 166,* 1620-1625.

Tate, D.F., Wing, R.R., & Winett, R.A. (2001). Using internet technology to deliver a behavioral weight loss program. *JAMA, 285,* 1172-1177.

Wadden, T.A., Crerand, C.E., & Brock, J. (2005). Behavioral treatment of obesity. *Psychiatric Clinics of North America, 28,* 151-170.

Wadden, T. A., & Foster, G. D. (2000). Behavioral treatment of obesity. *Medical Clinics of North America, 84,* 441-461.

Wadden, T. A., & Osei, S. (2002). The treatment of obesity: An overview. In T. A. Wadden & A. J. Stunkard (Eds.), *Handbook of obesity treatment* (pp. 229-248). New York, NY: Guilford Press.

Webber, K.H., Tate, D.F., & Bowling, J.M. (2008). A randomized comparison of two motivationally enhanced Internet behavioral weight loss programs. *Behavior Research and Therapy, 46,* 1090-1095.

Weight Watchers Publishing Group (1998). *Weight watchers new complete cookbook.* New York: Macmillan Press.

West, D.S., Gore, S.A., & Lueders, N.K. (2007). Behavioral obesity treatment translated. In J.D. Latner & G.T. Wilson (Eds.), *Self-help approaches for obesity and eating disorders* (pp. 243-264). New York: Guilford Press.

White, M.A., Martin, P.D., Newton, R.L., Walden, H.M., York-Crowe, E.E., Gordon, S.T., et al., (2004). Mediators of weight loss in a family-based intervention presented over the Internet. *Obesity Research, 12,* 1050-1059.

Williamson, D.A., Walden, H.M., White, M.A., York-Crowe, E., Newton Jr., R.L., Alfonso, A., et al., (2006). Two-year internet-based randomized controlled trial for weight loss in African-American girls. *Obesity, 14,* 1231-1243.

Wing, R. R. (2002). Behavioral weight control. In T. A. Wadden & A. J. Stunkard (Eds.), *Handbook of obesity treatment* (pp. 301-316). New York, NY: Guilford Press.

Wing, R.R., Papandonatos, G., Fava, J.L., Gorin, A.A., Phelan, S., McCaffery, J, et al., (2008). Maintaining large weight losses: the role of behavioral and psychological factors. *Journal of Consulting and Clinical Psychology, 76,* 1015-1021.

Wing, R.R., Pinto, A.M., Crane, M.M., Kumar, R., Weinberg, B.M., & Gorin, A.A. (2009). A statewide intervention reduces BMI in adults: Shape Up Rhode Island results. *Obesity, 17,* 991-995.

Wing, R.R., Tate, D.F., Gorin, A.A., Raynor, H.A., & Fava, J.L. (2006). A self-regulation program for maintenance of weight loss. *New England Journal of Medicine, 355,* 1563-1571.

Wing, R.R., Tate, D.F., Gorin, A.A., Raynor, H.A., Fava, J.L., & Machan (2007). "STOP Regain:" Are there negative effects of daily weighing?. *Journal of Consulting and Clinical Psychology, 75,* 652-656.

Wing, R. R., Venditti, E., Jakicic, J. M., Polley, B. A., & Lang, W. (1998). Lifestyle intervention in overweight individuals with a family history of diabetes. *Diabetes Care, 21*, 350-359.

Womble, L. G., Wadden, T. A., McGuckin, B. G., Sargent, S. L., Rothman, R. A., & Krauthamer-Ewing, E. S. (2004). A randomized controlled trial of a commercial internet weight loss program. *Obesity Research, 12*, 1011-1018.

In: Pathways to Obesity and Main Roads to Recovery
Editor: Piergiuseppe Vinai
ISBN: 978-1-61122-740-6

Chapter XIV

Cognitive-behavioral Treatment (CBT) for Obesity

***Jennifer R. Shapiro*[1] *and Cynthia M. Bulik*[2]**
[1]Santech, Inc., La Jolla, CA, USA
[2]University of North Carolina, Department of Psychiatry, Chapel Hill, NC, USA

Abstract

Obesity is an epidemic with associated health risks and mortalities. Current guidelines suggest to treat less severe forms of obesity with Cognitive Behavioral Therapy (CBT) and more intensive treatments (e.g., medication management or surgery) for more severe cases. The aims of this chapter are to review the history and advancement of CBT, describe how it is applied to weight management of overweight individuals and discuss benefits and limitations of this approach to obesity. Finally, future research ideas and innovative methods of enhancing CBT for obesity are illustrated.

Introduction

Over the past 30 years, obesity has become a widespread epidemic. Approximately 66% of American adults are overweight (body mass index [BMI] ≥ 25 kg/m^2) or obese (BMI ≥ 30 kg/m^2; Manson & Bassuk, 2003). Given that obesity is associated with increased risk of various medical comorbidities (e.g., diabetes, cardiovascular disease, pain, cancer), all-cause mortality, and psychological problems (Anderson & Wadden, 1999), it is critical to continue to develop and enhance various types of obesity treatment. Current effective treatments consist of surgical, residential treatment, medication management, cognitive-behavioral therapy (CBT), and self-help. This chapter will focus on the use of CBT for obesity treatment. Specifically, the aims are to describe CBT in general but also how CBT is applied to weight management, review the history and advancement of CBT, discuss the effectiveness of CBT for obesity, and explain the benefits of limitations of CBT for obesity. Finally, future research ideas and innovative methods of enhancing CBT for obesity will be illustrated.

What Is CBT?

Behavioral Theory

Behavioral Theory suggests that all behaviors are acquired through learning. Behavior modification is a form of treatment that helps individuals acquire new behaviors by using positive and negative reinforcement and punishment. Although behaviorism has demonstrated success in changing behaviors (e.g., classical or operant conditioning) in both animals and humans, it does not acknowledge the importance of critical non-observable factors such as choice, moods, thoughts, and feelings.

Cognitive Theory

Cognitive Theory, on the other hand (coined by Aaron Beck in the1960s), proposes that thoughts and feelings precede actions such that inaccurate thoughts drive unhealthy feelings and behaviors. Thoughts (specifically inaccurate and/or unhealthy "automatic thoughts" that enter our minds immediately and without evaluation), feelings, attitudes ("core beliefs") and behaviors are essentially stable cognitive patterns concerning oneself, others, and the future that are determined from previous experience (Beck, Rush, Shaw, & Emery, 1979; Beck, 1995). For example, individuals tend to repeatedly perceive events through "shaded sunglasses" and consistently interpret information based on their core beliefs, which are commonly erroneous. Cognitive therapy aims to alter negative and/or unhealthy thoughts and replace them with healthier accurate ones that that improve resultant negative feelings and behaviors.

Cognitive-Behavioral Therapy

CBT blends the individual assumptions of both cognitive and behavioral theories. On the one hand, these two theories may be theoretically incompatible, such that strict behavioral theory does not acknowledge the role of thinking in changing behavior. However, CBT uses cognitive techniques along with behavioral strategies to help people make healthy behavioral changes.

CBT is an active form of therapy in which the patient and therapist use a collaborative process to change unhealthy thoughts and behaviors. CBT focuses on current thinking, problematic behavior, precipitating factors, and developmental events. The approach is goal oriented, problem focused, structured, and requires active participation of the patient. The therapist uses the Socratic method (asking questions to illustrate points and stimulate ideas) to help patients identify their thought patterns and ultimately change distorted thinking, mood, and problematic behavior (Beck, Rush, Shaw, & Emery, 1979; Beck, 1995). Many CBT therapies (including those for depression, anxiety, psychosis, eating disorders, and obesity) have been traced back to Beck given that Cognitive Therapy essentially includes aspects of both cognitive and behavioral work. CBT typically includes education about the pathology, the CBT model, training in identification of automatic thoughts and core beliefs, and then evaluating such beliefs based on their veracity (by gathering evidence for and against the thought) with the ultimate goal of the patient being able to independently challenge their dysfunctional thoughts. In addition, behavioral aspects may include self-monitoring of certain behaviors, behavioral activation to increase pleasurable activities, skills training, and relaxation techniques.

Why Use CBT for Obesity?

Early Psychological Approaches

Psychologists have applied psychotherapeutic principles and techniques to the treatment of obesity since the 1950s. At that time, psychodynamic methods were used, which suggested that obesity was related to underlying difficulties with identifying, containing, and expressing thoughts, feelings, and needs (Moreno, Fuhriman, & Hileman, 1995). Accordingly, therapy helped patients identify and tolerate various problems that were masked by eating rather than directly working on the dietary and physical activity behaviors associated with obesity. Given this indirect mode of treatment, psychodynamic therapy was not particularly helpful for obesity. Research by Stunkard (1958) found that 12/100 patients treated via psychodynamic treatment lost more than 20 pounds and only two maintained their weight loss after two years.

History of Behavioral Treatment for Obesity

Given the poor treatment outcomes associated with psychological treatment for obesity in the 1960s, behavioral theorists began to conceptualize and treat obesity based on learning principles. Obesity was conceptualized as a failure of self-control due to the immediate reinforcing aspects of eating (e.g., taste) serving as more important than the long-term aversive consequences (weight gain, comorbidities; Ferster, Nurenberger, & Levitt (1962/1996)). Thus, treatment consisted of learning principles such as classical and operant conditioning to pair the negative consequences of eating *during* the actual eating episode.

Initial data demonstrated the effectiveness of the behavioral approach for weight management such that 80% of patients lost over 20 pounds, and 30% lost over 40 pounds in a rather short time frame (Stuart, 1967/1996). This set the stage for continued use of behavioral therapy for obesity.

Over time, continued research on behavioral treatment honed in on specific strategies including self-monitoring, contingency management, and stimulus control to help individuals manipulate their environment to increase healthy eating and decrease unhealthy eating.

(Abramson, 1977; Brownell & Jeffery, 1987; Brownell & Kramer, 1989). Various outcome data demonstrated an average weight loss of one pound per intervention week. Interventions increased in length from about ten weeks in 1960s to 16 to 20 weeks in the 1980s, and thus demonstrated greater weight losses over time. For a further review, see Anderson, Shapiro, & Lundgren (2001).

Current Cognitive-Behavioral Therapy for Obesity

As treatment lasted longer (up to 20 weeks), the aforementioned specific behavioral strategies of self-monitoring, contingency management, and stimulus control were enhanced by adding additional features such as nutritional information, physical activity, relapse prevention, social support (Brownell & Jeffery, 1987; Keefe & Blumenthal, 1980; Stunkard & Berthold, 1985), and specific tools adapted from CBT (thought restructuring, behavioral chaining, skill training, etc.). The combination of all of these additional tools supported a longer intervention and thus resulted in greater weight loss.

However, although weight loss is certainly the goal of treatment, weight is de-emphasized as it is not a behavior per se, but rather a result of behaviors that can be altered during treatment. The following strategies are some components of CBT for obesity:

Nutrition Education: Given that obesity is the result of positive energy balance when intake exceeds output, patients must understand healthy nutrition as well as unhealthy and unstructured eating, (e.g., emotional eating for any other reason than hunger including boredom, anger, frustration, excitement, etc.), succumbing to cravings, and eating disordered behaviors (food restriction, purging). A common mistake often seen in overweight individuals is food restriction during the day, which frequently results in larger meals at night or late-night snacking. In this component of treatment, patients are educated about healthy and balanced nutrition, portion control, and setting regular eating times throughout the day (e.g., three meals and two planned snacks).

Self-Monitoring: Self-monitoring of energy intake and expenditure is one of the most important facets of obesity interventions (Brownell, 1997) as it enables patients to become aware of their current eating patterns (type and amount of food), helps them learn about the nutritional value of foods, assists in planning meals, supports healthy food choices, and better ensures that they remain within their daily caloric needs as they are held accountable to themselves and their provider. Importantly, self-monitoring helps patients change their unhealthy patterns and observe their new healthier behaviors. Table 14.1 depicts an example of a self-monitoring template for obesity treatment.

Table 14.1. Daily Self-Monitoring Form. (Extracted from Shapiro & Bulik, 2007)

Time	Food, Drink, and Amount	B: Binge C: Craving P: Purge	Situation	Thoughts	Feelings and Intensity	Rate feelings and intensity (0—8)

Physical Activity: CBT for obesity recommends that patients gradually increase both lifestyle and structured exercise and also decrease their sedentary time spent in front of a computer or television. Physical activity is essential for weight loss but is also highly correlated with long-term weight management and decreased medical comorbidities. Current treatment guidelines recommend approximately 60 minutes of moderate-vigorous intensity physical activity on most days per week (or 300 minutes per week) for weight loss (USDHHS/ODPHP, 2008).

Cognitive-Restructuring: Cognitive techniques helps individuals identify negative and unhealthy thoughts related to food, eating, and weight, and develop more rational beliefs. Following general CBT, individuals learn to identify their automatic thoughts, challenge them, consider alternative views, determine the effect of the automatic thought on other thoughts, feelings, and behaviors, and identify typical thinking errors. For example, a thought such as, "I ate one cup of ice cream when I meant to only eat ½ cup according to the recommended serving size; I blew it and I should just eat the whole pint!" may lead to a behavior consistent with this thought. The individual may then feel out of control and act in a consistent way, ultimately eating the entire pint of ice cream, leading to further guilt and negative mood, and potentially creating a vicious cycle. CBT would teach the patient to identify such distorted thoughts and to replace them with more accurate and healthier alternatives, so that they do not experience the intense negative mood and behaviors. In the previous example, an alternative thought such as, "Although I ate more ice cream than I wanted, it is not the end of the world. I actually previously would have eaten even more than one cup. I am still in control and can put the rest away for another time" may help resist the continuation of the eating episode as this person may feel more in control. Over time, patients will learn to believe their more rational thoughts. In addition, since negative mood and stress can result in overeating, cognitive techniques are used to identify and challenge other negative thoughts, which may not be directly related to weight but result in negative mood and thus overeating for emotional reasons (e.g., My spouse is mad at me because she chose to go shopping with the girls rather than have a quiet night on the couch with me. I'm just going to stay home and feel sorry for myself and eat these hot dogs and French fries). Table 14.2 provides a list of common thinking errors.

Behavioral Chaining: CBT helps individuals identify triggers to their eating behavior. Triggers may be anything that leads to unhealthy eating, including negative thoughts, certain moods, various situations (social gatherings, interpersonal conflict, food advertisements, etc.). They also learn about the positive and negative consequences of their eating behavior. For example, while eating may serve a positive role such as reducing hunger and relieving loneliness, it may also serve a negative function such as weight gain, further depressed mood, and guilt. CBT assists individuals in slowing down and thinking about both the triggers as well as consequences prior to eating for non-nutrition purposes. Lining up a series of triggers, behaviors, and consequences results in a behavioral chain that illustrates the cascade of thoughts, feelings, and behaviors for the patient. Tools are provided to break the chain that empower the patient to change the course of events by breaking the chain at several points along the way.

Table 14.2. Thinking Errors. Table extracted from Shapiro & Bulik (2007)

All or Nothing Thinking (or black and white, polarized, or dichotomous thinking)	Viewing a situation in only two categories instead of on a continuum. E.g., If I have one piece of cake, I will lose control and have to eat the whole thing.
Overgeneralizing	Condemning oneself as a total person on the basis of a single event, or believing that if something turns out badly once, then it will always happen that way. E.g., My weight remained the same this week even though I followed my plan. I will never lose more weight.
Mental Filter (or Selective thinking)	Paying more attention to one negative detail instead of looking at the big picture. E.g., Even though I had 10 less binges this week than last, I am still angry at myself for the one that I had.
Rationalizing	Making excuses to justify behavior. E.g., It really is not a bad idea to eat the entire half-gallon of ice cream because I do need more calcium in my diet.
Catastrophizing (or fortune telling)	Predicting that things will turn out negatively. E.g., I don't think self-help will help me because nothing ever helps me to stop binge eating.
Mind Reading	Attempting to guess what others are thinking. E.g., If I eat the sandwich for lunch, my colleagues will think I eat too much.
Magical Thinking	Drawing links between unrelated events. E.g., If I lose weight I will be happy, successful, and get married.
Personal Ineffectiveness	Believing that you can do nothing to change the situation. E.g., I just have to eat sweets all day at work because every morning my coworker leaves pastries on the desk next to me.

Behavioral Strategies: Aside from challenging thoughts, CBT also incorporates various behavioral strategies to help resist unhealthy eating behavior. In addition to the stimulus control strategies listed in Table 14.3, CBT helps individuals strengthen cues for desired behavior (plan an afternoon activity instead of going home alone and eating) and avoid eating in response to various triggers (e.g., build in a pause between having thought to eat after an emotional conflict and the actual act of eating). This pause will allow one to practice thought restructuring, focusing on the consequences, or finding an alternative behavior. In addition, individuals practice engaging in alternative behaviors instead of eating and resist their cravings to learn that the urges will subside over time.

Table 14.3. Stimulus Control Techniques taken from Brownell (1997). Table extracted from Anderson, Shapiro, & Lundgren (2001)

Technique	Description and rationale
Do Nothing Else While Eating	This reduces the likelihood that eating will become paired with other behaviors such as watching television, reading, or working. Engaging in activities while eating also reduces one's awareness of caloric consumption.
Eat in One Place	This allows eating to become associated with one specific chair or table position, rather than many places within the home or office, reducing the chance of cravings at various locations. Individuals who work and eat at the same desk should turn or use another side of the desk to consume food.
Follow an Eating Schedule	Following an eating schedule helps control unnecessary caloric intake. This helps clients gain control over eating patterns and it reduces eating associated with external cues.
Shop From a List	Shopping from a food list reduces unnecessary impulse purchases.
Buy Foods That Require Preparation	Buying foods that require preparation avoids easy, prepared meals.
Remove Serving Dishes From Table	Removing food from the table makes the automatic response to have a second helping more difficult, so one must think about the consequences of taking a second helping.
Serve and Eat One Portion at a Time	Clients should wait five minutes after the urge to have a second helping before consuming more food. This technique is used to interrupt automatic eating and slows the eating process. Therefore, a person is less likely to continue eating when full.
Keep Problem Foods Out of Sight	Store problem foods higher on the shelf and healthier foods more readily accessible.
Control Behaviors at the Table	Clients are instructed to not clean their plates; put forks down between bites; pause during the meal; leave the table after eating.

Relapse Prevention: Relapse prevention is critical to maintain treatment gains. Since weight regain is quite common, patients must learn how to maintain their weight loss, engage in lifestyle healthy behavior changes for the long run, and continue to practice their skills learned in CBT so that occasional lapses (e.g., overeating on vacation or at a birthday party) do not turn into relapses (i.e., giving up hope and returning to old habits). Individuals are taught to identify and plan for high-risk situations so that they feel prepared to cope when they occur. Review cards can be created in which patients can take them out in time of need to remind them of positive self statements, coping responses, alternative behaviors, and phone numbers of support people.

When to Use CBT?

Treatment Matching

Current treatment guidelines suggest a stepped-care approach for the treatment of obesity taking BMI, comorbidities, and treatment cost into consideration. Specifically, for a BMI of 25 to 29.9, low-cost approaches include self-help, physician counseling, or organized self-help, while more moderately priced treatment consist of commercial programs (e.g., professional based CBT, Weight Watchers, etc.). For a BMI of 30, treatment recommendations are more expensive and include meetings with a registered dietitian, pharmacotherapy, or multi-disciplinary programs. The National Institutes of Health (NIH; 1998) supports the use of medication in conjunction with lifestyle therapy for patients with a BMI $\geq$ 30 or $\geq$ 27 if comorbidities are present as well as for those who are at greatest medical risk, have not responded to traditional weight management, have no contraindications to use of medication, understand the risk, and need long-term treatment. Finally, for those with a BMI of 39.9 and above, treatment recommendations include residential programs and/or surgery. The NIH recommends surgical methods for those who are severely obese (BMI $\geq$ 40 or $\geq$ 35 with comorbidities) or when less invasive methods have failed (NIH, 1998).

CBT for Obesity: Typical Protocol

CBT for obesity typically consist of 16-20 week programs and are usually offered in group formats. A well-known example is Kelly Brownell's LEARN approach (Brownell, 1997, 2004), which is used in many University based settings and offers the CBT components discussed in this chapter. However, in addition to group settings, patients could also meet with a psychologist for individual CBT for obesity.

What Are Benefits and Limitations of CBT?

Results and Benefits of CBT for Obesity

While some individuals are successful at losing significant amounts of weight (Klem, Wing, McGuire, Seagle, & Hill, 1997), research demonstrates that the majority of patients lose a modest 10 to 15% of their initial body weight (Wadden & Sarwer, 1999). Although modest, this amount of weight loss correlates with improvements in associated comorbidities and all cause mortality (National Heart, Lung, and Blood Institute, 1998).

In addition, CBT is helpful for individuals who meet diagnostic criteria for eating disorders associated with obesity. Approximately 5 to 8% of obese individuals meet criteria for Binge Eating Disorder (BED; Bruce and Agras, 1992; Bruce and Wilfley, 1996), however, 30 to 70% of obese individuals seeking weight-loss treatment meet criteria for BED (de Zwaan, 2001). BED is defined by eating a large amount of food, in a short period of time, and feeling out of control, as well as several other associated features (American Psychiatric Association, 1994). CBT has demonstrated success for BED by helping individuals target their triggers and manage their thoughts, feelings, and behaviors associated with binge eating. Group CBT for BED has been shown to be effective at reducing number of days binged, BMI, disinhibition, hunger, depression, and self-esteem (Wilfley et al., 2002).

Finally, results from the National Weight Control Registry, a study that investigated individuals who have lost at least 30 pounds through various methods and maintained this loss for at least one year, found that they key behaviors associated with success included continued exercise, healthy diet and maintaining a calorie range, and self-monitoring (Wing & Hill, 2001). In addition, other studies have found that continued patient-provider contact has been associated with successful maintenance of weight loss (Bjorvell & Rossner, 1992; Perri, 1998).

Limitations of CBT

Although CBT demonstrates positive short-term success, long-term outcome of weight-loss treatment remains problematic. Notably, this is often the case with any approach used to lose weight. According to a review, most patients (regardless of method of weight loss) had regained 35% to 50% of their weight loss one year after treatment (Wadden & Sarwer, 1999). However, given that obesity has previously been treated as an acute disorder, few of these studies provided long-term care for patients. On a promising note, obesity is now being conceptualized as a chronic medical disorder that requires long-term care (Brownell & Rodin, 1990).

In addition to poor long-term results and weight regain, CBT has several other limitations including moderate to high drop-out rates (Wonderlich, de Zwaan, Mitchell, Peterson, & Crow, 2003). Second, our society and built environment usually do not support weight loss. Individuals are constantly faced with palatable high-fat, high-calorie foods (e.g., fast food), and/or large portions (restaurant style) that are often less expensive and easier to prepare than healthier meals. Further, our environments are built to accommodate more sedentary activities and less physical activity contributing to further difficulty with weight loss. Given these environmental demands, patients must put in much effort to apply their CBT tools to develop an environment for themselves that supports their healthy changes. Third, given the average weight loss of 10 to 15%, patients often feel discouraged when they want to lose more weight or when their weight plateaus before they reach their goals. To counteract discouragement, it is recommended to help patients modify unreasonable expectations and increase body acceptance in the early stages of treatment (Wilson, 1996). Finally, there are limited specialty clinics offering CBT for obesity leaving many populations underserved and further, even when available, such treatment is often not covered by managed care unless it is associated with another psychiatric condition.

Summary and Future Directions

In sum, obesity is an epidemic with associated health risks and mortalities. Current guidelines suggest matching patients to treatment with often less severe forms of obesity being matched to CBT. However, CBT is also important for those treated with even the more serious treatments (residential, medication, surgery) to teach patients the skills to manage their triggers, cravings, and behaviors, even when it is physically more difficult for them to consume food.

Given that CBT made into self-help formats do show promise, further treatment development on more desirable, feasible, acceptable, and effective self-help tools are needed for use as a first-step intervention or for those who are unable to receive care elsewhere due to cost, time, long waiting lists, lack of specialty care, and other logistics or for those who are too ashamed or embarrassed to seek care.

The use of modern information technology (such as e-mail, the Internet, personal digital assistants, text messaging, and other technological advances) may assist in reaching such underserved populations and may help improve adherence to treatment and decrease drop out, thus enabling more patients to complete an adequate dose of treatment and ultimately maintain their weight losses.

Our team has developed a CD-ROM-based CBT program in which individuals can work through at their own pace and at a location of their choosing. The CD-ROM offers CBT tools and techniques and uses an interactive mode of delivery with real people educating, explaining, and providing examples throughout the program. Several individuals who binge-eat for different reasons are depicted and demonstrate how they use various CBT techniques during treatment. Our CD-ROM program follows a ten-week schedule and provides both nutritional and behavioral lessons. We recently conducted a randomized controlled trial consisting of a ten-week CD-ROM-based CBT program versus traditional group CBT versus wait list (WL) control in 66 overweight individuals with BED. Results showed that 68% of those in the CD-ROM condition completed the study compared to 59% in the group treatment. Moreover, 67% of those in the CD-ROM condition reported that they continued to use the CD-ROM at least once or twice within eight weeks after study completion. Finally, 75% of those who completed the ten-week waiting list condition chose to receive the CD-ROM over Group treatment. Preliminarily, no significant differences emerged across the active treatment groups on most outcome measures. However, there was a significantly greater decline in binge days in the two active groups relative to WL. CD-ROM appears to be an acceptable and at least initially preferred method of CBT delivery for overweight individuals with BED, and after enrollment, those using CD-ROM may have higher completion rates and continue to practice their skills than those in traditional face-to-face CBT treatment approaches (Shapiro, Reba-Harrelson, Dymek-Valentine, Woolson, Hamer, & Bulik, 2007).

In terms of weight loss, Tate, Wing, and Winett (2001) randomly assigned 91 overweight individuals to participate in either a six-month structured internet education or to internet behavior therapy, in which they received 24 weekly behavioral lessons via email, weekly online submission of self-monitoring forms with feedback, and an online bulletin board. A total of 65 individuals provided follow-up data and results showed that by six months, the behavior therapy group lost significantly more weight than the education group (4.1 kg versus

1.6 kg, respectively), had a greater proportion of individuals losing at least 5% of initial body weight (45% versus 22%, respectively), and had greater changes in waist circumference. This demonstrates that the use of internet and e-mail correspondence can be an effective method of behavioral weight loss treatment. Tate, Jackvony, and Wing (2003) also compared an internet weight reduction program alone versus the program plus behavioral counseling via email for one year in individuals at risk of type II diabetes. Results showed that, at one year, when compared to the internet intervention alone, the addition of email counseling led to a greater weight reduction (2.0 kg versus 4.4 kg loss, respectively), and greater decreases in percentage of initial body weight lost (2.2% versus 4.8%, respectively), BMI (0.8 versus 1.6, respectively), and waist circumference (4.4 cm versus 7.2 cm, respectively).

Over the past few years, our society has become even more technological. Individuals are not only seeking health information online in which the web-based treatments previously described are applicable, but individuals have become accustomed to more instantaneous contact, communication, and information (e.g., mobile phones, text messaging, social networking, phone applications). Thus, researchers have been applying CBT strategies to reach people anytime and anywhere. Shapiro and colleagues (2008) tested the preliminary acceptability of text messaging (SMS) to self-monitor behaviors associated with obesity in children aged 5 to 13. A total of 58 children (of all weight ranges, although many were in the overweight range) and a participating parent were randomized to one of three conditions: traditional paper-and-pencil self-monitoring (PP; N = 18), SMS (N = 18), or no-monitoring control (C; N = 22). All families participated in a three-session intervention in small groups (approximately five families), which were homogenous to treatment condition. The intervention was short in duration (three sessions) and designed to increase healthy eating and activity by addressing three simple targeted behaviors, including increasing physical activity, decreasing sugar-sweetened beverages, and decreasing screen time. Families in the C condition participated in the intervention sessions and were not expected to self-monitor thereafter. Families in the PP condition were given self-monitoring forms and instructed to record the three targeted behaviors daily for both parent and child. Families in the SMS condition were given a mobile phone and instructed to input their data via two text messages per day (one for parent and one for child). Each adult and child in the SMS group received an immediate, automatic feedback message based on how close he/she came to meeting his/her targeted goals. An algorithm was used to create feedback messages according to: 1) how many goals were met (none, some, all), and 2) enhancement or deterioration from the previous day. Families were aware that the responses were automated. Families began monitoring on day one of the program. After the three weekly intervention sessions, families were instructed to continue daily monitoring for eight weeks. Results show that SMS is feasible and acceptable by participants. First, during the initial interview, 100% of the children stated that they hoped they would be randomized to the SMS condition. Second, drop-out rates were substantially lower in the SMS condition (N = 5, 27.8%) versus PP (N = 10, 55.6%) or C (N = 11, 50%). Third, we found a substantial difference between the two groups with a total of 43% versus 19% total monitoring in both children and adults in the SMS and PP conditions, respectively.

Similarly, Patrick and colleagues (2009) randomly assigned overweight adults to receive either printed materials about weight control or a four-month intervention that included personalized SMS and multimedia service (MMS; images, longer messages, audio), printed materials, and brief monthly phone calls from a counselor. After 16 weeks, the intervention group lost significantly more weight than the control group.

Conclusion

CBT is an effective method for obesity treatment and weight management. Collectively, given the limitations associated with the delivery of CBT along with the promising results of technologically innovative and upgraded treatment delivery modalities, future treatment development should continue to enhance these approaches. Our society has become more technological and thus researchers and clinicians need to keep up with this movement or else their approaches will soon be outdated. For example, there are various iPhone applications that promote weight management by helping individuals self-monitor their daily energy balance on their iPhone. Other applications and programs are available for continued reminders and support during the day. Using these more novel approaches to treatment may be less shameful, expensive, or burdensome than seeking professional help, may result in increased adherence given the acceptability, ease and flexibility, and may thus ultimately lead to more lasting weight management. Finally, such novel approaches can also be used with the treatment matching guidelines (either as a first step treatment, in conjunction with more severe treatments such as obesity, or as a maintenance tool) so that individuals constantly have CBT tools at their disposal.

References

Abramson, E. E. (1977). Behavioral approaches to weight control: An updated review. *Behavior Research and Therapy, 15*, 355-363.

American Psychiatric Association. (1994). *Diagnostic and statistical manual of mental disorders (4th ed.).* Washington, DC: American Psychiatric Association.

Anderson, D. A, Shapiro, J. R., & Lundgren, J. D. (2001). The behavioral treatment of obesity. *The Behavior Analyst Today,* 2, 133-140.

Anderson, D. A., & Wadden, T. A. (1999). Treating the obese patient. Suggestions for primary care practice. *Archives of Family Medicine, 8*(2), 156-167.

Beck, J. S. (1995). *Cognitive Therapy: Basics and Beyond* (p. 119). New York: Guilford Press.

Beck, A. T., Rush, A. J., Shaw, B. F., & Emery, G. (1979). *Cognitive Therapy of Depression.* New York: Guilford Press.

Bjorvell, H., & Rossner, S. (1992). A ten-year follow-up of weight change in severely obese subjects treated in a behavioral modification programme. *International Journal of Obesity, 16*, 623-625.

Brownell, K. D. (1997). *The LEARN program for weight control* (7th ed.). Dallas, Tex: American Health Publishing.

Brownell K. (2004). *The LEARN Program for Weight Management* (10th Edition). Dallas, TX: American Health Publishing Companies.

Brownell, K. D., & Jeffery, R. W. (1987). Improving long-term weight loss: Pushing the limits of treatment. *Behavior Therapy, 18*, 353-374.

Brownell, K. D., & Kramer, M. (1989). Behavioral management of obesity. *Medical Clinics of North America, 73*, 185-201.

Brownell, K. D, & Rodin, J. (1990). *The weight maintenance survival guide.* Dallas: American Health Publishing.

Bruce, B., & Agras, W. S. (1992). Binge eating in females: A population-based investigation. *International Journal of Eating Disorders, 12*(4), 365-373.

Bruce, B., & Wilfley, D. (1996). Binge eating among the overweight population: a serious and prevalent problem. *Journal of the American Dietetic Association, 96*(1), 58-61.

de Zwaan M. (2001). Binge eating disorder and obesity. *International Journal of Obesity, 25,* S51-S55.

Ferster, C. B., Nurenberger, J. I., & Levitt, E. B. (1996). The control of eating. *Obesity Research, 4*, 401- 410. (Originally published in *Journal of Mathetics, 1*, 87-109. [1962])

Keefe, F. J., & Blumenthal, J. A. (1980). The life fitness program: A behavioral approach to making exercise a habit. *Journal of Behavior Therapy and Experimental Psychiatry, 11*, 31-34.

Klem, M. L., Wing, R. R., McGuire, M. T., Seagle, H. M., & Hill, J. O. (1997). A descriptive study of individuals successful at long-term maintenance of substantial weight loss. *American Journal of Clinical Nutrition, 66*, 239-246.

Manson, J. E., and Bassuk, S. S. (2003). Obesity in the United States: a fresh look at its high toll. *Journal of the American Medical Association, 289*(2), 229-230.

Moreno, J. K., Fuhriman, A. J., & Hileman, E. (1995). Significant events in a psychodynamic psychotherapy group for eating disorders. *Group, 19*, 56-62.

National Heart, Lung, and Blood Institute. (1998*). Clinical guidelines on the identification, evaluation, and treatment of overweight and obesity in adults: the evidence report.* (NIH Publication No. 98-4083). Bethesda, MD.

Patrick, K., Raab, F., Adams, M. A., Dillon, L., Zabinski, M., Rock, C. L., Griswold, W. G., Norman, G. J. (2009). A Text Message–Based Intervention for Weight Loss: Randomized Controlled Trial. *Journal of Medical Internet Research,11(1):e1*

Perri, M. G. (1998). The maintenance of treatment effects in the long-term management of obesity. *Clinical Psychology: Science and Practice, 5*, 526-543

Shapiro, J. R., Bauer, S., Kordy, H., Hamer, R. M., Ward, D., & Bulik, C. M. (2008). Use of Text Messaging for Monitoring Sugar-Sweetened Beverages, Physical Activity, and Screen Time in Children: A Pilot Study. *Journal of Nutrition and Education Behavior, 40:*385-391.

Shapiro, J. R., & Bulik, C. M. "CIBO e Computer, la Psicoterapia Cognitiva Dall'Approccio Classico All'auto Aiuto con L'utilizzo delle Tecnologie Informatiche." In P. Vinai & P. Todisco (Eds): *"Quando le emozioni diventano cibo, psicoterapia cognitiva del Binge Eating Disorder."* Cortina Milano. 2007.

Shapiro, J. R., Reba-Harrelson, L., Dymek-Valentine, M., Woolson, S., Hamer, R. M., & Bulik, C. M. (2007). Feasibility and acceptability of CD-ROM-based cognitive-behavioral treatment for binge eating disorder. *European Eating Disorders Review, 15* (3): 163-174.

Stuart, R. B. (1996). Behavioral control of overeating. *Obesity Research, 4*, 411-416. (Originally published in *Behavior Research and Therapy, 5*, 357-365. [1967])

Stunkard, A. J. (1958). The management of obesity. *New York State Medical Journal, 58*, 79-87.

Stunkard, A. J., & Berthold, H. C. (1985). What is behavior therapy? A very short description of behavioral weight control. *The American Journal of Clinical Nutrition, 41*, 821-823.

Tate, D. F., Jackvony, E. Z., Wing, R. R. (2005). Effects of internet behavioral counseling on weight loss in adults at risk for type 2 diabetes. *Journal of the American Medical Association, 289,* 1833—1836.

Tate, D. F., Wing, R. R., & Winett, R. A. (2005). Using internet technology to deliver a behavioral weight loss program. *Journal of the American Medical Association, 285,* 1172-1177.

USDHHS/ODPHP (U.S. Department of Health and Human Services' Office of Disease Prevention and Health Promotion). Physical Activity Guidelines for Americans (2008). Webise: http://www.health.gov/paguidelines/default.aspx (accessed: 3/19/2010).

Wadden TA & Sarwer DB. (1999). Behavioral treatment of obesity: New approaches to an old disorder. In D. Goldstein (Ed), *The Management of Eating Disorders* (pp 173-199). Totowa, NJ: Humana.

Wilfley, D. E., Welch, R. R., Stein, R. I., Spurell E. B., Cohen, L. R., Saelens B. E., Dounchis, J. Z., Frank, M. A., Wiseman, C. V., and Matt, G. E. (2002). A randomized comparison of group cognitive-behavioral therapy and group interpersonal psychotherapy for the treatment of overweight individuals with binge-eating disorder. *Archives of General Psychiatry, 59*, 713-721.

Wilson, G. T. (1996). Acceptance and change in the treatment of eating disorders and obesity. *Behavior Therapy, 27*, 417-439.

Wing, R. R., and Hill, J. O. (2001). Successful weight loss maintenance. *Annual Review of Nutrition, 21*, 323-341.

Wonderlich, S. A., de Zwaan, M., Mitchell, J. E., Peterson, C. & Crow, S. (2003). Psychological and dietary treatments of binge eating disorder: Conceptual implications. *International Journal of Eating Disorders, 34,* S58 - S73.

In: Pathways to Obesity and Main Roads to Recovery
Editor: Piergiuseppe Vinai
ISBN: 978-1-61122-740-6

Chapter XV

Pharmacotherapy

Roberta Situlin
Clinical Medicine and Medical Therapy Units, Hospital of Cattinara,
University of Trieste Italy

Abstract

Pharmacotherapy represents the second level of obesity management in patients at higher risk for overweight complications. The benefits of pharmacotherapy for weight control are, however, limited by side effects of different intensities, which reduce the compliance or may require discontinuation of treatment. Adverse effects induced by some categories of drugs have caused the withdrawal from the global or local markets of many agents, so there are few drugs nowadays approved for obesity control. The chapter focuses on characteristics mechanism of action, side effects and contraindications of each one.

Introduction

The conservative management of obesity is based, first of all, on diet, exercise and, at times, psychological support programs (Clinical Guidelines on the Identification, Evaluation, and Treatment of Overweight and Obesity in Adults, 1998; National Task Force on the Prevention and Treatment of Obesity, 2000; NICE clinical guideline. *Obesity*, 2006). The efficacy of these interventions on the achievement and maintenance of a meaningful weight loss is limited by the counter regulatory homeostatic mechanisms, activated by the induction of an energy deficit, and/or the recurrence of maladaptive behaviors. Pharmacotherapy, with agents that reduce food intake or nutrient absorption or increase energy expenditure, represents the second level of obesity management in patients at higher risk for overweight complications (Table 15.1) (Clinical Guidelines on the Identification, Evaluation, and

Treatment of Overweight and Obesity in Adults, 1998; National Task Force on the Prevention and Treatment of Obesity, 2000; NICE clinical guideline. *Obesity*, 2006).

Results from randomized, controlled clinical trials and meta-analysis have shown that pharmacotherapy, in association with lifestyle modifications, allows a modest greater weight loss, over that induced by energy restriction alone, and increases the percentage of patients reaching the 5 to 10 % weight-loss endpoints, recommended by clinical guidelines (Haddock et al., 2002; Li et al., 2005; Rucker et al., 2007; Neovius & Narbro, 2008). Such a level of weight reduction, however modest, is considered clinically significant, since it improves obesity-related consequences such as dyslipidemia, insulin resistance, and hypertension (Goldstein, 1992). Anti-obesity drugs may further improve the cardiovascular risk profile over the effects associated with weight reduction, per se (Rucker et al., 2007; Filippatos et al., 2005; Tziomalos et al., 2009; Hsieh et al., 2005; O'Meara et al., 2004; Siebenhofer et al., 2009). Pharmacotherapy agents are also used, with variable levels of efficacy, in obesity-related conditions such as type 2 diabetes mellitus (DMT2), polycystic ovary syndrome (PCOS) and non-alcoholic fatty liver disease (NAFLD)/non-alcoholic steato-hepatitis (NASH), or in eating disorders or iatrogenic overweight (Tziomalos et al., 2009; Norris et al., 2005; Lloret-Linares, 2008; Coutinho, 2009; Citrome, 2008; Ratziu, 2009; Viner, 2009). Continuous drug treatment is, at least partially, effective in weight maintenance after the weight loss phase (Haddock et al., 2002; Li et al., 2005; Rucker et al., 2007). The benefits of pharmacotherapy for weight control are, however, limited by side effects of different intensity, which reduce the compliance or may require discontinuation of treatment. Adverse effects induced by some categories of drugs have caused the withdrawal from the global or local markets of many agents.

Table 15.1. Indications for weight control pharmacotherapy

Ineffective, six months, trial of lifestyle modifications (diet and exercise)
Patients at higher risk from overweight complications including:
• Obese (BMI > 30 kg/m^2), even without associated clinical complications
• Overweight (BMI >27 kg/m^2), with two or more complications, including:
  • hypertension,
  • dyslipidemia,
  • insulin resistance or diabetes
• Subjects with visceral obesity, as indicated by:
  • a waist circumference >102 cm in males,
  • a waist circumference >88 cm in females,
  (even with a normal body weight, but having two or more of the above mentioned complications).
 	
Absence of contraindications and adequate tolerance of the prescribed drug
Weight loss of at least 2 kg in the first four weeks and for at least three months

Examples include, in chronological order: thyroid hormones (causing hyperthyroidism), amphetamines (for the risk of addiction), fenfluramine and the association fenfluramine-phentermine (responsible for pulmonary hypertension and heart valvular diseases), rimonabant (for the risk of psychosis) and just very recently, in Europe, sibutramine (because of a higher incidence of cardiovascular events) (Seghatol & Rigolin, 2002; Christensen, 2007; FDA, 2009; FDA, 2010).

Furthermore, some patients have contraindications to the pharmacological treatment, others are *non responders*, because of inadequate lifestyle modifications or other factors. Drop-out rates from pharmacotherapy are high because of costs, side-effect intolerance, dissatisfaction with results, discrepancy between health and esthetical or self-esteem goals, and greater availability of more effective bariatric surgery (Haddock et al., 2002; Li et al., 2005; Rucker et al., 2007; Foster et al., 1997) Drugs now approved for obesity control are limited to few agents (Table 15.2).

To expand the pharmacotherapy opportunities, compounds approved for the treatment of other conditions, but not for obesity, are prescribed off label, while new drugs and combinations of agents are under intensive investigation to improve the medical management of obesity (Tables 15.2 and 15.3) (Bays, 2004; Zanella et al., 2009).

Table 15.2. Agents for obesity treatment

Approved by the FDA for long-term overweight treatment				
Agents	**Mechanism of action**	**Main applications**	**Doses**	**Main adverse effects**
Sibutramine	5 HT, DOPA and NE reuptake inhibitor	Obesity, especially with frequent hunger and lack of satiety; Obesity with DMT2	10–15 mg once a day	Increased heart rate and blood pressure, dry mouth, stipsis, insomnia
Orlistat	Gastric and pancreatic lipase inhibitor	Obesity; Obesity with reduced GT; Obesity with DMT2	120 mg 2/day or 3/d, at meals	Malabsorption, steatorrhea
Approved by the FDA for other indication and prescribed off-label for overweight treatment				
Topiramate	Glutamate kainite receptor antagonist, GABA activity enhancer Monoamine activity enhancer	Obesity with frequent hunger; BED; Obesity with DMT2; Obesity from psychiatric drugs Obesity; Obesity from psychiatric drugs	200-400 mg/day	Insomnia, Paresthesias Memory and concentration deficits Taste distortion
Zonisamide			400-600mg/day	Fatigue, somnolence, taste distortion, creatinine increase
Bupropion	NE and DOPA reuptake inhibitor	Obesity with depression; Obesity from antidepressants (SSRIs)	300-400 mg/day	Insomnia, seizures (low risk with controlled release formulations)
Metformin	Mild anorexigenic effect	Obesity with reduced GT, or metabolic syndrome; Obesity with DMT2, also in association with anti-obesity drugs	850 mg/bid	Stomach upset, diarrhea, lactic acidosis

Table 15.3. Possible future drugs for obesity treatment

Agents	Mechanism of action
Agents active on neuropeptide receptors – Melanocortin, MC3 and MC4 receptor agonists (fragments from cleaved POMC) – Neuropeptide Y, NPY, (Y1 and Y5) receptor antagonist – Melanin-concentrating hormone (MCH) receptor antagonists – MK-0364, cannabinoid-1 receptor inverse agonists, taranabant, and CP-945598 cannabinoid-1 receptor antagonists – Serotonin 2C receptor agonists (5-HT2C), lorcaserin	– Increase POMC anorexigenic effects – Inhibit NPY orexigenic effects – Reduce hunger and feeding behavior – Inhibit feeding – Regulate satiety and metabolic rate
Hormones secreted by adipocytes or agents active on their regulatory mechanisms – Leptin – Agents active on leptin signaling pathways: – Suppressors of cytokine signaling-3 protein (SOCS3) and inhibitors of tyrosine phosphatase-1B protein (PTP-1B) – Analogues of the recombinant human ciliary neurotrophic factor, CTNF – Oleoyl estrone – Adiponectin	– In the maintenance phase, to control higher appetite and lower energy expenditure – Reduce leptin resistance – Independent activation of the JAF/STAT leptin receptors – Reduces adipocyte size and number – -Reduces fat accumulation, increases fatty acid oxidation in skeletal muscle, improves insulin sensitivity
Agents active on GI tract neurohormone receptors, (peripherally or in the CNS) or increasing neurohormone concentrations – Cholecystokinin –alfa receptor agonists – Peptide YY 3-3,6 PYY and TM30338, synthetic analogues of PPY – Central acting incretin mimetic drugs – Glucagon-like peptide-1 (GLP-1) agonists (exenatide, extracted from lizard) and synthetic amylin analogues, (pramlintide) – Dipeptidyl peptidase IV (DPP-IV) inhibitors	– Inhibit gastric emptying, increase satiety – Inhibit NPY neurons, reduce gastric motility, increase satiety and meal termination – Suppress appetite, increase satiety, insulin secretion and sensibility – Lower GLP inactivation
Agents regulating lipid metabolism – AOD9404 synthetic C–terminal fragments of human growth hormone (hGH) – Stearoyl-coenzyme A desaturase, SCD, inhibitors – Inhibitors of fatty acid synthase and stimulators of carnitine palmitoyltransferase (CPT1) C75 – 11 beta-hydroxy steroid dehydrogenase type 1 – (11- betaHSD1) inhibitors	– Increase lipolysis without hyperglycemia or cell proliferation – Decrease lipid storage, increase fatty acid oxidation – Decrease lipogenesis and lipid storage, increase fatty acid oxidation – Decrease lipid storage and improve insulin resistance
Nutrient absorption – Lipoic acid (LA) – Lipase blocker, cetilistat	– Inhibits intestinal sugar transport, antioxidant action – Reduces triglyceride absorption, with higher tolerability than orlistat
Combined agents Phentermine plus topiramate; Bupropion plus naltrexone (opioid-receptor antagonist); Bupropion plus zonisamide; Sibutramine plus oleoyl estrone, Ezetimibe plus orlistat	

Drugs Approved for Obesity Treatment

Drugs Reducing Food Intake

Agents that increase the availability of noradrenergic (NE), dopaminergic (DOPA) and serotoninergic (5-HT) neurotransmitters, regulating hunger and satiety, have been introduced for the treatment of obesity since many years (Haddock et al., 2002; Yanovski & Yanovski 2002). The drugs either increase the release of neurotransmitters from the synapsis (for example, phentermine and diethylpropion, active on NE, and fenfluramine, on 5HT); or inhibit the neurotransmitter reuptake at the synaptic cleft (mazindol, active on NE, and sibutramine, on both 5HT and NE); or act as receptor agonists (for example, the alfa-1 NE agonist, phenopropanolamin). Drugs approved for the short-term treatment of obesity, no longer than three months, include agents with a low, but potential, risk of abuse such as diethylpropion and phentermine (included in the Drug Enforcement Administration, DEA, schedule IV) and benzphetamine and phendimetrazine (in DEA schedule III). Phentermine is the most used product: at doses of 15 to 30 mg/day, it causes a greater weight loss than the placebo, however the development of tachyphylaxis and tolerance within few weeks limits its use (Haddock et al., 2002; Li et al., 2005; Yanovski & Yanovski, 2002). Side effects are characteristic of sympathomimetic drugs and include dry mouth, stipsis, insomnia, restlessness, euphoria and increased heart rate and blood pressure. Another group of appetite suppressants are the antagonists of the cannabinoid-1 receptor (CB_1). Among these, *rimonabant* caused weight loss with a significant improvement in the metabolic profile and cardiovascular risk factors (Christensen et al., 2007). Introduced in 2006, the drug was officially withdrawn in 2009, by the European Medicines Agency, EMEA, because of psychiatric side effects, including anxiety, depression and increased suicidal or psychosis risk.

Sibutramine

Characteristics, Mechanism of Action and Availability

Sibutramine is a monoamine reuptake inhibitor active on the central nervous system with adrenergic, serotoninergic, and dopaminergic effects (Haddock et al., 2002; Bray et al., 1999). The inefficiency of the drug, developed for the treatment of depression, as mood regulator and the associated anorexigenic effects shifted the indication to obesity control. The enhancement of satiety seems to be more relevant than hunger suppression; furthermore, the drug increases thermo genesis in animal models and, at least partially, in humans (Bray et al., 1999; Mitchell et al., 2003; Hansen et al., 1999). Sibutramine, available since 1998, is approved by the FDA for adults, but it is off label for adolescents, younger than 16 years, or children. In Europe and UK, sibutramine has been suspended by EMEA from February 2010 (FDA 2009, FDA 2010).

Efficacy

Sibutramine is indicated for weight reduction and weight-loss maintenance. The drug, in the range of 10 to 15 mg/day in conjunction with diet, caused, at one year, an average weight loss of 4.2 to 4.5 kg over that observed in the diet and placebo control group (Li et al., 2005; Rucker et al., 2007). Furthermore, a higher percentage of the treated patients (55% vs. 27% and 28 vs. 10%) reached respectively a weight loss of 5 and 10%, and 10 to 30% more patients maintained 80 to 100% of the initial weight loss in the long term (Rucker et al., 2007). The drug introduced after a weight loss of at least 6 kg, induced in four weeks by a very low-calorie diet, VLCD, caused a further weight decrease (−5.2 kg vs. + 0.5 kg in controls) and, at one year, 75% of the treated patients maintained 100% of the weight loss, vs. 42% in controls (Apfelbaum et al., 1999). In the Sibutramine Trial of Obesity Reduction and Maintenance, STORM, 43% of the patients on continuous treatment maintained 80% of the weight loss, at two years, vs. 16% in controls (James et al., 2000). The addition of group lifestyle modification sessions to sibutramine plus low calorie diet, LCD, at one year, caused an average weight loss of 12 % vs. 5 and 6.7% respectively, in controls on drug plus diet or on lifestyle counseling, plus diet, suggesting the relevance of the patient education and psychological support during medical treatment (Wadden et al., 2000). In type 2 diabetic obese patients, the drug caused a weight loss between 2.8 and 5.3 kg, over the placebo group and improved the glycemic control in subjects on sibutramin only or on sulphonylurea, metformin or pioglitazone (Rucker et al., 2007; Filippatos et al., 2005; Tziomalos et al., 2009; Norris et al., 2005; Lloret-Linares et al., 2005; Coutinho 2009; Fujioka et al., 2000; Serrano-Rios 2002; McNulty et al., 2003; Derosa et al., 2008). In these studies, fewer patients with DMT2, compared with non-diabetic obese, reached the 5 and 10% weight loss endpoints. In obese patients, with or without diabetes mellitus, sibutramine improves lipid profile by reducing triglyceride and increasing HDL cholesterol levels and lowers serum uric acid concentration (Rucker et al., 2007; Filippatos et al., 2005; James et al., 2000; Fujioka et al., 2000; McNulty et al., 2003). The drug tends to increase blood pressure, both in normotensive and hypertensive patients; however, the effect may be offset by a meaningful weight loss of 5 or 10% (Rucker et al., 2007; Siebenhofer et al., 2009; Fujioka et al., 2000; McNulty et al., 2003). Sibutramine has been used effectively in obese adolescents; however, side effects seem to be higher at this age (Coutinho, 2009; Viner et al., 2009; Berkowitz et al., 2006). Some positive results were shown in PCOS, NASH and binge eating; however, the data need further validation (Tziomalos et al., 2009; Ratziu & Zelber-Sagi, 2009). The efficacy in the control of overweight issues induced by antipsychotic agents is controversial (Citrome et al., 2008).

Treatment Doses, Side Effects and Contraindications

Treatment should be started with 10 mg, once daily, and if weight loss is <2 kg, in four weeks, and tolerance is good, the dose can be increased to 15 mg/day. Intake should be interrupted with a weight loss <5%, in the first four weeks, after the higher dose, or if loss is <5% after three months, or with a weight regain of 3 kg or more. The most common side effects of the drug, related mostly to its adrenergic effects, include dry mouth, stipsis, insomnia, increased heart rate (on the average by four to seven beats/minute) and diastolic blood pressure (by 2 to 3 mm Hg) (Bray et al., 1999; James et al., 2000; Fujioka et al., 2000). These changes are more frequent in the first 7 to 12 weeks of therapy. Some patients and adolescents may develop more relevant changes (Berkowitz et al., 2006). Therefore, surveillance of blood pressure and pulse rate needs to be scheduled. Treatment should be interrupted in previously normotensive patients with heart rate >100 b/min, at rest, or increased blood pressure >145/90, in two consecutive occasions, or in previously well-controlled hypertensive subjects with blood pressure increasing >145/90. Sibutramine is contraindicated with eating disorders (anorexia and bulimia nervosa), major depression or maniac conditions, alcohol or drug abuse, uncontrolled hypertension, existing pulmonary hypertension, heart valve damage, coronary heart disease, chronic renal failure, severe arrhythmias, previous myocardial infarction, stroke or TIA, hyperthyroidism, seizures, pheocromocytoma, intake of monoamine oxidase inhibitors, antidepressant or anorectic drugs. In November 2009, the FDA, on the basis of preliminary data from the SCOUT trial (Sibutramine Cardiovascular Morbidity/Mortality Outcomes in Overweight or Obese Subjects at Risk of a Cardiovascular Event) reported a 11.4% incidence of cardiovascular events (heart attack, stroke, resuscitated cardiac arrest, or death) in subjects with a history of cardiovascular disease, on sibutramine treatment, vs. 10% in the placebo arm. Diabetic patients with a cardiovascular disease history showed the highest rates of complications (13.9% vs. 11.9%). The FDA, while waiting for the full SCOUT trial report, has requested the manufacturer to modify the drug label with the addition of "history of cardiovascular disease" among the CONTRAINDICATIONS to the sibutramine treatment, while EMEA has suspended the drug (FDA, 2009; FDA, 2010). The association of SSRIs with sibutramine can induce hypotension, diarrhea and skin flushing (serotonin syndrome). Erythromycin and ketoconazole may increase the plasma levels of the drug.

Drugs Reducing Fat Absorption

Orlistat

Characteristics, Mechanism of Action and Availability

Orlistat is a specific inhibitor of the gastric and pancreatic lipases, causing a dose-dependent reduction in the intestinal absorption of triglycerides (Hvizdos & Markham, 1999). Treatment combining 120 mg of orlistat, two to three times daily, at meals, with a moderately low-calorie diet, contributing 30% of the total energy as fat, lowers triglyceride absorption by 30% (Hvizdos & Markham, 1999). Furthermore, the drug decreases cholesterol absorption, by 25%, and reduces free fatty acid levels, thus modulating insulin sensitivity (Mittendorfer et al., 2001; Kelley et al., 2004). Orlistat is approved by the FDA for the treatment of obese subjects, adults and adolescents, from the age of 12 years.

Efficacy

Orlistat is effective over placebo on weight loss, waist circumference reduction, weight-loss maintenance, glycemic control, diabetes prevention and treatment, and improvement of cardiac risk factors such as dyslipidemia, blood pressure and inflammation markers (Li et al., 2005; Rucker et al., 2007; Hsieh et al., 2005; O'Meara et al., 2004; Norris et al., 2005; Sjostrom et al., 1998; Davidson et al., 1999). Trials with one year of treatment showed an average weight loss of 2.7 to 2.9 kg, with 21% and 12% more patients on the drug reaching a weight loss >5 and 10%, respectively (Li et al., 2005; Rucker et al., 2007). Data on weight maintenance are generally positive (Rucker et al., 2007). The introduction of the drug in obese subjects who had lost at least 8% of their basal weight on a six-month LCD, was associated, at one year, with a lower weight regain than in controls (32.8 vs. 58.7 %) (Hill et al., 1999). Orlistat treatment, in association with lifestyle counseling, continued for three years, in subjects who had lost a relevant amount of weight (14.4 kg) with an eight-week VLCD, was associated with a maintenance of 2.4 kg over controls (weight gain of 4.6 kg vs. 7.0 kg) (Richelsen et al., 2007). The drug is effective also in obese adolescents (19). The XENDOS study (XENical in the Prevention of Diabetes in Obese Subjects) showed, at four years, a 37.3% reduction in the incidence of diabetes, in the treated group (orlistat plus lifestyle modification), compared to controls (lifestyle modification only), mediated by an improvement in glucose tolerance (Torgerson et al., 2004). In obese patients with DMT2, on oral antidiabetic drugs (sulfonylurea or metformin) or insulin, orlistat, at one year caused a weight loss in the range of 1.9 to 2.9 % above controls, reduced the requirement of antidiabetic medications and improved the glycemic profile (Rucker et al., 2007; Hsieh et al., 2005; O'Meara et al., 2004; Norris et al., 2005; Lloret-Linares et al., 2009; Kelley et al., 2004; Sjostrom et al., 1998; Hill et al., 1999; Hollander et al., 1998; Miles et al., 2002; Jacob et al., 2009). Independent pharmacological lipid-lowering effects on total and LDL cholesterol and triglyceride levels and improvement in HDL concentration in obese, with or without diabetes, have been shown in most cases (Rucker et al., 2007; Hsieh et al., 2005; O'Meara et al., 2004; Sjostrom et al., 1998; Hill et al., 1999). The usefulness of the drug in obesity-related conditions such as PCOS, NASH, BED or iatrogenic obesity is not clearly defined (Coutinho, 2009; Citrome et al., 2008; Ratziu et al., 2009).

Doses, Side Effects and Contraindications

Treatment doses are 120 mg, bid or tid, immediately before or during meals or within one hour from eating. Orlistat has no systemic effects since absorption from the intestine is minimal. Symptoms are induced by the unabsorbed lipids, with borborygmi, flatulence, abdominal cramps, increased stool frequency, steatorrhea, and in the worst cases, rectal oily discharge and fecal incontinence. The frequency and intensity of symptoms are higher during the first few weeks and often improve afterward. Side effects increase with fat intake >30% of total energy. Orlistat may decrease the absorption of fat soluble vitamins with a higher risk of deficiency for vitamin D. Multivitamin supplementation is generally prescribed. Orlistat may cause vitamin K depletion, thus increasing the risks associated with warfarin treatment. The plasma levels of cyclosporine may be lowered by the co administration with orlistat. Special caution and monitoring should, therefore, be applied to patients on these drugs, or orlistat should not be prescribed. The drug is contraindicated in subjects with cholestasis and malabsorption syndromes and in pregnancy and breastfeeding.

Drugs Approved for Treatment of other Conditions and off Label for Obesity

Antiepileptic Drugs

Topiramate and Zonisamide

Zonisamide (a sulfonamide) and topiramate (a beta-fructopyranose sulfamate) are drugs approved for the treatment of selected seizure disorders and the prophylaxis of migraines. The associated weight loss induced by the drugs suggested their use for obesity control.

Zonisamide probably acts through monoamine activity enhancement, thus decreasing appetite. Treatment, combined with a LCD, for 16 weeks, caused a weight loss of 5 kg over the placebo (5.9 kg vs. 0,9kg), and 57% of the patients vs. 10% of controls reached a weight loss of at least 10%. Patients who continued treatment up to 32 weeks had an additional weight loss of 3.1 kg over controls (Gadde et al., 2004). Side effects include fatigue, somnolence and early, modest, creatinine increase. Topiramate acts mainly as antagonist of the glutamate kainite receptor, possibly decreasing glutamate orexigenic effects, and as GABA (γ-amino butyric acid) system enhancer, and it may also inhibit adipocyte lipogenesis (Astrup et al., 2004). Other mechanisms, not fully explained, are most likely involved. The drug, at doses of 96, 192, and 256 mg/day, for 60 weeks, caused a weight loss of 7.0, 9.1, and 9.7%, respectively, vs. 1.7% in the placebo group (Wilding et al., 2004). Blood pressure and glucose tolerance improved. Topiramate is effective also in weight and glycemic control in diabetic obese patients, as mono therapy or in association with metformin (Eliasson et al., 2007; Rosenstock et al., 2007; Toplak et al., 2007). Controlled release compounds seem to be safer. The drug improves weight control in patients with binge eating possibly through a mood-stabilizing effect and a better impulse control (Toplak et al., 2009). Side effects, which occur mostly at the beginning of treatment, include memory, attention or language difficulties, paresthesias, psychomotor slowing, depression and, rarely, suicidal ideation (Astrup et al., 2004). Topiramate should not be combined with phenytoin, which increases its plasma levels or carbamazepine, which increases its elimination. The drug lowers the serum levels of digoxin and contraceptives and increases those of phenytoin. The carbonic anhydrase inhibition induced by both drugs may cause taste changes and hyperchloremic acidosis, requiring regular serum bicarbonate monitoring and contraindicating the use with other carbonic anhydrase inhibitors, such as acetazolamide, or with agents predisposing to acidosis.

Antidepressants

Bupropion

The drug is a NE and DOPA reuptake inhibitor with no significant effects on serotonin. Beside controlling depression and being useful in smoking cessation, bupropion causes a dose-dependent weight loss possibly through appetite regulation and lower food craving. At doses of 400 mg/day, the drug induced a weight loss of about 3.7% above placebo, in six months; 37% and 26% more treated patients reached a weight loss of 5 and 10%, compared to controls. Continuing treatment for another 24 weeks at a dose not lower than 300 mg/day, maintained a weight loss of 5% (Anderson et al., 2002). The drug could be particularly indicated in obese patients with depression or in substitution for SSRIs drugs, responsible for weight gain, but is contraindicated in subjects with seizures or bulimia nervosa (Jain et al., 2002). Side effects include insomnia and seizures.

Anti Diabetics

Metformin

Metformin is a biguanide approved for the treatment of type 2 diabetes mellitus both in adults and adolescents. The drug has mild, not fully explained, anorexigenic properties, and improves glucose tolerance without the weight gain effects induced by insulin, sulfonyureas or thiazolidinediones. The drug can be particularly indicated in adults, adolescents and children as monotherapy, or in association with other antiobesity drugs, in obese diabetic subjects and in non-diabetic obese, with glucose intolerance, to improve the metabolic control and prevent diabetes mellitus or the metabolic syndrome. (Seanz et al., 2005; Knowler et al., 2002; Orchard et al., 2005; Knowler et al., 2009; Park et al., 2009). In obese subjects with DMT2 metformin monotherapy, compared to diet alone, and to diet plus other antidiabetic agents, caused significant improvements in HbA1c, glycemic control, overweight (with a modest loss), dyslipidemia, and diastolic blood pressure (Orchard et al., 2005). In the Diabetes Prevention Program, the drug, at 2.8 years, caused a weight loss of 2 kg, (4% of the initial weight), reduced the incidence of diabetes by an average of 31% and the development of the metabolic syndrome by 17% and maintained some of the weight loss at four years, significantly above controls (Orchard et al., 2005; Knowler et al., 2002). At ten years, the incidence of diabetes was reduced by 18% (Knowler et al., 2009). The efficacy of metformin in patients with PCOS and NASH or iatrogenic obesity, from antipsychotic drugs, is not clearly defined (Tang et al., 2009; Björkhem-Bergman et al., 2010). Common side effects are stomach upset and diarrhea. The risk of lactic acidosis increases at higher doses. Metformin is contraindicated with renal dysfunction.

Conclusion

Pharmacotherapy for obesity helps more patients to achieve and maintain a moderate weight loss and some metabolic and clinical benefits over simple lifestyle modifications. Currently available anti-obesity agents, however, are fewer; not all patients are eligible or responders or compliant to the treatment while the long-term efficacy and safety of the drugs are unknown. Many new options are currently being investigated. Benefits on mortality and cardiovascular morbidity or on obesity related diseases need further evaluation.

References

A.A. V.V. (2006) Obesity: the prevention, identification, assessment and management of overweight and obesity in adults and children. *NICE clinical guideline* CG043.

Anderson, J.W. & Greenway, F.L. & Fujioka, K. & Gadde, K.M. & McKenney, J. & O'Neil, P.M. (2002). Bupropion SR enhances weight loss: a 48-week double-blind, placebo-controlled trial. *Obes Res, 10*(7), 633–641.

Apfelbaum, M. & Vague, P. & Ziegler, O. & Hanotin, C. & Thomas, F. & Leutenegger, E. (1999). Long-term maintenance of weight loss after a very-low-calorie diet: a randomized blinded trial of the efficacy and tolerability of sibutramine. *Am J Med, 106*(2), 179-84.

Astrup, A. & Toubro, S. (2004). Topiramate: a new potential pharmacological treatment for obesity. *Obes Res, 12 Suppl,* 167S-73S.

Bays, H.E. (2004). Current and investigational antiobesity agents and obesity therapeutic treatment targets. *Obes Res, 12 (8)*, 1197–121.

Berkowitz, R.I. & Fujikova, K. & Daniels, S.R. & Hopping, A.G. & Owen, S. & Perry, A.C. et al., (2006). Effects of sibutramine treatment in obese adolescents. A randomized trial. *Ann Intern Med, 145(2),* 81-90.

Björkhem-Bergman, L. & Asplund, A.B. & Lindh, J.D. (2010). Metformin for weight reduction in non-diabetic patients on antipsychotic drugs: a systematic review and meta-analysis. *J Psychopharmacol. Jan 15,* [Epub ahead of print]

Bradley, D.P. & Kulstad, R. & Schoeller, D.A. (2010). Exenatide and weight loss. *Nutrition, 26(3),* 243-249.

Bray, G.A. & Blackburn, G.L. & Ferguson, J.M. (1999). Sibutramine produces dose-related weight loss. *Obes Res, 7 (2)*, 189–198.

Christensen, R. & Kristensen, P.K. & Bartels, E.M. & Bliddal, H. &, Astrup, A. (2007). Efficacy and safety of the weight-loss drug rimonabant: a meta-analysis of randomized trials. *Lancet, 17, 370(9600),*1706-13.

Citrome, L. & Vreeland, B. (2008). Schizophrenia, obesity, and antipsychotic medications: what can we do? *Postgrad Med,120(2),*18-33.

Coutinho, W. (2009). The first decade of sibutramine and orlistat: a reappraisal of their expanding roles in the treatment of obesity and associated conditions. *Arq Bras Endocrinol Metabol., 53,* 262-70.

Davidson, M.H. & Hauptman, J. & Di Girolamo, M. et al., (1999). Weight control and risk factor reduction in obese subjects treated for 2 years with orlistat: a randomized controlled trial, *JAMA, 281 (3),* 235–242.

Derosa, G. & D'Angelo, A. & Salvadeo, S.A. & Ferrari, I. & Gravina, A. & Fogari, E. & Maffioli, P. & Cicero, A.F. (2008). Sibutramine effect on metabolic control of obese patients with type 2 diabetes mellitus treated with pioglitazone. *Metabolism, 57*(11), 1552-7.

Eliasson, B. & Gudbjörnsdottir, S. & Cederholm, J. & Liang, Y. & Vercruysse, F. & Smith, U. (2007). Weight loss and metabolic effects of topiramate in overweight and obese type 2 diabetic patients: randomized double-blind placebo-controlled trial. *Int J Obes, 31(7),* 1140-1147.

FDA (2009). Early communication about an ongoing safety review of Meridia (sibutramine hydrochloride), November 2009.

FDA (2010). *Follow-up to the November 2009 early communication about an ongoing safety review of sibutramine, marketed as meridia,* 21 January 2010.

Filippatos, T.D. & Kiortsis, D.N. & Liberopoulos, E.N. & Mikhailidis, D.P. & Elisaf, M.S. (2005). A review of the metabolic effects of sibutramine. *Current medical research and opinion*, 21(3), 457-68.

Foster, G.D. & Wadden, T.A. & Vogt, R.A. & Brewer, G. (1997). What is a reasonable weight loss? Patients' expectations and evaluations of obesity treatment outcomes. *J Consult Clin Psychol, 65(1),*79-85.

Fujioka, K. & Seaton, T.B. & Rowe, E. & Jelinek, C.A. & Raskin, P. & Lebovitz, H.E. & Weinstein S.P. (2000). Sibutramine/Diabetes Clinical Study Group. Weight loss with sibutramine improves glycaemic control and other metabolic parameters in obese patients with type 2 diabetes mellitus. *Diabetes Obes Metab, 2(3),* 175-87.

Gadde, K.M. & Franciscy, D.M. & Wagner, H.R. & Krishnan, K.R. (2003). Zonisamide for weight loss in obese adults: a randomized controlled trial. *JAMA, Apr 9, 289(14),* 1820-5.

Goldstein, D.J. (1992). Beneficial health effects of modest weight loss. *International journal of obesity and related metabolic disorders: journal of the International Association for the Study of Obesity, 16(6)*, 397-415.

Haddock, C. & Poston, W.S. & Dill, P.L. (2002). Pharmacotherapy for obesity: a quantitative analysis of four decades of published randomized clinical trials. *International journal of obesity and related metabolic disorders: journal of the International Association for the Study of Obesity, 26.* 262–273.

Hansen, D.L. & Toubro, S. & Stock, M.J. & Macdonald, I.A. & Astrup, A. (1999). The effect of sibutramine on energy expenditure and appetite during chronic treatment without dietary restriction. *Int J Obes Relat Metab Disord, 23(10),* 1016-24.

Hill, J.O. & Hauptman, J. & Anderson, J.W. & Fujioka, K. & O'Neil, P.M. & Smith, D.K. & Zavoral, J.H. & Aronne, L.J. (1999). Orlistat, a lipase inhibitor, for weight maintenance after conventional dieting: a 1-y study. *Am J Clin Nutr, 69(6),* 1108-16.

Hollander, P.A. & Elbein, S.C. & Hirsch, I.B. & Kelley, D. & McGill, J. & Taylor, T. & Weiss, S.R. & Crockett, S.E. & Kaplan, R.A. & Comstock, J. & Lucas, C.P. & Lodewick, P.A. & Canovatchel, W. & Chung, J. & Hauptman, J. (1998). Role of orlistat in the treatment of obese patients with type 2 diabetes. A 1-year randomized double-blind study. *Diabetes Care, 21 (8),* 1288-94.

Hsieh, C.J. & Wang, P.W. & Liu, R,T, & Tung, S.C. & Chien, W.Y. & Chen, J.F. (2005). Orlistat for obesity: benefits beyond weight loss. *Diabetes Research and Clinical Practice, 67(1)*, 78-83.

Hvizdos, K.M. & Markham, A. (1999). Orlistat: a review of its use in the management of obesity. *Drugs, 58,4,* 743–760.

Jacob, S. & Rabbia, M. & Meier, M.K. & Hauptman, J. (2009). Orlistat 120 mg improves glycaemic control in type 2 diabetic patients with or without concurrent weight loss. *Diabetes Obes Metab, 11(4)*, 361-371.

Jain, A.K. & Kaplan, R.A. & Gadde, K.M. et al., (2002). Bupropion SR vs. placebo for weight loss in obese patients with depressive symptoms. *Obes Res, 10,* 1049–1056.

James, W.P. & Astrup, A. & Finer, N. & Hilsted, J. & Kopelman, P. & Rossner, S. et al., (2000). Effect of sibutramine on weight maintenance after weight loss: a randomized trial. STORM Study Group. Sibutramine Trial of Obesity Reduction and Maintenance. *Lancet, 356(9248)*, 2119-25.

Kelley, D.E. & Kuller, L.H. & McKolanis, T.M. et al., (2004). Effects of moderate weight loss and orlistat on insulin resistance, regional adiposity, and fatty acids in type 2 diabetes. *Diabetes Care, 27,* 33–40.

Knowler, W.C. & Barrett-Connor, E. & Fowler, S.E. & Hamman, R.F. & Lachin, J.M. & Walker, E.A. & Nathan, D.M. (2002). Diabetes Prevention Program Research Group. Reduction in the incidence of type 2 diabetes with lifestyle intervention or metformin. *N Engl J Med, 7; 346(6)*, 393-403.

Knowler, W.C. & Fowler, S.E. & Hamman, R.F. & Christophi, C.A. & Hoffman, H.J. & Brenneman, A.T. & Brown-Friday, J.O. & Goldberg, R. & Venditti, E. & Nathan, D.M. (2009). Diabetes prevention program research group, 10-year follow-up of diabetes incidence and weight loss in the diabetes prevention program outcomes study. *Lancet, 14, 374(9702)*, 1677-1686.

Leombruni, P. & Lavagnino, L. & Fassino, S. (2009). Treatment of obese patients with binge eating disorder using topiramate: a review. *Neuropsychiatr Dis Treat, 5*, 385-92.

Li, Z. & Maglione, M. & Tu, W. & Mojica, W. & Arterburn, D. & Shugarman, L.R. (2005). Meta-analysis: pharmacologic treatment of obesity. *Annals of Internal Medicine, 142(7)*, 532-46.

Lloret-Linares, C. & Greenfield, J.R. & Czernichow, S. (2008). Effect of weight-reducing agents on glycaemic parameters and progression to Type2 diabetes: a review. *Diabet Med.;25(10),* 1142-50.

McNulty, S.J. & Ur, E. & Williams, G. (2003). A randomized trial of sibutramine in the management of obese type 2 diabetic patients treated with metformin. *Diabetes Care, 26(1),* 125-131.

Miles, M. & Leiter, L. & Hollander, P. et al., (2002). Effect of orlistat in overweight and obese patients with type 2 diabetes treated with metformin, *Diabetes Care, 25*, 1123–1128.

Mitchell, J.E. & Gosnell, B.A. & Roerig, J.L. & De Zwaan, M. & Wonderlich, S.A. & Crosby, R.D. et al., (2003). Effects of sibutramine on binge eating, hunger, and fullness in a laboratory human feeding paradigm. *Obes Res, 11(5),* 599 602.

Mittendorfer, B. & Ostlund, R.E. & Patterson, B.W. & Klein, S. (2001). Orlistat inhibits dietary cholesterol absorption. *Obes Res, 9(10)*, 599-604.

National Institute of Health. (1998). Clinical Guidelines on the Identification, Evaluation, and Treatment of Overweight and Obesity in Adults: The Evidence Report. *Obesity Research, 6 Suppl 2,* 51S-209S.

National Task Force on the Prevention and Treatment of Obesity (2000). Overweight, obesity, and health risk. *Archives of Internal Medicine, 160(7)*, 898-904.

Neovius, M. & Narbro, K. (2008). Cost-effectiveness of pharmacological anti-obesity treatments: a systematic review. *International Journal of Obesity, 32 (12)*, 1752-63

Norris, S.L. & Zhang, X. & Avenell, A. & Gregg, E. & Schmid, C.H. & Lau, J. (2005), Pharmacotherapy for weight loss in adults with type 2 diabetes mellitus. *Cochrane Database Syst Rev., 18*, CD004095.

O'Meara, S. & Riemsma, R. & Shirran, L. & Mather, L. & Riet G. (2004). A systematic review of the clinical effectiveness of orlistat used for the management of obesity. *Obesity reviews: an official journal of the International Association for the Study of Obesity, 5(1)*, 51-68.

Orchard, T.J. & Temprosa, M. & Goldberg, R. & Haffner, S. & Ratner, R. & Marcovina, S. & Fowler, S. (2005). Diabetes Prevention Program Research Group. The effect of metformin and intensive lifestyle intervention on the metabolic syndrome: the Diabetes Prevention Program randomized trial. *Ann Intern Med, 19, 142(8)*, 611-619.

Park, M.H. & Kinra, S. & Ward, K.J. & White, B. & Viner, R.M. (2009) Metformin for obesity in children and adolescents: a systematic review. *Diabetes Care, 32(9)*, 1743-175.

Ratziu, V. & Zelber-Sagi, S. (2009). Pharmacologic therapy of non-alcoholic steatohepatitis. *Clin Liver Dis, 13(4),* 667-88.

Richelsen, B. & Tonstad, S. & Rössner, S. & Toubro, S. & Niskanen, L. & Madsbad, S. & Mustajoki, P. & Rissanen, A. (2007). Effect of orlistat on weight regain and cardiovascular risk factors following a very-low-energy diet in abdominally obese patients: a 3-year randomized, placebo-controlled study. *Diabetes Care, 30 (1)*, 27-32.

Rosenstock, J. & Höllander, P. & Gadde, K.M. & Sun, X. & Strauss, R. & Leung, A. OBD-202 Study Group. (2007). A randomized, double-blind, placebo-controlled, multicenter study to assess the efficacy and safety of topiramate controlled release in the treatment of obese type 2 diabetic patients. *Diabetes Care*, 30(6), 1480–1486.

Rucker, D. & Padwal, R. & Li, S.K. & Curioni, C. & Lau, D.C. (2007). Long-term pharmacotherapy for obesity and overweight: updated meta-analysis. *British Medical Journal, 335,(7631)*, 1194-9.

Seanz, A. & Fernandez-Esteban, I. & Mataix, A. & Ausejo, M. & Roque, M. & Moher, D. (2005). Metformin as monotherapy for type 2 diabetes mellitus. *Cochrane Database Syst Rev, CD002966.*

Seghatol, F.F. & Rigolin, V.H. (2002). Appetite suppressants and valvular heart disease. *Curr Opin Cardiol, 17 (5),*486–492.

Serrano-Rios, M. & Melchionda, N. & Moreno-Carretero, E. (2002). Role of sibutramine in the treatment of obese Type 2 diabetic patients receiving sulphonylurea therapy. *Diabet Med, 19(2),* 119-24.

Siebenhofer, A. & Horvath, K. & Jeitler, K. & Berghold, A. & Stich, A.K. & Matyas, E. & Pignitter, N. & Siering, U. (2009), Long-term effects of weight-reducing drugs in hypertensive patients. *Cochrane Database Syst Rev., 8,* CD007654.

Sjostrom, L. & Rissanen, A. & Andersen, T et al., (1998). Randomized placebo-controlled trial of orlistat for weight loss and prevention of weight regain in obese patients. European Multicentre Orlistat Study Group. *Lancet, 352, 9123,* 167–172.

Tang, T. & Lord, J.M. & Norman, R.J. & Yasmin, E. & Balen, A.H. (2009). Insulin-sensitizing drugs for polycystic ovary syndrome *Cochrane Database Syst Rev., 8,* CD003053.

Toplak, H. & Hamann, A. & Moore, R. & Masson, E. & Gorska, M. & Vercruysse, F. & Sun, X. & Fitchet, M. (2007). Efficacy and safety of topiramate in combination with metformin in the treatment of obese subjects with type 2 diabetes: a randomized, double-blind, placebo-controlled study. *Int. J Obesity, 31*, 138–146.

Torgerson, J.S. & Hauptman, J. & Boldrin, M.N. & Sjostrom, L. (2004). XENical in the prevention of diabetes in obese subjects (XENDOS) Study: a randomized study of orlistat as an adjunct to lifestyle changes for the prevention of type 2 diabetes in obese patients. *Diabetes Care, 27 (1*), 155-61.

Tziomalos, K. & Krassas, G.E. & Tzotzas, T. (2009). The use of sibutramine in the management of obesity and related disorders: an update. *Vasc Health Risk Manag., 5(1),* 441 52.

Viner, R.M. & Hsia, Y. & Tomsic, T. & Wong, I.C. (2010). Efficacy and safety of anti-obesity drugs in children and adolescents: systematic review and meta-analysis. *Obes Rev, 11,* 593-602.

Wadden, T.A. & Berkowitz, R.I. & Womble, L.G. & Sarwer, D.B. & Phelan, S. & Cato, R.K. & Hesson, L.A. & Osei, S.Y. & Kaplan, R. & Stunkard, A.J. (2005). Randomized trial of lifestyle modification and pharmacotherapy for obesity. *N Engl J Med, 17, 353(20),* 2111-20.

Wilding, J. & Van Gaal; L. & Rissanen, A. & Vercruysse, F. & Fitchet, M. OBES-002 Study Group (2004). A randomized double-blind placebo-controlled study of the long-term efficacy and safety of topiramate in the treatment of obese subjects. *Int J Obes Relat Metab Disord, 28(11)*, 1399-410.

Yanovski, S.Z. & Yanovski, J.A. (2002). Obesity. *N Engl J Med, 21;346(8),* 591-602.

Zanella, M.T. & Flexa Ribeiro, F. (2009). Emerging drugs for obesity therapy. *Arq Bras Endocrinol Metab, 53(2),* 271-80.

In: Pathways to Obesity and Main Roads to Recovery
Editor: Piergiuseppe Vinai
ISBN: 978-1-61122-740-6

Chapter XVI

Bariatric Surgery: Indications and Procedures

Luca Busetto
Department of Medical and Surgical Sciences, University of Padova, Italy

Abstract

The reduction of the surgical risks, new technical skills, and the recognition of the clinical benefits produced by the sustained weight loss are at the basis of the exponential increasing of bariatric surgery in the last years. A wide array of bariatric techniques have been proposed; those nowadays utilized can be divided, according to their mechanism of action, in three broad groups: restrictive procedures, in which the gastric volume is reduced (vertical banded gastroplasty and gastric banding), procedures in which a by-pass of the distal stomach and duodenum is added to the gastric restriction (gastric by-pass) and surgical techniques in which the exclusion of a larger part of the small intestine is added to the gastric restriction (bilio-pancreatic diversion, duodenal switch). Risk/benefit profile of any procedure such as indications and contraindications to bariatric surgery among adults and adolescent patients are discussed in the chapter.

Introduction

The use of bariatric surgery increased exponentially in the last years. The larger use of bariatric surgery in the clinical management of severe obesity may be driven by an increasing acceptance of this type of therapy in the medical and surgical community. The reduction of the surgical risks, associated with newer technical skills, and the recognition of the clear clinical benefits produced by the sustained weight loss obtained by bariatric surgery on the global health of the morbid obese patient are at the basis of this change.

Several studies demonstrated in the last years the beneficial effects of bariatric surgery not only in terms of weight loss, but also in terms of reduction of the excess morbidity and mortality observed in morbid obese patients. The most important of these studies is certainly the Swedish Obesity Subjects (SOS) study, a prospective controlled study of more than ten years of follow-up in which the outcomes of 2,000 morbid obese patients treated with several types of procedure (gastric banding, vertical banded gastroplasty and gastric by-pass) have been compared with the outcomes of 2,000 well-matched morbid obese controls treated with conventional medical treatment. Globally considered, patients in the surgical group had a ten-year weight loss corresponding to 16.1% of baseline body weight, whereas in the medical group, a small 1.6% increase in body weight was observed (Sjöström et al., 2004). This huge difference in weight loss translated into a substantial difference in obesity-associated metabolic co-morbidities. The percentage of patients who had a ten-year remission of type 2 diabetes, hypertriglyceridemia and low HDL-cholesterol levels was significantly higher in the surgical than in the control group (Sjöström et al., 2004). In patients free from metabolic abnormalities at baseline, the number of new cases of type 2 diabetes was lower in the surgical patients than in controls: new type 2 diabetes appeared in 25% of non-diabetic patients in the control group and in 7% of non-diabetic patients in the surgical group (relative risk of type 2 diabetes in the surgical group: 0.25; 95% CI: 0.17-0.38) (Sjöström et al., 2004). Clinical benefits were not limited to metabolic co-morbidities in the SOS study. Surgical group had also a more significant improvement of respiratory problems (exertional dyspnoea and sleep disorders) (Karason et al., 2000), a better working capacity with fewer days of absence (Narbro et al., 1999), and a better self-reported quality of life (Karlsson et al., 1998). Finally, total mortality was also lower in the surgical group of the SOS study. Patients in the surgical group had a 24.6% reduction in ten-year total mortality compared to patients in the medical group (relative risk of death in the surgical group: 0.76; 95%CI: 0.59 to 0.99) (Sjöström, Narbro, Sjöström, 2007). The low number of events prevented a statistically meaningful analysis about the different causes of death, but both cardiovascular and cancer deaths appeared to be reduced. A reduction in the incidence of new cases of cancer has been recently reported in the female surgical patients enrolled in the SOS study (Sjöström, Gummesson, Sjöström, 2009).

Indications for Bariatric Surgery

General indications for bariatric surgery have been for the first time formalized in a Consensus Development Conference Statement sponsored by the National Institutes of Health in Bethesda in (1991). Those indications have been substantially confirmed by many published guidelines afterward and in particular by the inter-disciplinary European guidelines on surgery of severe obesity formulated in 2007, by a joint committee formed by IFSO (International Federation for the Surgery of Obesity), IFSO-EC (International Federation for the Surgery of Obesity—European Chapter), EASO (European Association for Study of Obesity) and ECOG (European Childhood Obesity Group)(Fried, Hainer, Basdevant, 2007). According to this document, adult patients (18 to 60 years) have an indication for bariatric surgery if they have a BMI >40 kg/m^2 or in a they have a BMI 35 to 40 kg/m^2, and they are suffering from a co-morbidity for which surgically induced weight loss is expected to confer a clinical benefit (such as metabolic disorders, cardio-respiratory disease, severe joint disease, obesity-related severe psychological problems). BMI criterion may be the current BMI or a documented previous BMI of this severity. Therefore, surgery may be performed in patients with a lower BMI value if this BMI is the result of an intensified weight-loss treatment before surgery (pre-operative weight loss is frequently indicated for the reduction of the surgical risk) or in patients who exhibited a substantial weight loss in a conservative treatment program but started to gain weight again.

Bariatric Surgery among Adolescents Patients

More stringent criteria have been proposed for the use of bariatric surgery in adolescents with severe obesity (Fried, Hainer, Basdevant, 2007)). Patients must have failed to lose weight or to maintain long-term weight loss with appropriate non-surgical medical care, and they must to comply with long-term follow-up after surgery.

Bariatric surgery can be considered if the patient:

1. Has a BMI >40 kg/m^2 (or 99.5° percentile for respective age) and at least one co-morbidity,
2. Has followed at least six months of organized weight reducing attempts in a specialized centre
3. Shows skeletal and developmental maturity
4. Is capable of committing to comprehensive medical and psychological evaluation
5. Is willing to participate in a postoperative multidisciplinary treatment program.
6. Can access surgery in a unit with specialist pediatric support.

In patients aged more than 60 years, the risk/benefit profile of bariatric surgery is less clear and indication should be considered individually, usually with the primary objective to improve quality of life and not to increase lifespan (Fried, Hainer, Basdevant, 2007).

Contraindications

Finally, contraindications to bariatric surgery are as follows (Fried, Hainer, Basdevant, 2007).

1. Absence of a period of identifiable medical management
2. Patient who is unable to participate in prolonged medical follow-up
3. Non-stabilized psychotic disorders, severe depression and personality disorders
4. Alcohol abuse and/or drug dependencies
5. Diseases threatening life in the short term
6. Patients who are unable to care for themselves and have no long-term family or social support.

Procedures

In the history of bariatric surgery, a wide array of bariatric techniques have been proposed and subsequently abandoned, because of poor long-term results or excessive rates of side effects and complications. The procedures that passed this process of selection and that are nowadays utilized in modern bariatric surgery may be divided, according to their mechanism of action, in three broad groups:

1. Restrictive procedures, in which the gastric volume is reduced. The mechanism of action is purely based on the earlier generation of satiety and the limitation of the introduction of food (vertical banded gastroplasty and gastric banding).
2. Procedures in which a by-pass of the distal stomach and duodenum is added to the gastric restriction. The mechanism of action involves modifications in the secretion of hormones produced by the stomach and the first intestinal tract that regulate eating behavior (gastric by-pass).
3. Procedures in which the exclusion of a larger part of the small intestine is added to the gastric restriction. The mechanism of action is mainly based on the malabsorption of nutrients (bilio-pancreatic diversion, duodenal switch).

Any single procedure may produce different results and has specific complications. Any procedure has, therefore, particular risk/benefit profile.

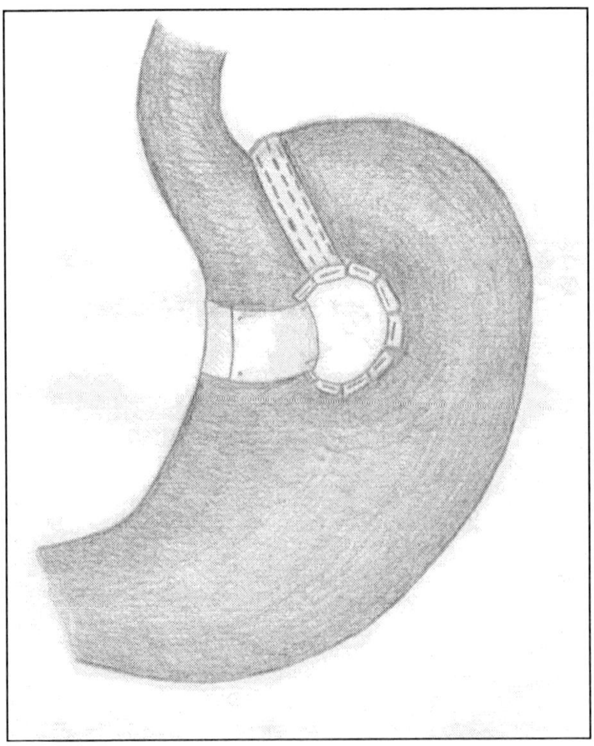

Figure 16.1. Vertical Banded Gastroplasty.

Vertical Banded Gastroplasty (VBG)

VBG is the oldest restrictive procedure. It was been developed in the early 1980s, by Mason (1982). Key element of the procedure is the creation of a very small proximal gastric pouch (15 to 20 cc), communicating with the rest of the stomach through a very narrow stoma. The gastric pouch is created with the use of mechanical staplers, and the stoma diameter is fixed and reinforced with the application of a small band. In the classic technique described by Mason, the gastric pouch is separated from the rest of the stomach by a multiple suture line (Figure 16.1). In the technique later introduced by Mac Lean, the gastric pouch is definitely divided from the rest of the stomach (Mac Lean, Rhode, Forse, 1990). VBG is now currently performed laparoscopically (Londroth et al., 1996).

Peri-operative mortality is very low (0.1%) (Buchwald, 2004). In the first year after surgery, VBG patients may lose 60 to 70% of their excess weight (EWL: 60 to 70%) (Buchwald, 2004)), but the durability of weight loss is more questionable. Body weight usually stabilizes after the first year, and the new body weight may be maintained only if patients are able to cope with the changes of eating behavior that are requested by gastric restriction. Anyway, ten years after surgery, 40% of patients still have an EWL >50% (Doherty, 2001). The most frequent and typical complication of VBG, occurring in more than 10% of cases, is the dehiscence of the gastric partition line with the formation of a new passage between the gastric pouch and the rest of the stomach (gastro-gastric fistula). Treatment of this complication requires a new surgical procedure. Other complications are represented by stoma stenosis (2%) with malnutrition and frequent food regurgitation that may require endoscopic dilatation or redo surgery, and pouch dilatation with loss of the early satiety and weight regain (Doherty, 2001). VBG has been now practically abandoned in favor of gastric banding.

Adjustable Gastric Banding (LAGB)

LAGB, firstly introduced by Kuzmak in late 1980s (Kuzmack, 1986), is today the most frequently performed restrictive procedure worldwide and the most frequently performed bariatric procedure at all in Europe. This procedure does not require the section or the removal of any organ, and it is fully reversible both at the functional and at the anatomical level. As in VBG, the key element of the procedure is the creation of a very small proximal gastric pouch communicating with the rest of the stomach through a very narrow stoma. In the case of LAGB, however, the pouch is created not suturing the stomach, but simply putting around it a silicone-made round band. The band has an inflatable section, and it is connected by a tube to a small port that is positioned subcutaneously in the abdominal wall (Figure 16.2). This system provides the possibility to regulate the level of restriction after surgery, simply inflating or deflating the band, by adding or removing a few ml of saline solution through the access port.

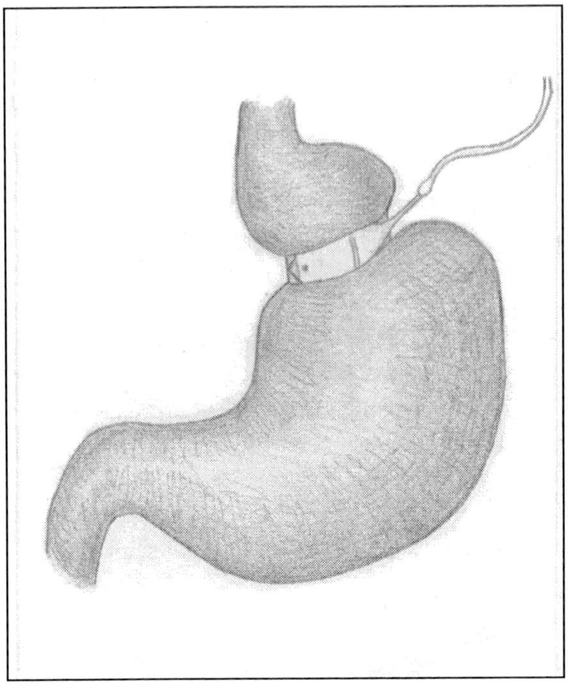

Figure 16.2. Adjustable Gastric Banding.

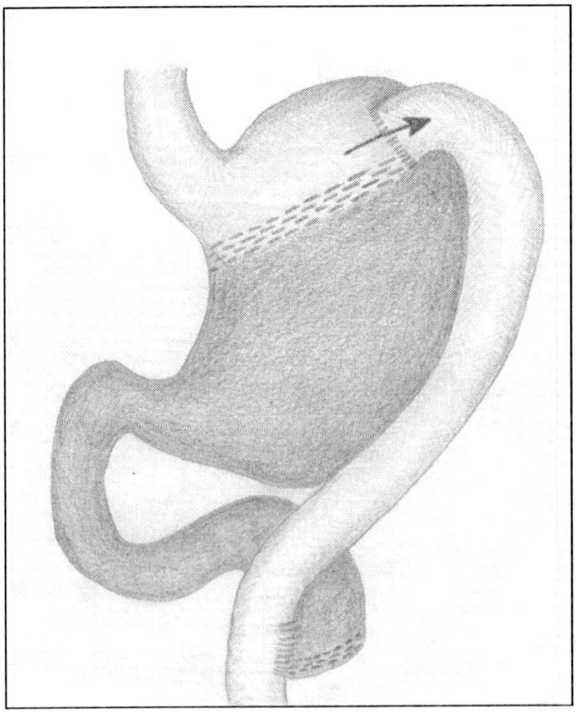

Figure 16.3. Roux-en-Y Gastric Bypass.

The placement of LAGB is routinely performed by laparoscopy (Cadiere, 1994), with very few operatory complications and a very low peri-operative mortality rate of 0.1%

(Buchwald, 2004). LAGB patients may have a %EWL of 40 to 50% (Buchwald, 2004), with a generally good weight maintenance also in the very long term (Favretti et al., 2007). However, a tendency to weight regain may be observed in a minority of LAGB patients (Favretti et al., 2009). The most frequent and specific complication of the LAGB is represented by pouch dilatation. This complication may be usually treated conservatively, by a temporary complete deflation of the banding (Busetto et al., 2003). Redo surgery (band removal or band repositioning) may be required in case of slippage of the band through the stomach or in case of erosion of the gastric wall and migration of the band into the gastric lumen. Total rate of these complications is reported to be relatively low (about 5%) in the best hands (Favretti et al., 2007). Minor surgery may be required by problems at the level of the regulation system, such as deconnection of the port or port twisting.

Roux-en-Y Gastric Bypass (RYGB)

RYGB was been introduced in the late 1960, by Mason (Mason, Ito, 1967). Many technical variants have been proposed over time. RYGB is the most frequently performed procedure in the United States.

Key element of the procedure is the creation of a very small proximal gastric pouch (30 ml) not communicating with the rest of the stomach, but directly connected to a jejunal loop (Figure 16.3). The distal part of the stomach, the duodenum and the first part of the jejunum remain by-passed to the transit of food and are anastomized to the alimentary tract at a variable distance from the stomach. Distal stomach, duodenum and the biliary tract are not further accessible with the usual endoscopic techniques after surgery. In the most classical variants of RYGB, no malabsorption of food is involved.

Weight loss is produced partly by a restrictive mechanism and partly by changes in the secretion of gastro-enteral hormones with known effects of food-intake regulation and glucose metabolism (GLP-1, ghrelin)(12). RYBG may be performed laparoscopically by advanced laparoscopic surgeons (Wittgrove, Clark, 1997).

Peri-operative mortality is about 0.5% (Buchwald et al., 2004). Short-term %EWL after RYGB is reported to range between 60% and 75% (Buchwald et al., 2004). A tendency to weight regain may be observed in longer series, with long-term %EWL leveling to 50% (Pories et al., 1995). Weight regain may be partly caused by dehiscence of the gastric partition line or dilatation of the gastro-jejunal anastomosis. RYGB patients may develop nutritional deficiencies in iron, folates and vitamin B12 (Halverson, 1986). Routine supplementation is strongly recommended (Mechanick, 2008). The popularity of RYGB has been recently refueled by the observation that this type of procedure may have more pronounced effects on type 2 diabetes than restrictive procedures. Modifications in the levels of GLP-1 and other incretins are considered to be the basis of the specific metabolic effect of RYGB (Pories, 1995).

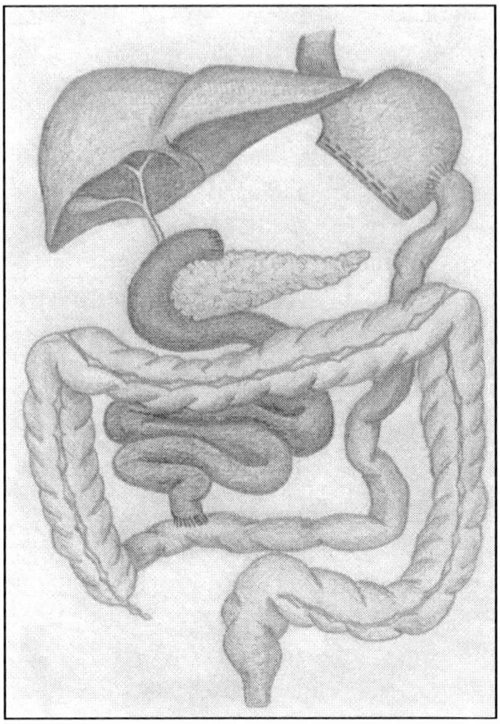

Figure 16.4. Bilio-Pancreatic Diversion.

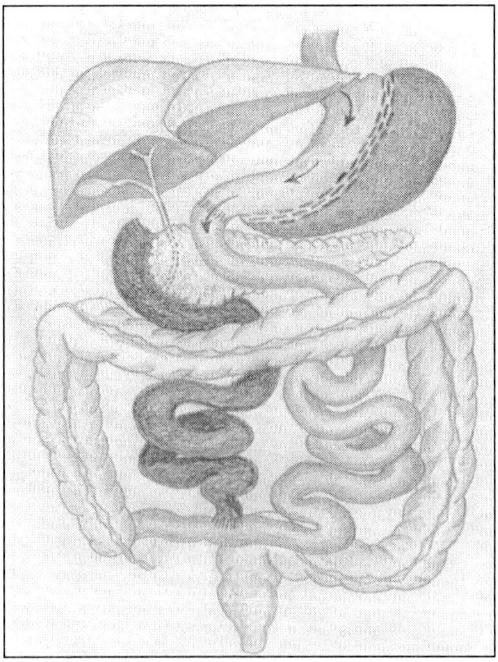

Figure 16.5. Bilio-Pancreatic Diversion with Duodenal Switch.

Bilio-pancreatic Diversion (BPD)

BPD was been introduced in bariatric surgery by Scopinaro in the late 1970s (Scopinaro et al., 1979), and represents the prototype for malabsorptive procedures. Key elements of the procedures are a partial distal gastric resection and the creation of a long Roux-en-Y loop with an alimentary tract of 200 cm and a common limb of only 50 cm (Figure 16.4). This profound anatomical rearrangement of the digestive system causes a selective malabsorption of lipids and complex carbohydrates that consents a profound very stable weight loss. Alcohol and simple sugars are normally absorbed, and the rare cases of weight regain may be usually explained by uncontrolled alcohol or sugar intakes. BPD may be done laparoscopically (Scopinaro, Marinari, Camerini, 2002).

Peri-operative mortality is 1.1% (Buchwald et al., 2004). BPD patients have a %EWL over 70% (Buchwald et al., 2004), very stable in the long-term (Scopinaro et al., 1998). The impressive effects of BPD on body weight are paid off by the negative consequences of malabsorption. Routine supplementation with calcium, iron and vitamins is mandatory (Mechanick et al., 2008). The most severe nutritional complication is represented by protein malnutrition, which may require hospitalization and parenteral nutrition and, in rare cases, may be lethal if not adequately treated (Scopinaro et al., 1998). The incidence of protein malnutrition has been reduced from 15 to 3% by modifications of the surgical technique (Scopinaro et al., 1998). Severe thiamine deficiencies with neurologic sequelae and cases of Wernicke-Korsakoff encephalopathy have been also reported (Scopinaro et al., 1998). Finally, we do not have clear information about the impact of calcium and vitamin D malabsorption on bone mass and the risk of fractures over the long term. Chronic diarrhea with steatorrhea, flatulence and the higher incidence of proctological complications may be considered minor problems, but they may have profound effects on the quality of life of BPD patients.

Bilio-Pancreatic Diversion with Duodenal Switch (DS-BPD)

DS-BPD was been firstly developed by Hess and Marceau in 1988 (Hess and Hess, 1998; Marceau et al., 1998) in order to reduce the side effects of classic BDP. Key elements of DS-BPD are a sleeve vertical gastrectomy with the creation of a gastric remnant of about 150 to 200 ml and a bilio-pancreatic diversion with a duodenal switch, a 150 cm alimentary tract and a 100 cm common limb (Figure 16.5).

Weight loss is similar to classic BDP, but the preservation of a functional pylorus seems to consent a better control of diarrhea. Moreover, the use of a duodenum-entero anastomosis instead of a gastro-entero anastomosis may have important effects on the rate of anastomotic ulcers. In 1999, Gagner first performed DS-BPD laparoscopically (Gagner, Patterson, 2000) and in order to reduce the surgical risk in super-obese patients later proposed the execution of the procedure in two surgical steps (first sleeve gastrectomy and second duodenal switch) (Regan et al., 2003). As an unexpected consequence, many authors observed that sleeve gastrectomy seems to produce a weight loss and is at least in the short term more pronounced that the weight loss expected by a simple restrictive procedure. This observation caused the emergence of laparoscopic *Sleeve Gastrectomy (LSG)* as an isolated bariatric procedure (Deitel, Crosby, Gagner, 2007). Long-term results of LSG are still under scrutiny.

At this moment, there is insufficient evidence-based data to suggest how to assign a patient to any particular bariatric. The choice of the procedure is, therefore, frequently based on the use of not proved subjective criteria and on surgeon's technical preferences and skills.

The Role of the Multidisciplinary Team

European guidelines (Fried, Hainer, Basdevant, 2007) clearly state that a decision to offer surgery should follow a comprehensive inter-disciplinary assessment. Such assessment should optimally be provided by a multidisciplinary team experienced in obesity management and bariatric surgery that includes the obesity physician, the surgeon, the anesthetist, a psychologist or psychiatrist, a nutritionist and/or dietitian, and a nurse practitioner/social worker. Indeed, patients indicated for bariatric surgery should undergo not only the routine preoperative assessment required for any major abdominal surgery, but also they should receive a more complex preoperative management that includes a careful assessment of general health and nutritional status, a clear and extensive explanation of the dietary changes that are required after surgery, the optimization of the treatment of the obesity-related co-morbidities in order to reduce the risks of the surgical procedure, and the assessment of motivation and willingness to adhere to follow-up programs. The preoperative evaluation should also ensure that the patient is fully informed on the benefits, consequences and risks of the surgical options and the necessity of lifelong follow-up, that the patient understands the potential (limited) outcomes of surgery, and that the patient can give truly informed consent including a statement on risks of the surgery and acceptance behavior modification of lifestyle and of follow-up. It is quite obvious that such complex evaluation and management may be better performed by a dedicated integrated multidisciplinary team than in the usual clinical setting.

After bariatric surgery, all patients require regular lifelong qualified surveillance and follow-up. Regular clinical follow-up has clear clinical aims: all possible short- and long-term surgical complications and events directly related to the operation should be treated, and long-term post-surgery follow-up and management of obesity and obesity-related diseases and operation-related non-surgical nutritional consequences should be provided. However, probably the most important task after surgery is to provide to the patients support in order to reinforce their adherence to those lifestyle changes that are critical in long-term weight-loss maintenance after bariatric surgery. The ideal setting for such a comprehensive approach is an inter-disciplinary integrated team and/or clinic.

Conclusion

Bariatric surgery is at present the most effective treatment for morbid obese patients. Long-term weight loss provided by surgery has proven important positive effects on the morbidity and mortality of patients with severe obesity. Several surgical options are now available, and all of them have demonstrated long-term efficacy and acceptable risks and side effects. However, bariatric surgery remains a complex and demanding therapy that should be provided by qualified and dedicated multidisciplinary teams.

References

Buchwald, H., Avidor, Y., Braunwald, E., et al., (2004). Bariatric Surgery. A systematic review and meta-analysis. *JAMA, 292*, 1724-1737

Busetto, L., Segato, G., De Marchi, F., et al., (2003). Post-operative management of laparoscopic banding. *Obes Surg, 13*, 121-127

Cadiere, G.B., Bruyns, J., Himpens, J., et al., (1994). Laparoscopic gastroplasty for morbid obesity. *Br J Surg, 81*, 1524-1525.

Deitel, M., Crosby, R.D., Gagner, M., (2008). The First International Consensus Summit for Sleeve Gastrectomy (SG), New York City, October 25-27,. *Obes Surg, 18*, 487-96.

Doherty, C. (2001). Vertical banded gastroplasty. *Surg Clin N America, 81*, 1097-1112

Favretti, F., Ashton, D., Busetto, L., Segato, G., De Luca, M., (2009). The gastric band: first-choice procedure for obesity surgery. *World Journal of Surgery,* 33, 2039-2048.

Favretti, F., Segato, G., Ashton, D., et al., (2007). Laparoscopic adjustable gastric banding in 1,791 consecutive obese patients: 12-year results. *Obesity Surgery,. 17*, 168-175.

Fried, M., Hainer, V., Basdevant, A., (2007). Inter-disciplinary European guidelines on surgery of severe obesity. *Int J Obes., 31*, 569–77.

Gagner, M., Patterson, E.,(2000). Laparoscopic biliopancreatic diversion with duodenal switch: a case series of 40 consecutive patients. *Obes Surg., 10*, 514-523.

Halverson, J.D., (1986). Micronutrient deficiencies after gastric bypass for morbid obesity. *Am Surg., 11*, 594-598.

Hess, D.S., Hess, D.W., (1998). Biliopancreatic diversion with a duodenal switch. *Obes Surg. 8,* 267-282.

Karason, K., Lindroos, A.K., Stenlöf, K., Sjöström, L., (2000). Relief of cardiorespiratory symptoms and increased physical activity after surgically induced weight loss. *Arch Intern Med., 160,* 1797-802.

Karlsson, J., Sjöström, L., Sullivan, M., Swedish, (1998). Obese Subjects (SOS)—an intervention study of obesity. Two-years follow-up of health-related quality of life (HRQL) and eating behavior after gastric surgery for severe obesity. *Int J Obes., 22*, 113-26.

Kuzmac, L.I. (1989) Gastric banding. In: Deitel, M. (ed) *Surgery for the morbidly obese patient.* (pp 225–259) Philadelphia, PA. Lea & Febiger.

Londroth, H., Dalenback, J., Haglind, E., et al., (1996). Vertical banded gastroplasty by laparoscopic technique in the treatment of morbid obesity. *Surg Laparosc Endosc., 6*, 102-107.

Mac Lean, L.D., Rhode, B.M., Forse, R.A.,(1990). Late results of vertical banded gastroplasty for morbid and super obesity. *Surgery., 107*, 20-27.

Marceau, P., Hould, F.S., Simard, S., et al. (1998). Biliopancreatic diversion duodenal switch. *World J Surg., 22*, 947-954.

Mason, E.E., Ito, C., (1967). Gastric by-pass in obesity. *Surg Clin N Amer,47*:1345-1352.

Mason EE. (1982) Vertical banded gastroplasty for morbid obesity. *Arch Surg. 91,* 701-706.

Mechanick, J.I., Kushner, R.F., Sugerman, H.J., et al., (2008). American Association of Clinical Endocrinologist, the Obesity Society, and American Society for Metabolic and Bariatric Surgery medical guidelines for clinical practice for the peri-operative nutritional, metabolic, and nonsurgical support of the bariatric surgery patient. *Endocr Pract., 14,* 1-83.

Narbro, K., Ågre, N.G., Jonsson, E., et al., (1999). Sick leave and disability pension before and after treatment of obesity: A report from the Swedish Obese Subjects (SOS) study. *Int J Obes., 23*, 619-24.

National Institutes of Health Consensus Development Conference draft Statement Gastrointestinal surgery for severe obesity. (1991).*Obes Surg., 1*, 257-66.

Pories, W.J., Swanson, M.S, Mac Donald, K.G., et al., (1995). Who would have thought it? An operation proves to be the most effective therapy for adult onset diabetes mellitus. *Ann Surg., 222*, 339-352.

Regan, J.P., Inabnet, W.B., Gagner, M., Pomp, A,. (2003). Early experience with two-stage laparoscopic Roux-en-Y gastric bypass as an alternative in the super-super obese patient. *Obes Surg., 13*, 861-4.

Scopinaro, N., Adami, G.F., Marinar,i G.M., et al., (1998). Biliopancreatic diversion. *World J Surg.,* 22, 936-946.

Scopinaro, N., Gianetta, E., Civalleri, D., Bonalumi, U., Bach,i V., (1979). Biliopancreatic bypass for obesity: II. Initial experience in man. *Br J Surg., 66*, 618-620.

Scopinaro, N., Marinari, G.M., Camerini, G., (2002). Laparoscopic standard biliopancreatic diversion: technique and preliminary results. *Obes Surg., 12*, 362-365.

Sjöström, L., Gummesson, A., Sjöström, C.D., (2009). Effects of bariatric surgery on cancer incidence in obese patients in Sweden (Swedish Obese Subjects Study):a prospective, controlled intervention trial *Lancet Oncol., 1,* 653-62.

Sjöström, L., Lindroos, A.K., Peltonen, M., et al., (2004). Lifestyle, Diabetes, and Cardiovascular Risk Factors 10 Years after Bariatric Surgery. *N Engl J Med., 351*, 2683-93.

Sjöström, L., Narbro, K., Sjöström, C.D., (2007). Effects of bariatric surgery on mortality in Swedish obese subjects. *N Engl J Med., 357,* 741-52.

Wittgrove, A.C., Clark, G.W., (1997). Laparoscopic gastric by-pass: a four year prospective study of 230 patients followed from 3 to 42 months. *Obes Surg, 7,* 285-286.

In: Pathways to Obesity and Main Roads to Recovery
Editor: Piergiuseppe Vinai
ISBN: 978-1-61122-740-6

Chapter XVII

Treatment of Binge Eating Disorder

***James E. Mitchell*[1] *and Kristine Steffen*[2]**
[1]Neuropsychiatric Research Institute University of North Dakota School of Medicine and Health Science, ND, USA
[2]Neuropsychiatric Research Institute University of North Dakota School of Medicine and Health Science, ND, USA

Abstract

The treatment of BED has progressed substantially since the original introduction of this diagnosis in the DSM-IV. Both pharmacotherapy and psychotherapy approaches appear to play a role. Cognitive behavioral techniques seem to be the treatment of choice currently. While these are highly effective in reducing or eliminating binge eating behavior, the result in terms of weight loss is usually modest at best. As the field moves forward, increasing emphasis needs to be placed on effective strategies for the treatment of overweight and obesity, which are major health problems for many of these individuals.

Introduction

Despite the fact that binge eating disorder (BED) has not yet achieved the status of an official psychiatric diagnosis, it was included as an example of Eating Disorder Not Otherwise Specified (EDNOS) and in the appendices to the DSM-IV as a disorder for further study. However, a large literature has been developed on this condition since the publication of the DSM-IV. In particular, a substantial treatment literature has developed. As will be seen in the pages ahead, this literature suggests that both pharmacotherapy and psychotherapy can play important roles in the treatment of individuals with BED, and the relative indications for each type of intervention are yet clearly delineated. However, a point of considerable importance in the BED literature concerns the issue of weight loss. Most patients presenting for treatment with BED are highly desirous of weight loss, as many of them have problems with being overweight or obesity. Although there was initial optimism that if we could successfully teach patients to not binge eat they would lose substantial amounts of weight, the subsequent treatment literature has not borne this out. Indeed, the amount of weight loss in most treatment studies that specifically target binge eating has been modest at best. Therefore, the treatment of BED in some ways has reached the same impasse as the field of obesity treatment, in that none of our interventions thus far have been shown to result in substantial and sustained weight loss, except in the case of severe obesity where bariatric surgery clearly has a lasting impact.

Nonetheless, substantial progress has been made in addressing the issue of BED treatment, and that literature will be briefly reviewed. After reviewing those studies, we will then turn to a more detailed analysis of cognitive behavioral therapy (CBT) for BED. This therapy appears to be the best established form of psychotherapy for those with BED. It has been manualized by a number of authors and can be delivered in relatively brief treatment packages that result in highly significant decrements in the frequency of binge eating behavior.

Pharmacotherapy

Various agents have been tried in the treatment of those with BED. Recently a meta-analysis of this area has appeared (Reas & Grilo, 2008). Many of these agents were tried following their demonstration of efficacy in patients with bulimia nervosa (BN); but others have been tried because of their clear impact on obesity and weight. Agents used empirically have included antidepressants, particularly the SSRIs, anticonvulsants, and more traditional anti-obesity agents.

SSRIS

Relative to fluvoxamine, the results have been mixed. An earlier study by Hudson et al., (1998) suggested positive results, while a more recent trial by Pearlstein et al., (2003) found that the active drug did not separate from placebo on the major outcome variables.

There has been one placebo-controlled treatment trial of escitalopram, finding that the drug was superior to placebo in reducing body weight and modestly effective in reducing binge eating frequency (Guerdjikova et al., 2008) and another suggested efficacy for citalopram (McElroy et al., 2003). One randomized trial suggested efficacy for sertraline (McElroy et al., 2000). Trials using fluoxetine have been inconsistent (Arnold, et al., 2002; Grilo, et al., 2005). Therefore, overall there is some suggestion that SSRI antidepressants have a positive effect on the symptoms experienced by individuals with BED but these findings have been inconsistent, and there have been no long-term follow-up studies.

Anti-convulsants

Relative to traditional anticonvulsant medications, two trials have suggested that topiramate results in greater reduction in frequency of target symptoms such as binge eating behavior compared to placebo, and weight loss was also significant (McElroy et al., 2003; McElroy et al., 2004; McElroy, 2007). However, significant adverse events were encountered by patients on topiramate, including headache, taste perversion and cognitive problems. A single trial with zonisamide has been reported, and there were positive effects on binge eating and weight; however, the drug agent was not well tolerated (McElroy et al., 2006). A recent controlled trial failed to show significant differences between lamotrigine and placebo on binge eating frequency and weight change, although weight reduction was numerically greater with lamotrigine versus placebo (Guerdjikova et al., 2009). While the high placebo response rate in this study may have prevented the drug from demonstrating superiority over placebo, the trial was able to show that lamotrigine was well tolerated in patients with BED.

Anti-obesity Agents

There are three trials that have been published suggesting that sibutramine, the FDA approved agent for obesity that has both norepinepherine and serotonin reuptake inhibition effects, is effective in decreasing binge eating and inducing weight loss (Appolinario et al., 2003; Milano et al., 2005Wilfley et al., 2008). Sibutramine has been associated with some significant adverse events including insomnia and dry mouth, increased heart rate and elevation in blood pressure in a minority of patients.

Other Agents

The norepinephrine reuptake inhibitor atomoxetine is currently marketed for ADHD. It was also shown in one study to be superior to placebo in inducing weight loss and in decreasing binge day frequency in those with BED (McElroy et al., 2007).

Comparison Trials

A related question is whether pharmacotherapy improves outcome in patients receiving structured psychotherapy interventions. Three studies have examined this issue and the results of all three suggest that medication augmentation with the SSRIs fluvoxamine or fluoxetine does not add to the effectiveness of psychotherapy on most major outcome variables, although one study did find modestly greater improvement on depressive symptoms when patients were also treated with medication (Devlin et al., 2005; Grilo et al., 2005; Ricca et al., 2001).

In addition to the antidepressant trials, there have also been trials examining whether the addition of topiramate or orlistat provide additional weight loss, or other benefit, to psychotherapy in treating those with BED. One controlled trial suggested that when added to

CBT, topiramate is more likely to enhance remission from binge eating and induce weight loss (Claudino et al., 2007). Grilo et al., (2005) has also examined whether or not the addition of orlistat to CBT improved outcome (Grilo et al., 2005) and Golay et al., (2005) examined the addition of orlistat to a mildly hypocaloric diet. However, orlistat did not appear to significantly improve the reduction in frequency of binge eating seen with these other interventions.

In summary, there does appear to be a role for medication in the treatment of those with BED, but their proper role has yet to be elucidated.

Psychotherapy

One central question that was of concern early in this treatment literature is whether or not dietary restriction to induce weight loss would exacerbate binge eating. This question now appears to have been answered, with the result that binge eating is not exacerbated by such an intervention (Gladis et al., 1998). Therefore, weight loss treatment may be safe and appropriate for these patients.

Much of the psychotherapy literature on BED has focused on CBT, analogous to the treatment of BN. The National Institute for Clinical Excellence Guidelines published in Great Britain (NICE, 2004) suggests that modified CBT is the treatment of choice for BED. The treatment literature in this area has grown enormously and suggests excellent effects on binge eating frequency and rates of remission with good preservation of improvement over time (Fairburn et al., 1993; Wilson et al., 2007; Wilfley et al., 1993; Agras et al., 1997; Wilfley et al., 2002). Also, CBT has been shown to be more effective than either fluoxetine or placebo (Grilo et al., 2005). Of note, other psychotherapy techniques have also been shown to have merit including interpersonal psychotherapy (IPT) which has yielded results essentially identical to those with CBT in two trials (Wilfley et al., 1993; Wilfley, 2002), as well as dialectic behavior therapy (DBT) , which appears quite promising (Telch et al., 2001). There is also some evidence that behavioral weight-loss treatment itself impacts positively on the symptoms of BED (Gladis et al., 1998) but overall, the results regarding behavioral weight loss and very low-calorie diets must be interpreted as mixed. There is also a growing substantial literature that suggests that guided self-help approaches may be effective for BED, although additional literature is needed in this regard (Grilo et al., 2005; Grilo, 2008).

Assessment

Prior to treatment, every patient should undergo a routine psychiatric evaluation and a medical evaluation as well. The psychiatric evaluation should focus on current and past eating problems, weight history, co-morbid psychopathology, and an assessment of social support. The medical evaluation should include a careful examination for medical co-morbidities that are frequently seen in patients with BED because of their obesity. These can include hypertension, obstructive sleep apnea, cardiovascular disease, diabetes and several forms of cancer. Many of these patients require ongoing medical management because of these medical co-morbidities. It is also very useful for patients to undergo a nutritional assessment prior to treatment, with recommendations for a balanced eating plan and a hypo-caloric diet plan if weight loss is desired.

Consideration should also be given to the membership of the treatment team. This depends in large part on the nature of the intervention. Manual-based psychotherapies require a therapist with specialized training, be it in CBT, IPT or DBT. Pharmacological interventions will require a physician knowledgeable about BED and the psychopharmacology of this condition.

Not uncommonly, it is also useful to involve the family or caregivers in the evaluation or treatment of patients with BED. This may be part of the evaluation process where additional information is obtained from others, or as part of treatment where educational sessions can be offered for family members and caregivers. Not uncommonly, the treatment of BED will result in a significant impact on other family members and sometimes friends, and preparing individuals who will be affected in advance will clearly improve the process.

Cognitive Behavior Therapy for BED

What follows is a brief discussion of a CBT program for BED. The program can be administered in either a group or individual format and is designed to be delivered in 14 sessions over a 16-week period, with weekly visits for 12 weeks and then sessions every other week.

The first session in this program provides in-depth psycho-education about BED including epidemiology, diagnostic criteria and the consequences of this disorder. The goals of treatment are emphasized, including interruption of binge eating and the establishment of regular healthy eating patterns. Also the concept of cognitive restructuring and the need for better coping strategies are introduced. There is also a handout on things patients can expect when they change their eating behavior. In particular, it is emphasized that sometimes mood may worsen temporarily when behavior changes. Patients also complete a handout where they list reasons for stopping the binge eating behavior and reasons against stopping it. This is an effective way of dealing with ambivalence about stopping the behavior, since most patients are somewhat ambivalent when they begin the treatment. It is stressed that this is not necessarily a negative prognostic sign. In terms of homework assignments, patients complete a written task regarding alternatives to binge eating.

The second session introduces the concept of cues and consequences. Various cues are discussed, including social, situational, physiological and mental cues as are various consequences, including social, situational, feelings and thoughts. Contained between these is a response set with an emphasis on thoughts, feelings and behaviors. Emphasis is placed on the model that short-term positive consequences reinforce BED behaviors while long-term negative consequences are frequently ignored. Emphasis is placed on shifting to a focus on longer term consequences. There is also a section on strategies for change, including rearranging cues by avoidance and restricting the stimulus field, as well as strengthening cues for desired behavior. Methods for changing responses for cues (such as building in a pause or engaging in alternative behaviors) are discussed. Homework focuses on completing Rearranging Cues and Consequences worksheets.

Session 3 focuses again on cues and consequences with a strong emphasis on developing a healthier eating pattern. Patients are asked to begin eating three meals and two snacks a day and to try to include all types of foods in their diet. They are also given an introduction to meal planning.

In the fourth session, emphasis is placed on the response set of thoughts, feelings and behaviors. Automatic thoughts are examined. Emphasis is placed on differentiating thoughts from feelings. Also, a handout is provided on styles of thinking, including overgeneralization, catastrophizing, dichotomous thinking and rationalization.

In session 5, the focus is on thought restructuring. Two models are offered. The first is to challenge maladaptive thoughts by questioning them, and the second is challenging problematic thoughts by testing them prospectively. Specific examples are offered. There is also a discussion about underlying beliefs about food and eating behavior.

In the sixth sessions, emphasis is placed on cues and chains. The cue-response set is shown to be part of a chain, and emphasis is placed on developing strategies for interrupting the chain as early as possible. Subjects are given Chain Worksheets to complete at home prior to the next session.

In session 7, there is discussion about impulsivity, self-control and mood enhancement. Subjects are asked to delineate areas where they have particular problems with impulsivity, mainly as it relates to food. There is also strong emphasis on mood enhancement involving increasing pleasant events in the person's life and planning for these in advance. Subjects also complete a "reward list" of people, places, things, activities and rewards that they would like to introduce into their lives.

In session 8, there is a strong emphasis on examining body image. There is a discussion on cultural and family influences on body image. There is also a strong emphasis on finding elements in one's physical self that are positive and that have been ignored. Also there is an exercise on developing affirmations.

The ninth session focuses on self-esteem issues. In particular there. is a strong examination of thoughts about self and how to challenge and change these. Patients also complete a Self-concept Inventory where they examine their functioning in a variety of areas of life.

The tenth session focuses on stress management and problem solving. Stress response is delineated in some detail, looking at both positive responses and negative responses. Suggestions for stress management are offered. Also, there is a handout and discussion on learning to handle mistakes.

Session eleven focuses on assertiveness. Assertiveness versus aggressiveness are defined, as is passive behavior. Patients also list possible assertive self statements and examine their thoughts regarding assertive and non-assertive behaviors.

Session twelve focuses on the issue of weight loss. If subjects are overweight or obese, there is discussion about sensible ways to restrict caloric intake to induce gradual weight loss. Emphasis is placed on avoiding "fad" diets. A great deal of emphasis is placed on developing a regular exercise pattern that can be effectively maintained over time.

Sessions 13 and 14 focus on relapse prevention strategies. Emphasis is placed on understanding a lapse versus a full relapse. Subjects develop a relapse prevention plan that they can implement in the case of a lapse. Subjects also outline additional changes that they would like to make in the months ahead.

Conclusion

This approach is highly structured. Patients are told at the outset and reminded throughout the treatment that other issues that surface may not be adequately dealt with in this kind of intervention, and that they may need additional therapy for other problems at a later time. When a group format is used, emphasis is placed on patients who are making good progress, and generally the groups develop a great deal of cohesion and support for the members.

References

Agras, W.S., Telch, C.G., Arnow, B., Eldredge, K., Marnell, M. (1997). One-year follow-up of cognitive-behavioral therapy for obese individuals with binge eating disorder. *Journal of Consulting and Clinical Psychology, 65*, 343-347.

Appolinario, J.C., Bacaltchuck, J., Sichieri, R., Claudino, A.M., Godoy-Matos, A., Morgan, C., et al., (2003). A randomized, double-blind, placebo-controlled study of sibutramine in the treatment of binge-eating disorder. *Archives of General Psychiatry, 60,* 1109-1116.

Arnold, L.M., McElroy, S.L., Hudson, J.I., Welge, J.A., Bennett, A.J., Keck, P.E. (2002). A placebo-controlled, randomized trial of fluoxetine in the treatment of binge-eating disorder. *Journal of Clinical Psychiatry, 63,*1028-1033.

Claudino, A.M., de Oliveria, I.R., Appolinario, J.C., Cordas, T.A., Duchesne, M., Sichieri, R, et al., (2007). Double-blind, randomized, placebo-controlled trial of topiramate plus cognitive-behavior therapy in binge-eating disorder. *Journal of Clinical Psychiatry, 68,* 1324-1332.

Devlin, M.J., Goldfein, J.A., Petkova, E., Jiang, H., Raizman, P.S., Wolk, S., et al., (2005). Cognitive behavioral therapy and fluoxetine as adjuncts to group behavioral therapy for binge eating disorder. *Obesity Research, 13,* 1077-1088.

Fairburn, C.G., Marcus, M.D., Wilson, G.T. (1993). Cognitive behavior therapy for binge eating and bulimia nervosa: A comprehensive treatment manual. In C.B. Fairburn, & G.T. Wilson, (Eds), *Binge eating: Nature, assessment and treatment* (pp.361-404). New York: Guilford Press.

Gladis, M.M., Wadden, T.A., Vogt, R., Foster, G., Kuehl, R.H., Bartlett, S.J. (1998). Behavioral treatment of obese binge eaters: Do they need different care? *Journal of Psychosomatic Research, 44*, 375-384.

Golay, A., Laurent-Jaccard, A., Habicht, F., Gachoud, J.P., Chabloz, M., Lammer, A., et al., (2005). Effect of orlistat in obese patients with binge eating disorder. *Obesity Research, 13*, 1701-1708.

Grilo CM. (2008). Guided self-help for binge eating disorder. In J. Latner, & G.T. Wilson, (Eds), *Self-help for obesity and binge eating*. New York. Guilford Press.

Grilo, C.M., Masheb, R.M. (2005). A randomized controlled comparison of guided self-help cognitive behavioral therapy and behavioral weight loss for binge eating disorder. *Behavior Research and Therapy, 43,* 1509-1525.

Grilo, C.M., Masheb, R.M., Salant, S.L. (2005). Cognitive behavioral therapy guided self-help and orlistat for the treatment of binge eating disorder: A randomized, double-blind, placebo-controlled trial. *Biological Psychiatry, 57*, 1193-1201.

Grilo, C.M., Masheb, R.M., Wilson, G.T. (2005). Efficacy of cognitive behavioral therapy and fluoxetine for the treatment of binge eating disorder: A randomized double-blind placebo-controlled comparison. *Biological Psychiatry, 57*, 301-309.

Guerdjikova, A.I., McElroy, S.L., Kotwal, R., Welge, J.A., Nelson, E., Lake, K., et al., (2007). High-dose escitalopram in the treatment of binge-eating disorder with obesity: a placebo-controlled monotherapy trial. *Human Psychopharmacology, 23,* 1-11.

Guerdjikova, A.I., McElroy, S.L., Welge, J.A., Nelson, E., Keck, P.E., Hudson, J. (2009). Lamotrigine in the treatment of binge-eating disorder with obesity: a randomized, placebo-controlled monotherapy trial. *International Clinical Psychopharmacology, 24,* 150-8.

Hudson, J.I., McElroy, S.L., Ramond, N.C., Crow, S., Keck, P.E., Jr., Carter, W.P., et al., Fluvoxamine in the treatment of binge-eating disorder: a multicenter placebo-controlled, double-blind trial. *American Journal of Psychiatry, 155,* 1756-1762.

McElroy, S.L., Arnold, L.M., Shapira, N.A., Keck, P.E., Rosenthal, N.R., Karim, M.R. et al., (2003). Topiramate in the treatment of binge eating disorder associated with obesity: a randomized, placebo-controlled trial. *American Journal of Psychiatry, 160,* 255-261.

McElroy, S.L., Casuto, L.S., Nelson, E.B., Lake, K.A., Sotullo, C.A., Leck, P.E. Jr, et al., (2000). Placebo-controlled trial of sertraline in the treatment of binge eating disorder. *American Journal of Psychiatry, 157,* 1004-1006.

McElroy, S.L., Guerdjikova A, Kotwal R, Welge JA, Nelson EB, Lake KA, et al., (2007). Atomoxetine in the treatment of binge-eating disorder: a randomized placebo-controlled trial. *Journal of Clinical Psychiatry, 68,* 390-398.

McElroy, S.L., Hudson, J.L., Capece, J.A., Beyers, K., Fisher, A.C., Rosenthal, N.R. (2007). Topiramate for the treatment of binge eating disorder associated with obesity: a placebo-controlled study. *Biological Psychiatry, 61,* 1039-1048.

McElroy, S.L., Hudson, J.L., Malhotra, S., Welge, J.A., Nelson, E.B., Keck, P.E. Jr. (2003). Citalopram in the treatment of binge eating disorder: a placebo-controlled trial. *Journal of Clinical Psychiatry, 64,* 807-813.

McElroy, S.L., Kotwal, R., Guerdjikova, A.I., Welge, J.A., Nelson, E.B., Lake, K.A. et al., (2006). Zonisamide in the treatment of binge eating disorder with obesity: a randomized controlled trial. *Journal of Clinical Psychiatry, 67*, 1897-1906.

McElroy, S.L., Shapira, N.A., Arnold, L.M., Keck, P.E., Rosenthal, N.R., Wu, S.C. et al., (2004). Topiramate in the long-term treatment of binge-eating disorder associated with obesity. *Journal of Clinical Psychiatry, 67*, 1897-1906.

Milano, W., Petrella, C., Casella, A., Capasso, A., Carrino, S., Milano, L. (2005). Use of sibutramine, an inhibitor of the reuptake of serotonin and noradrenaline, in the treatment of binge eating disorder: a placebo-controlled study. *Advances in Therapy, 22,* 25-31.

National Institute for Clinical Excellent (2004). Eating disorders—Core interventions in the treatment and management of anorexia nervosa, bulimia nervosa and related eating disorders (Clinical Guidelines No. 9). Available from www.nice.org.uk/guidance/CG9)

Pearlstein, T., Spurell, E., Hohlstein, L.A., Gurney, V., Read, J., Fuchs, C. et al., (2003). A double blind, placebo-controlled trial of fluvoxamine in binge eating disorder: a high placebo response. *Archive of Women's Mental Health, 6,* 147-151.

Reas, D.L., Grilo, C.M. (2008). Review and meta-analysis of pharmacotherapy for binge eating disorder. *Obesity, 16,* 2024.

Ricca, V., Mannucci, E., Mezzani, B., Moretti, S., Di Bernardo, M., Bertelli, M. et al., (2001). Fluoxetine and fluvoxamine combined with individual cognitive-behavior therapy in binge eating disorder: a one-year follow-up study. *Psychotherapy and Psychosomatics, 70*, 98-306.

Telch, C.F., Agras, W.S., Linehan, M.M. (2001). Dialectical behavior therapy for binge eating disorder. *Journal of Consulting and Clinical Psychology, 69*, 1061-1065.

Wilfley, D.E., Agras, W.S., Telch, C.F., Rossiter, E.M., Schneider, J.A., Cole, A.G. et al., (1993). Group cognitive-behavioral therapy and group interpersonal psychotherapy for the nonpurging bulimia individual: A controlled comparison. *Journal of Consulting and Clinical Psychology, 61*, 296-305.

Wilfley, D.E., Crow, S.J., Hudson, J.I., Mitchell, J.E., Berkowitz, R.I., Blakesley, V. et al., (2008). Efficacy of sibutramine for the treatment of binge eating disorder: a randomized multicenter placebo-controlled double-blind study. *American Journal of Psychiatry, 165*, 4-6.

Wilfley, D.E., Welch, R.R., Stein, R.I., Spurrell, E.B., Cohen, L.R., Saelens, B.E. et al., (2002). A randomized comparison of group cognitive-behavioral therapy and group interpersonal psychotherapy for the treatment of overweight individuals with binge eating disorder. *Archives of General Psychiatry, 59*, 713-721.

Wilson, G.T., Grilo, C.M., Vitousek, K.M. (2007). Psychological Treatment of Eating Disorders. *American Psychologist, 62*, 199-216.

In: Pathways to Obesity and Main Roads to Recovery
Editor: Piergiuseppe Vinai
ISBN: 978-1-61122-740-6

Chapter XVIII

Treatment of Night Eating Syndrome

Kelly C. Allison[1] and Amy Sgrenci Langsam[2]
[1]Psychology in Psychiatry, Center for Weight and Eating Disorders, University of Pennsylvania School of Medicine, Philadelphia, PA, USA
[2]Clinical Psychology, LaSalle University, Philadelphia, PA, USA

Abstract

There is little research to date on treatments for night eating syndrome (NES), with more studies addressing pharmacotherapy than psychotherapy. Four reports, one of them a randomized controlled trial, of selective serotonin reuptake inhibitors have shown efficacy for NES. One pilot study of cognitive behavior therapy that has been developed for NES has also shown promise. The CBT treatment approach is described. Both of these treatments show significant decreases in the percent of food consumed after the evening meal and the number of nocturnal ingestions, along with modest weight loss. Reports have highlighted the need to disseminate effective treatments to care providers, as many sufferers describe that their healthcare professionals do not take their complaints seriously or do not know how to treat it.

Introduction

Night eating syndrome (NES), a form of disordered eating discovered over 50 years ago, was originally defined by three features: morning anorexia, evening hyperphagia (a quarter or more of daily food intake consumed after 18:00 hrs), and insomnia (Stunkard, Grace, & Wolf, 1955). NES was perceived to be related to stress and was reported among obese individuals who had difficulty losing weight (Stunkard et al., 1955). In the late 1990s, there was renewed interest in NES, likely due to the rise of obesity rates in the United States and other developed countries. At this time, the presence of nocturnal ingestions was noted (Birketvedt et al., 1999). Vinai and colleagues discuss the development of current diagnostic criteria (Allison et al., 2010) in Chapter VI of this volume. Research on the treatment of NES is limited and includes more pharmacotherapy trials than psychotherapy trials. We will review these treatment approaches that have been developed for NES. More specifically, this chapter will address the importance of continuing research in the treatment of NES, existing treatments, an outline of cognitive behavioral therapy (CBT) for NES, why CBT is recommended, and the effects and limitations of current treatments.

Importance of Providing Treatments for NES

Goncalves, Moore, Stunkard, & Allison (2009) examined patients' perspectives and satisfaction with their doctors' treatments for night eating (NE). The study included 103 patients who completed an internet-based questionnaire to assess their perceptions of their doctors' knowledge and treatment of NE. The authors also compared reports of treatment satisfaction for NE to satisfaction of their treatment for a headache by the same doctors. Sixty-one percent of the participants were "not at all satisfied" with their treatment of NE, reporting doctors had low recognition and high levels of dismissal of their NE signs and symptoms. Of patients who had been treated for both NE and headaches by the same doctor, 76% were "not at all satisfied" with their NE treatment, while only 29% were "not at all satisfied" with their treatment of headaches. The study concluded that doctors do not frequently identify or treat NE, which results in patient dissatisfaction with their care (Goncalves et al., 2009).

This study's results provide evidence that awareness of the diagnosis of NES needs to be raised among healthcare providers, treatments need to be further studied, and effective treatments for NES need to be dispersed more widely to medical and mental health providers.

Clinical Vignette

As many people who have NES suffer alone because of embarrassment over their nightly rituals, we provide a clinical description of one woman's story to illustrate the distress and impairment that accompany the disorder. All identifying information has been changed or disguised.

Alexis presented for treatment at the age of 60—almost 40 years after her night eating symptoms began. She recounted that she began waking up during the night in graduate school, at about the same time that she was also struggling with depression. She felt an internal drive to eat something in the middle of the night and started preparing cookie dough, which she would eat raw. Even after her depression subsided, her nightly eating continued. At the time of her evaluation, she was waking to eat at least four times each night. She tried to limit the foods that were available in her home, but she still felt motivated to eat something each time she awoke.

Although she was highly successful in her professional life, Alexis struggled with an unstable marital relationship. Also, since her 40s, she had developed some health problems that interfered with her sleep. These health issues eventually forced her to stop working, which increased her depressive symptoms as well. All of these factors seemed to exacerbate the night eating behaviors. Thus, she described her forays into the kitchen each night as very enjoyable. The nightly food-seeking behaviors seemed to function as a time for her to be free, which she felt rarely during the day. She also believed that she would not be able to fall back to sleep unless she satisfied that overwhelming urge to eat.

If she were at a hotel or on a vacation, and a variety of foods were available, she would ingest an objectively large amount of food, such as a large bag of potato chips or a container of peanuts. She has also gone to lengths to access food that has been locked away at night, such as climbing out of one window to enter a locked room through another window.

She felt that she could not talk about her night eating behaviors with others because they did not understand how serious the behaviors were and how much they were affecting her life. She exercised several times per week and ate a controlled-calorie, high-protein diet during the day. It was not until the evening when her control melted away, and her pleasurable food-seeking behaviors began. Each morning, she awoke feeling overly full and feeling disgusted with herself.

We will review the treatments for NES that have been studied that may have some benefit for Alexis and others with NES.

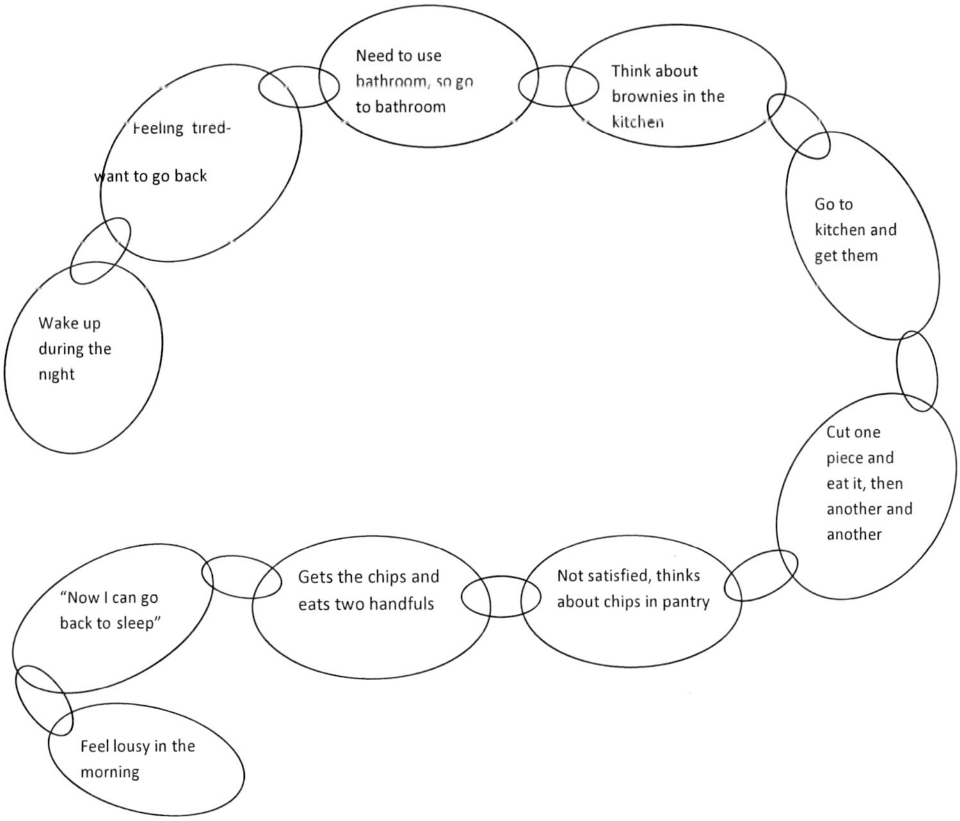

Figure 18.1. My Behavioral Chain for NES.

Psychopharmacological Treatments

Research has suggested that selective serotonin reuptake inhibitors (SSRIs) are an effective treatment for NES. Miyaoka and colleagues (2003) conducted four case studies and found that each of these patients suffering from NES was successfully treated with paroxetine or fluvoxamine. Similarly, a 12-week open-label trial of sertraline with 17 night eating participants led to significant reductions of core NES features, including nocturnal awakenings (60% decrease), nocturnal ingestions (67% decrease), and percentage of caloric intake after dinner (50% decrease) (O'Reardon, Stunkard, & Allison, 2004). In participants whose NES remitted, weight decreased by a mean of 4.8 kg, but it increased slightly in the remaining 12 participants by a mean of 0.6 kg. The sertraline dosage varied, starting at 50 mg and increasing up to 200 mg, as needed and as tolerated. A third open-label study included 50 individuals with NES who were receiving treatment (sertraline) from their own physicians while being assessed and monitored by Stunkard, Allison, Lundgren, et al., (2006). Again, they found similar results, including a reduction in nocturnal ingestions (70% decrease), reduction in calories consumed after dinner (66% decrease), and weight loss among overweight and obese participants (-2.2 kg).

The only published randomized double-blind pharmacotherapy trial for NES included 34 patients randomized to eight weeks of either sertraline (N = 17) or placebo (N= 17) (O'Reardon, Allison, Martino et al., 2006). Dosing was similar to the previous studies mentioned, starting at 50 mg and increasing up to 200 mg, as needed and as tolerated. Participants taking sertraline reported significantly greater percent reductions than the placebo group, respectively, on the same core NES indicators: number of awakenings (74% vs. 14%), nocturnal ingestions (81% vs. 14%), and total scores on the Night Eating Symptom Scale (NESS) (57% vs. 16%).

Topiramate has also been shown to be an effective treatment for NES in open-label reports. One study found that topiramate reduced night eating episodes and produced weight loss in two patients with NES and two patients with Sleep-related Eating Disorder (SRED) (Winkelman, 2003). Moreover, a case series found that six sertraline non-responders who were subsequently treated with topiramate significantly decreased their total score on the NESS, the amount of calories they consumed after dinner, and their weight (- 4.6 kg over 12 weeks, $p <. 05$), in addition to non-significant reductions in nocturnal ingestions (Allison, 2005). However, the side-effect profile of topiramate is often more severe than those of SSRIs. Nevertheless, these findings suggest the need for randomized controlled trials testing topiramate for persons with NES.

It is important to note that many healthcare providers try to treat the insomnia related to NES first. The rationale behind this is logical, thinking that if one could provide a treatment to get the patient to sleep through the night, then the problem of eating would be solved. Yet, those treatments often are comprised of benzodiazepines and hypnotics, particularly zolpidem, which typically reduce awareness for the nocturnal ingestions so that persons experience parasomnic nocturnal eating episodes similar to those in SRED (see Howell, Schenck & Crow, 2009). Persons with NES typically still rise from bed to seek food while taking these agents, but the hypnotics may act to reduce awareness and further diminish control over nocturnal ingestions. To date, little success has been found using these medications for NES and, therefore, seem to be contraindicated (O'Reardon, Stunkard, & Allison, 2004; Morgenthaler & Silber, 2002; Schenck et al., 2005).

Psychosocial Treatments

Behavioral treatment for NES has been studied and has shown mixed results (Coates, 1978; Williamson, Lawson, Bennet, & Hinz, 1989). Pawlow, O'Neil, and Malcolm (2003) conducted the first and only controlled treatment study of progressive muscle relaxation (PMR) for NES. The study compared a group that received one week of abbreviated PMR group versus a control group that was instructed to sit quietly for an equal amount of time. The PMR group increased their morning hunger and significantly decreased their evening hunger ratings compared to the control group. Additionally, the PMR group reported significant reductions of stress, anxiety, and depression. Recognizing NES as a stress-related disorder (Stunkard et al., 1955; Allison et al., 2004), PMR appears valuable, yet more research is needed for conclusive findings.

Cognitive Behavioral Therapy for NES

A CBT program for NES was developed (Allison, Lundgren, Moore, O'Reardon & Stunkard, 2010) based on manuals developed for treating binge eating (Fairburn, Marcus, & Wilson, 1993) and behavioral weight loss (Brownell, 2004). These empirically validated manuals were modified specifically for targeting the signs and symptoms of NES. The program focuses on shifting the circadian pattern of food intake to earlier in the day, while concurrently breaking the habituated response of eating to induce sleep—both initially and during the night. The daily eating patterns of individuals with NES is quite different than those of persons without NES. Specifically, daytime meals are delayed and are smaller until mid-afternoon (Boston, Moate, Allison, Lundgren, & Stunkard, 2008). Their ingestions show wide variability in general; they may have small snacks during the day instead of meals, either because they are not physically hungry, or because they are consciously restricting their intake knowing they will be unable to control their intake later that night. Recommending structured meals and snacks throughout the day is necessary to break the cycle of night eating, however, this alone is not sufficient. The treatment also targets cognitions related to night eating and teaches behavioral strategies, such as stimulus control and the use of physical barriers to reduce the accessibility of food.

In the initial pilot study (Allison et al., 2010), significant reductions were found in four major outcome measures at the end of treatment using mixed model regression analyses. These measures included scores on the NESS, percent of caloric intake consumed after dinner, number of awakenings, and number of nocturnal ingestions. Fourteen participants completed the treatment out of the 25 enrolled. Completer analyses generated greater improvements than the mixed model results, reducing nocturnal ingestions from 5.6 to 0.5 per week ($p <. 01$) and decreasing the percentage of caloric intake after dinner from 36% to 22% ($p <. 05$). The mixed model analysis also displayed significant weight losses, with a decrease of 3.1 kg ($p < .01$). These significant results demonstrate the need for a larger, randomized controlled trial of CBT with NES.

CBT of NES: Summary of Manual for Treatment

The program consists of ten individual therapy sessions that are conducted weekly during the first eight weeks and bi-weekly for the last two sessions. Clinical experience suggests that the effort spent keeping sleep and food records 24 hours a day is more work than many individuals expect for treatment; therefore, discussing this commitment early on is beneficial. Each session begins with a review of the previous session's homework that includes food and sleep logs, Night Eating Assessments (NEAs; Allison & Stunkard, 2007), and thought records (Allison, Stunkard & Thier, 2004).

The first phase of treatment includes sessions one through four. This phase focuses on developing the therapeutic alliance, explaining CBT, and educating the patient on the fundamental CBT techniques.

In the first session, the clinician and patient detail the patient's typical eating and sleeping routines for the 24-hour day. NES is explained as a delay or shift in the usual pattern of eating by describing how the body is typically "set up" to eat during the day and sleep during the night. Yet, in NES patients, the drive to eat has been conditioned to take place at an unusual time, which disrupts the usual pattern of sleep. From the start of treatment, patients are asked to monitor their food intake, physical activity, and sleep behaviors. They begin to record in a diary daily when and what they eat throughout the day and night, any physical activity, and what times they sleep. During this first session, patients are introduced to NEAs. These forms consist of visual analog scales on which patients are to rate the degree of several mood states, such as physical hunger, anxiety, cravings, feeling compelled to eat, physical agitation, boredom, and depressed mood. The NEAs are to be completed after the kitchen is "closed" time (also to be discussed and set during the first session), including repetitive eating or "grazing" before bedtime and nocturnal ingestions. NEAs are used to increase awareness for the impetus behind eating at night and are to be kept at the bedside or in the kitchen where the patient will best remember to complete them. Patients are asked to start structuring regular meal and snack times and bedtimes in their daily lives. The eventual goal is for patients to eat three meals and two to three snacks per day.

The next session focuses on behavioral techniques used to create barriers to eating after their evening meal. Examples may include putting locks on cabinets, brushing teeth immediately after their evening meal or snack, or putting a sign up on their refrigerator as a reminder not to eat after a certain time of night. Additionally, behavioral chains are introduced during the second session. This chain is completed by the patient highlighting each step in the process of evening and/or nighttime eating. An example of a behavioral chain is included in Figure 1. Next, the patient and therapist assess the "weakest links" of the chain that need to be broken to end the cycle (Allison et al., 2004). It is important to make the patient aware that this nightly eating process is not as automatic as it may appear, and that individuals with NES make active decisions every time about food choices during the night.

Calorie restriction is introduced in the third session for patients who are overweight or obese. Patients begin to monitor their calories they are consuming each day in their daily food and sleep logs. The goal is to consume more calories earlier in the day and reduce the caloric intake between dinner and bedtime and during nocturnal ingestions, using physical barriers and changing the food environment. Dysfunctional thought records are introduced in the fourth session, which is a tool designed to challenge the underlying automatic thoughts that act as stimuli for the after dinner and nocturnal ingestions (Allison et al., 2004; Allison & Stunkard, 2009). The records can help with resisting cravings or coping due to anxiety or insomnia. As stressful events during the day likely influence nighttime eating, it is essential for patients to examine their thoughts that are related to any distressing events that may be impacting a patient's emotional resources. Then, through examination of the thought records, the patient and therapist work together to propose alternative thoughts and solutions for those situations.

Sessions five through eight continue to focus on the relationships between cognitions, emotions, and behaviors. Other areas discussed include stress reduction through progressive muscle relaxation (based on the successes of the trial on PMR by Pawlow et al., 2003) and deep breathing (taught in session), sleep hygiene (e.g., fall asleep without the television on all night, not eating in the bedroom, setting standard morning awakening time and bedtime), and the importance of a healthy amount of exercise.

The final two sessions are held every other week and are designed to increase the patient's self-efficacy so that they feel mastery over how they are controlling their nighttime eating behaviors. During these sessions, the clinician helps the patient with anticipated stressors or triggers for night eating and discusses relapse prevention. If needed, additional sessions can be continued as booster sessions in order to prevent relapse, or for continued weight loss or weight maintenance, as appropriate.

Limitations and Recommendations for Future Research

In summary, little research has tested pharmacological and psychotherapeutic approaches for treating NES. At least four studies show success with the SSRI, sertraline, and other studies are currently underway testing other serotonin agents. More rigorous testing of topiramate is also required.

To date, only one pilot study has tested the CBT approach outlined here. Larger, controlled trials are needed to confirm the preliminary results. It seems that the CBT approach may need to be tailored to individuals' needs with regard to their weight status. The current treatment incorporates behavioral weight-loss techniques that are applicable and usually desired by patients who are overweight and obese. For patients who are normal weight, they typically present with more traditional eating disordered behaviors, such as severe daytime restriction and excessive exercise (Lundgren, Allison, O'Reardon, & Stunkard, 2008), which they use to compensate for their nighttime eating. Attention to these compensatory behaviors needs to be addressed in this group instead of the behavioral weight-loss component.

Persons with NES are clearly in need of a) treatments that are effective and b) healthcare providers who recognize the disorder and are aware of these treatments. We have reviewed the starting points for realizing these goals and call for further research to expand our knowledge of effective treatments for those who suffer from NES.

References

Allison, K. (2005, September). *Treatment of the night eating syndrome*. Symposium talk presented at the annual meeting of the Eating Disorders Research Society, Toronto, Canada.

Allison, K.C., Lundgren J.D., Moore R.H., O'Reardon J.P., Stunkard A.J. (2010) Cognitive behavior therapy for night eating syndrome: a pilot study. *American Journal of Psychotherapy*, *64*, 91-106.

Allison, K.C., & Stunkard, A.J. (2007) Self-help for night eating syndrome. In J. Latner & G. T. Wilson (Eds.), *Self-help for obesity and binge eating* (pp. 310-324). New York: Guilford Press.

Allison, K.C., Stunkard, A.J., & Their, S.L. (2004). *Overcoming night eating syndrome: A step-by step guide to breaking the cycle*. Oakland, CA: New Harbinger.

Birketvedt, G.S., Florholmen, J., Sundsfjord, J., Osterud, B., Dinges, D., Bilker, W., & Stunkard, A.J. (1999). Behavioral and neuroendocrine characteristics of the night-eating syndrome. *Journal of the American Medical Association, 282,* 657-663.

Boston, R.C., Moate, P.J., Allison, K.C., Lundgren, J.D., & Stunkard, A.J. (2008). Modeling circadian rhythms of food intake by means of parametric deconvolution: Results from studies on the night eating syndrome. *American Journal of Clinical Nutrition, 87,* 1672-7.

Brownell, K.D. (2004). *The LEARN program for weight management, 10th edition*. Dallas: LEARN—The Lifestyle Company.

Coates, T.J. (1978). Successive self-management strategies towards coping with night eating. *Journal of Behavior Therapy and Experimental Psychiatry, 9,* 181-183.

Fairburn, C.G., Marcus, M.D., & Wilson, G.T. (1993). Cognitive behavioral therapy for binge eating and bulimia nervosa: A comprehensive treatment manual. In C. G. Fairburn & G. T. Wilson (Eds.), *Binge eating: Nature, assessment, and treatment* (pp. 361-404). New York: Guilford Press.

Goncalves, M.D., Moore, R.H., Stunkard, A.J., & Allison, K.C. (2009). The treatment of night eating: The patient's perspective. *European Eating Disorders Review, 17,* 184-190.

Howell, M.J., Schenck, C.H., & Crow, S.J. (2009). A review of nighttime eating disorders. *Sleep Medicine Reviews, 13*, 23-34.

Lundgren, J.D., Allison, K.C., O'Reardon, J.P., & Stunkard, A.J. (2008). A descriptive study of non-obese persons with night eating syndrome and a weight-matched comparison group. *Eating Behaviors, 9,* 352-359.

Miyaoka, T., Yasukawa, R., Tsubouchi, K., Miura, S., Shimizu, Y., Sukegawa, T., Maeda, T., Mizuno, S., Kameda, A., Uegaki, J., Inagaki, T., & Horiguchi, J. (2003). Successful treatment of nocturnal eating/drinking syndrome with selective serotonin reuptake inhibitors. *International Clinical Psychopharmacology, 18*, 175-177.

Morgenthaler, T.I. & Silber, M.H. (2002). Amnestic sleep-related eating disorder associated with zolpidem. *Sleep Medicine, 3*, 323-327.

O'Reardon, J.P., Allison, K.C., Martino, N.S., Lundgren, J.D., Heo, M., & Stunkard, A.J. (2006). A randomized placebo controlled trial of sertraline in the treatment of the night eating syndrome. *American Journal of Psychiatry, 163,* 893-898.

O'Reardon, J.P., Stunkard, A.J., & Allison, K.C. (2004). A clinical trial of sertraline in the treatment of the night eating syndrome. *International Journal of Eating Disorders, 35*, 16-26.

Pawlow, L.A., O'Neil, P.M., & Malcolm, R.J. (2003). Night eating syndrome: Effects of brief relaxation training on stress, mood hunger and eating patterns. *International Journal of Obesity and Related Metabolic Disorders, 27,* 970-978.

Schenck, C.H., Connoy, D.A., Castellanos, M., Johnson, B., Werner, R., Wills, L., et al., (2005). Zolpidem-induced sleep-related eating disorder (SRED) in 19 patients. *Sleep, 28*, A259.

Stunkard, A.J., Allison, K.C., Lundgren, J.D., Martino, N.S., Heo, M., Etemad, B., & O'Reardon, J.P. (2006). A paradigm for facilitating pharmacotherapy at a distance: sertraline treatment of the night eating syndrome. *Journal of Clinical Psychiatry, 67,*1568-1572.

Stunkard, A.J., Grace, W.J., & Wolff, H.G. (1955). The night-eating syndrome: a pattern of food intake among certain obese patients. *American Journal of Medicine, 19,* 78-86.

Williamson, D. A., Lawson, O.D., Bennett, S.M., & Hinz, L. (1989). Behavioral treatment of night bingeing and rumination in an adult case of bulimia nervosa. *Journal of Behavior Therapy and Experimental Psychiatry, 20,* 73-77.

Winkelman, J.W. (2003). Treatment of nocturnal eating syndrome and sleep-related eating disorder with topiramate. *Sleep Medicine, 4,* 243-246.

In: Pathways to Obesity and Main Roads to Recovery
Editor: Piergiuseppe Vinai
ISBN: 978-1-61122-740-6

Chapter XIX

Sleep-related Eating Disorder: Relationship to Amnesia and a Review of its Treatment

Michael J. Howell[1] and Carlos H. Schenck[2]
[1]Department of Neurology Department of Medicine University of Minnesota, MN, USA
[2]Department of Psychiatry University of Minnesota, MN, USA

Abstract

Sleep related eating disorder (SRED) is characterized by a disruption of the nocturnal fast with episodes of feeding after an arousal from nighttime sleep. The recurrent eating occurs with varying degrees of diminished awareness, including amnesia. SRED is recognized as a parasomnia (i.e., a behavioral disorder accompanying sleep) and is often associated with other sleep disorders, particularly Sleepwalking, Restless Leg Syndrome (RLS) and Obstructive Sleep Apnea (OSA) (American Academy of Sleep Medicine, 2005). Importantly, amnestic SRED has been linked with sedating medications, in particular the widely prescribed benzodiazepine receptor agonists such as zolpidem (Morgenthaler & Silber, 2002). Zolpidem-associated SRED is particularly common among patients who have sleep initiation and maintenance difficulties related to RLS.

Introduction

We will introduce this chapter with a review of the physiology that maintains the normal overnight fast. We will then provide a historical description of abnormal nocturnal eating with diminished consciousness, including a review of medication-induced SRED. Then we will discuss recent insights regarding the relationship between amnesia and SRED. Finally, we will conclude with a review of nocturnal eating therapies. Please see Table 19.1 for definitions used in this chapter.

Normal Metabolic Physiology during Sleep

Under normal physiological conditions, there is a continuous absence of food intake for approximately half of every 24 hours. Energy homeostasis is maintained through the sleep period by alterations in glucose metabolism and by appetite suppression (see Table 19.2). This is in contrast to a prolonged (voluntary or involuntary) fast during wakefulness, which results in hypoglycemia and increased appetite (Morgenthaler & Silber, 2002).

Nighttime changes in glucose utilization and tolerance helps maintain stable energy stores. First, diminished motor activity during sleep decreases peripheral metabolism. Second, brain metabolism of glucose is decreased during sleep, particularly during NREM sleep (Boyle et al., 1994). Third, insulin is rapidly disposed of during sleep, resulting in higher glucose levels (Van Cauter et al., 1991). Fourth, Growth Hormone is released at the onset of sleep, stimulating gluconeogėnesis and inhibiting glucose reuptake (Van Cauter et al., 2000). Finally, cortisol secretion during the middle of the sleep period stimulates gluconeogenesis, promotes lipolysis, and the mobilization of amino acids and ketones (Spiegel et al., 1999).

Sleep changes in hormone secretion promote satiety and suppresses appetite. In particular, leptin, a peptide hormone secreted by adipocytes, inhibits hunger centers in the hypothalamus. Leptin peaks soon after sleep onset, helping to suppress feeding behavior (Simon et al., 1998).

Historical Descriptions

The first descriptions of isolated nocturnal eating were noted in association with sleepwalking. In 1981, nocturnal eating while sleepwalking was reported in a 35-year-old woman with schizoaffective disorder (Nadel, 1981). In 1990, three patients with somnambulistic eating were described who ate abnormal foods, such as raw bacon, with subsequent amnesia (Whyte, 1990). In 1991, a series of 19 patients with nocturnal eating was reported (Schenck et al., 1991). This condition was named sleep-related eating disorder (SRED) and was then classified as a parasomnia in the International Classification of Sleep Disorders (American Academy of Sleep Medicine, 2005). Subsequent series have helped define the clinical spectrum of SRED (Schenck et al., 1993; Winkelman, 1998; Vetrugno et al., 2006). The phenomenology of SRED, and the personal ordeals suffered by affected patients, as well as the gratifying response to therapy, has been documented in a book with case histories (Schenck, 2005), and in a documentary film (Schenck, 2007).

Table 19.1.

Night eating	Eating after the last meal and prior to final awakening
Evening hyperphagia	Excessive eating after the last meal and prior to falling asleep
Nocturnal eating	Eating that occurs after an arousal from sleep prior to final awakening

Table 19.2. Energy homeostasis during sleep

Decreased glucose utilization	Impaired glucose tolerance	Appetite suppression
Decreased motor activity Decreased cerebral glucose activity	GH secretion at sleep onset Insulin disposal increased	Increased leptin

SRED and Benzodiazepine Receptor Agonists

Many of the early reports noted that amnestic nocturnal eating was associated with sedating psychotropic medications. In fact, the first case of amnestic nocturnal eating in 1981, was associated with a combination of chlorpromazine, amitriptyline, and methyprylon (Nadel, 1981). Subsequently, SRED has been reported with triazolam, lithium, olanzapine, and risperidone (Schenck & Mahowald, 1994; Paquet, 2002; Lu et al., 2004).

Benzodiazepine receptor agonists (BRA) have been associated with initiating and exacerbating nocturnal eating. The first case report of amnestic nocturnal eating related to zolpidem use was described in member of the armed services in 1999. Four days after starting zolpidem, the 46-year-old male described sleep walking with meal preparation and no recollection of events. The behavior immediately ceased following discontinuation of the agent (Harazin & Berigan, 1999). A series of zolpidem-associated SRED was reported in 2002. Five middle-aged patients were described, two of whom already had intermittent episodes of conscious nocturnal eating prior to starting zolpidem. All five patients were on various neuropsychiatric agents, and interestingly, all had a history of RLS. Soon after initiating zolpidem, each patient described amnestic nocturnal eating that stopped with discontinuation of zolpidem (Morgenthaler & Silber, 2002).

Subsequent case studies have documented the diverse spectrum of amnestic SRED with zolpidem. One case report described a 51-year-old female with RLS who noted empty food-packages in the morning soon after she started taking zolpidem. She later discerned that she had been eating sandwiches on several occasions (Sansone & Sansone, 2008). Recently, a case of SRED with zolpidem was noted in a 45-year-old male insomnia patient. After ten days of treatment, he was missing on two occasions after going to bed. Both times, he was found eating "sweets" at his place of business. After driving his car over two kilometers, he had climbed into his place of business through the shutter instead of using the door (Dang et al., 2008). This type of complex yet inappropriate behavior is not unusual in sleepwalkers. All of the above SRED cases ceased after discontinuing zolpidem.

Recently, uncontrollable nocturnal eating occurred in a 40-year-old female after taking a 15 mg dose of zolpidem (normal dose 5 to 10 mg) (Tsai et al., 2007). This case illustrates the dose effect of zolpidem and amnestic nocturnal eating. In our published abstract on 19 patients with amnestic SRED induced by zolpidem, most patients were taking 10 to 20 mg zolpidem (Schenck et al., 2005). In our experience, amnestic SRED often occurs when, in a desperate attempt to induce sleep, patients escalate dose with or without a new prescription.

Extended-release formulations of zolpidem have also been implicated in SRED. A 46-year-old female presented with new symptoms suggestive of OSA after gaining 50 pounds. She claimed that her weight gain was secondary to amnestic nocturnal eating that began 12 months earlier after starting extended-release zolpidem for insomnia. The patient was switched to the medication eszopiclone, also a BRA, and her amnestic eating behavior subsequently stopped (Najjar, 2007). Another report describes two women (70 and 75 years old) who developed amnestic nocturnal eating only after switching from immediate-release to extended-release zolpidem. Both patients also had RLS that was reported to be under good control with anti-RLS agents. Events resolved in both patients after switching back to the immediate-release formulation (Chiang & Krystal, 2008).

Recent publications have demonstrated the prevalence of zolpidem-associated SRED and speculated upon potential underlying neuronal mechanisms. In a cross-sectional study of a psychiatric population, 14 of 22 patients with SRED had been exposed to zolpidem. Interestingly, four of the 22 had been exposed to zopiclone, a less frequently prescribed BRA (Lam et al., 2008), suggesting that amnestic nocturnal eating is a feature of the entire BRA class and not merely the agent zolpidem. BRAs induce sleep and amnesia through enhancement of GABA activity at alpha1 GABA A receptors. It has been suggested that the complex behavior noted with some BRAs is in part related to increasing binding affinity (Dolder & Nelson, 2008). However, more pharmokinetic research is needed.

Importantly, a substantial number of cases of BRA-associated amnestic nocturnal eating are seen in the setting of patients with RLS (2,20,25). RLS is a condition distinct from, but often clinically confused with, insomnia. Difficulty initiating and maintaining sleep is a major presenting complaint in patients with RLS. We speculate that inappropriate diagnosis and treatment of RLS as primary or conditioned insomnia is a crucial underlying step in the pathogenesis of many amnestic SRED cases.

SRED and Amnesia

The presence of impaired consciousness has historically been a distinguishing feature of SRED. In the original series of SRED cases, 32 of 38 patients claimed at least partial impairment in awareness (Schenck et al., 2003). In another case series, 21 of 23 patients had incomplete consciousness and/or amnesia for the behavior (Winkelman, 1998).

Conversely, a subsequent study demonstrated full awareness during nocturnal eating episodes. In this recent clinical and PSG study, all 26 patients claimed full alertness after nocturnal eating in a sleep lab. However the authors did not report whether the subjects typically had full awareness during nocturnal eating at home (Vetrugno et al., 2006). This is an important distinction, as the level of consciousness may be different in a sleep laboratory compared to a more familiar (i.e., home) sleeping environments. Also, in SRED, awareness will vary night-to-night and sometimes between episodes of the same night (Winkelman, 2006). Reduced awareness and subsequent amnesia is not a required diagnostic criterion for SRED in the International Classification of Sleep Disorders—2nd version (American Academy of Sleep Medicine, 2005), even though most SRED patients do not claim full consciousness while engaged in nocturnal eating.

The spectrum of amnesia noted in SRED reports may be explained by co-morbid sleepwalking or OSA and by the use of sedating medication. The first case reports of nocturnal eating with amnesia were associated with a co-morbid sleepwalking disorder or use of a psychotropic medication (Nadel, 1981; Whyte, 1990; Schenck & Mahowald, 1994). Moreover, the majority of patients in the original series were taking sedating medication or had a previous history of sleepwalking. This was not unexpected considering the patients were gathered at a tertiary sleep disorders center (Schenck et al., 2003). Furthermore, in a survey of 92 nocturnal eating subjects, over 80% of participants claimed full awareness of their behavior, and none had a history of sleepwalking. If participants had a history of sleepwalking they were very likely (73%) to be at least partially unaware of the behavior (de Zwaan et al., 2006). In the PSG study cited above, none of the 26 patients having full awareness of eating in the sleep lab were taking sedating medications, and only one had a history of sleepwalking (Vetrugno et al., 2006).

SRED is commonly associated with other sleep disorders, in particular parasomnias such as sleepwalking. In the original reported series of 38 patients with SRED, sleepwalking was noted in 23, RLS in five, OSA in four, and narcolepsy in four (Schenck et al., 2003). In another study noted above, of 23 SRED patients, 18 had a history of a parasomnia (Winkelman, 1998). In our experience, sleepwalking without eating often precedes SRED. Then, once nocturnal eating occurs, it may become the predominant or exclusive sleepwalking behavior.

Treatment

The first goal in treating dysfunctional nocturnal eating is to identify and correct any co-morbid sleep disorders and eliminate suspected inducing agents. SRED is commonly associated with other sleep disorders, in particular parasomnias such as sleepwalking. In the original reported series of 38 patients with SRED, sleepwalking was noted in 23, RLS in five, OSA in four, and narcolepsy in four (Schenck et al., 2003). In the study noted above, of 23 SRED patients, 18 had a history of a parasomnia (Winkelman, 1998). In our experience, sleepwalking without eating often precedes SRED. Then, once nocturnal eating occurs, it may become the predominant or exclusive sleepwalking behavior.

The nocturnal eating of SRED can often be controlled by suppressing co-morbid RLS and PLMD. Dopaminergics, opiods, and benzodiazepines are agents typically employed in the treatment of RLS and PLMD. In our original case series, combinations of these medications have effectively eliminated nocturnal eating associated with RLS and PLMD (Schenck et al., 2003). Interestingly, dopamine dysfunction has been linked to RLS, PLMD, as well as SRED.

Table 19.3. Medications associated with SRED

Zolpidem-immediate release
Zolpidem-sustained release
Zopiclone
Triazolam
Midazolam
Risperidone
Olanzapine

Table 19.4. Drugs used in SRED treatment

Medication class	Agent	Authors and year	Study Design	Primary Diagnosis (# of subjects)	Results (Responders/total subjects)*
Dopaminergics	Carbidopa /levodopa	Schenck et al., 1993	case series	SRED (12)	(10/12) temporary remission in 2/12.
	bromocriptine	Schenck et al., 1993	case series	SRED (3)	(2/3) temporary remission in 1/3.
	pramipexole	Provini et al., 2005	pilot double blind, placebo, crossover	SRED (11)	decreased nocturnal activity as measured by actigraphy, no change in number of awakenings or ingestions
antiseizure	topiramate	Winkelman, 2003	open label trial	SRED (2) NES (2)	(4/4) mean weight loss 11.1 kg over 8.5 months
	topiramate	Martinez-Salio et al., 2007	case report	SRED (1)	(1/1) 2 year follow up
	topiramate	Schenck et al., 2006	case series	SRED (17)	(12/17) mean weight loss of 9.2 kg among responders after 1.8 years;
	topiramate	Winkelman, 2006	open label trial	SRED (25)	(17/25) mean weight loss 11.1 kg over mean 11.6 months; 21/25 adverse events and 7/17 responders d/c'd after 1 year
Serotonergics	fluoxetine	Schenck et al., 1993	case series	SRED (3)	(2/3)
	fenfluramine	Spaggiari et al., 1994	case series	Noct. eating syndrome *(7)	(6/7) mean weight loss 11.1 kg over 8.5 months
	paroxetine fluvoxamine	Miyaoka et al., 2003	case series	nocturnal eat./drink. syndrome *(4)	paroxetine (3/3) fluvoxamine (1/1)
	sertraline	O'Reardon et al., 2004	Open label trial	NES (17)	Compared to baseline patients had less awakenings and nocturnal ingestions after starting sertraline ($p<.01$)
	sertraline	O'Reardon et al., 2006	double blind, placebo controlled	NES (34)	Compared to placebo: sertraline subjects had 81% less nocturnal ingestions compared to 14% less for placebo Overweight and Obese Sertraline subjects lost more weight compared to similar placebo subjects (2.9kg vs. 0.3kg)

* Responders defined as elimination of nocturnal eating or diminished nocturnal eating with other clinical improvement such as weight loss.

** terminology not frequently employed.

SRED associated with OSA is often effectively treated with continuous positive airway pressure (CPAP), the standard treatment for sleep disordered breathing. In both reported cases of SRED with OSA, CPAP eliminated the nocturnal eating (Schenck & Mahowald, 1994). In our ongoing series of SRED patients with co-morbid OSA, approximately 50% of SRED cases were controlled with CPAP, with the other 50% of patients required separate pharmacotherapy.

SRED co-morbid with sleepwalking can be effectively treated with dopaminergic therapy. In our original case series, eight sleepwalking patients with SRED were effectively treated with bromocriptine and/or clonazepam (Schenck et al., 2003). However, cumulative publications have indicated that benzodiazepines, the standard treatment for sleepwalking, are typically ineffective as monotherapy.

Discontinuing the offending medication is the best treatment for drug-induced SRED (Morgenthaler & Silber, 2002; Sansone & Sansone, 2008; Dang et al., 2008; Tsai et al., 2007; Schenck et al., 2005; Chiang & Krystal, 2008) (see Table 19.3). Rarely, patients who did not have nocturnal eating prior to exposure will have persisting episodes after cessation. It is not certain whether this is a temporary phenomenon or, whether the offending agent is lowering a threshold in patients who were predisposed to nocturnal eating.

At this time, three classes of pharmacotherapies have been studied and appear to be potentially effective in treating nocturnal eating. In SRED, the antiseizure medication topiramate and dopaminergics have both demonstrated promising results. Nocturnal eating associated with Night Eating Syndrome (NES) has responded well to sertraline (Please see the precedent chapter for details regarding treatment of NES). However, research on the therapy of SRED is still in its infancy, and further investigations, in particular randomized controlled trials, are necessary.

Dopaminergic agents may be effective in the treatment of SRED even in the absences of RLS/PLMD. The original case series noted that either bedtime levodopa or bromocriptine were effective in eliminating nocturnal eating, especially in patients with associated RLS (Schenck et al., 2003). The mechanism by which dopamine agents may suppress nocturnal eating is unknown; however, they demonstrate appetite suppression in animal models (Martin-Iverson & Dourish, 1989). Recently, pramipexole, a dopamine agonist, was investigated in a small, double-blind, placebo-controlled crossover trial. Pramipexole was well tolerated in all patients, including those without RLS or PLMD. On pramipexole, subjects noted improved sleep, and reduced nighttime activity was documented with actigraphy. There was no improvement in the number or duration of awakenings (Provini et al., 2005). The main side effects of dopamine agonist include: sedation, orthostasis, nausea, manic episodes, paranoia, psychosis, and, hallucinations.

Early studies indicate that the anti-seizure medication topiramate may be an effective treatment for nocturnal eating in SRED. An open label trial of topiramate in four patients with nocturnal eating demonstrated positive results. The agent was well tolerated, nocturnal eating diminished, and weight loss (mean of 11.1kg) was noted in all four individuals over 8.5 months (Winkelman 2003). A case report with similar results was recently published. This 28-year-old obese male had a ten-year history of nocturnal eating episodes that were eliminated with topiramate. It was also reported that the agent was well tolerated over a two-year follow up (Martinez-Salio et al., 2007). In a case series that we published as an abstract, of 17 SRED patients treated with topiramate, 12 were treatment responsive. The agent was well tolerated, and over 1.8 years, there was a mean weight loss of 9.2 kg among the treatment responders (Schenck, 2006). Another chart review of 25 follow-up SRED patients reported that 68% of SRED patients were treatment responders. Further, over one year, 28% of patients lost more than 10% of their body weight. Adverse events were high, however, and 41% of patients discontinued the medication (Winkelman, 2006). The main side effects of topiramate include: weight loss, paresthesias, renal calculus, cognitive dysfunction, and orthostasis.

Modulation of central nervous system serotonin may lead to effective treatment of nocturnal eating. In 1994, an investigation reported that all six nocturnal eating patients treated with the serotonin agent fenfluramine had a pronounced reduction in caloric intake and episode frequency (Spaggiari et al., 1994). Another report described complete eradication of nocturnal eating in four subjects as early as two weeks after initiation of an SSRI (Miyaoka et al., 2003). Nocturnal eating in patients diagnosed with the NES has been controlled with SSRI's (O'Reardon et al., 2004; O'Reardon et al., 2006) (For greater detail regarding the treatment of NES, please see chapter XVIII). SSRI's may be effective in treating nocturnal eating in patients with SRED, however, more research is needed. In the original case series, fluoxetine was effective in two of three SRED patients (Schenck et al., 2003).

Conclusion

The nocturnal eating of SRED occurs when there is a break in the nighttime fast. Initial investigation into nocturnal eating should attempt to identify co-morbid sleep disorders and to eliminate inducing agents. In particular, sleepwalking, OSA, RLS, and PLMD are treatable and commonly associated with nocturnal eating. SRED is associated with psychotropic medication, most notably the BRA zolpidem, but with other sedative hypnotics as well. Polysomnography with a seizure montage at an accredited sleep laboratory is needed to identify and treat co-morbid sleep disorders.

At this time, three types of pharmacotherapies have been studied and appear to be potentially effective. In SRED, the antiseizure medication topiramate and dopaminergics have both demonstrated promising results. Nocturnal eating associated with the NES has responded well to sertraline.

References

American Academy of Sleep Medicine. (2005) International Classification of Sleep Disorders: Diagnostic and Coding Manual. 2nd Edition ed. Westchester. IL: American Academy of Sleep Medicine;.

Boyle, P.J., Scott, J.C., Krentz, A.J., Nagy, R.J., Comstock, E., Hoffman, C. (1994) Diminished brain glucose metabolism is a significant determinant for falling rates of systemic glucose utilization during sleep in normal humans. *J. Clin. Invest., 93,* 529-535.

Chiang, A., Krystal, A. (2008). Report of two cases where sleep-related eating behavior occurred with the extended-release formulation but not the immediate-release formulation of a sedative-hypnotic agent. *J. Clin. Sleep Med., 15,* 155-156.

Dang, A., Garg, G., Rataboli, P.V. (2008) Zolpidem induced nocturnal sleep-related eating disorder (NSRED) in a male patient. *Int. J. Eat. Disord., 23,* 385-6.

de Zwaan, M., Roerig, D.B., Crosby, R.D., Karaz, S., Mitchell, J.E. (2006) Nighttime eating: a descriptive study. *Int. J. Eat. Disord., 39,* 224-232.

Dolder, C.R., Nelson, M.H. (2008). Hypnosedative-induced complex behaviors: incidence, mechanisms and management. *CNS Drugs, 22,* 1021-1036.

Harazin, J., Berigan, T.R. (1999) Zolpidem tartrate and somnambulism. *Mil. Med., 164*, 669-670.

Lam, S.P., Fong, S.Y., Ho, C.K., Yu, M.W., Wing, Y.K. (2008). Parasomnia among psychiatric outpatients: a clinical, epidemiologic, cross-sectional study. *J. Clin. Psychiatry, 69,* 1374-1382.

Lu, M.L., Shen, W.W. (2004) Sleep-related eating disorder induced by risperidone. *J. Clin. Psychiatry, 65,* 273-274.

Martinez-Salio, A., Soler-Algarra, S., Calvo-Garcia, I., Sanchez-Martin, M. (2007) Nocturnal sleep-related eating disorder that responds to topiramate. *Rev. Neurol., 15,* 276-279.

Martin-Iverson, M.T., Dourish, C.T. (1988) Role of dopamine D-1 and D-2 receptor subtypes in mediating dopamine agonist effects on food consumption in rats. *Psychopharmacology (Berl), 96*, 370-374.

Miyaoka, T., Yasukawa, R., Tsubouchi, K., Miura, S., Shimizu, Y., Sukegawa, T., et al., (2003) Successful treatment of nocturnal eating/drinking syndrome with selective serotonin reuptake inhibitors. *Int. Clin. Psychopharmacol., 18*, 175-177.

Morgenthaler, T.I., Silber, M.H. (2002) Amnestic sleep-related eating disorder associated with zolpidem. *Sleep Med. Jul, 3(4),* 323-327.

Nadel, C. (1981) Somnambulism, bed-time medication and over-eating. *Br. J. Psychiatry, 139,* 79.

Najjar, M. (2007). Zolpidem and amnestic sleep-related eating disorder. *J. Clin. Sleep Med., 15,* 637-638.

O'Reardon, J.P., Allison, K.C., Martino, N.S., Lundgren, J.D., Heo, M., Stunkard, A.J. (2006) A randomized, placebo-controlled trial of sertraline in the treatment of night eating syndrome. *Am J Psychiatry, 163*, 893-898.

O'Reardon, J.P., Stunkard, A.J., Allison, K.C. (2004) Clinical trial of sertraline in the treatment of night eating syndrome. *Int J Eat Disord., 35,* 16-26.

Paquet, V., Strul, J., Servais, L., Pelc, I., Fossion, P. (2002) Sleep-related eating disorder induced by olanzapine. *J.Clin.Psychiatry, 63,* 597.

Provini, F., Albani, F., Vetrugno, R., Vignatelli, L., Lombardi, C., Plazzi, G., et al., (2005). A pilot double-blind placebo-controlled trial of low-dose pramipexole in sleep-related eating disorder. *Eur. J. Neurol., 12,* 432-436.

Sansone, R.A., Sansone, L.A. (2008) Zolpidem, somnambulism, and nocturnal eating. *Gen. Hosp. Psychiatry, 30,* 90-91.

Schenck, C.H., Connoy, D.A., Castellanos, M., Johnson, B., Wills, L., Cramer-Bornemann, M.A., Mahowald, M.W. (2005) Zolpidem-induced Sleep-Related Eating Disorder (SRED) in 19 patients. *Sleep, 28,*:a259.

Schenck, C.H., Hurwitz, T.D., Bundlie, S.R., Mahowald, M.W. (1991) Sleep-related eating disorders: polysomnographic correlates of a heterogeneous syndrome distinct from daytime eating disorders. *Sleep, 14,* 419-431.

Schenck, C.H., Hurwitz, T.D., O'Connor, K.A., Mahowald, M.W. (1993) Additional categories of sleep-related eating disorders and the current status of treatment. *Sleep, 16,* 457-466.

Schenck, C.H., Mahowald, M.W. (1994) Review of nocturnal sleep-related eating disorders. *Int. J. Eat. Disord., 15,* 343-356.

Schenck, C.M. (2006) Topiramate therapy of sleep-related eating disorder (SRED). *Sleep, 29,* a268.

Schenck, CH. (2005). Paradox Lost: midnight in the battleground of sleep and dreams. 1st ed.: Extreme-Nights, LLC, Minneapolis, MN; (www.parasomnias-rbd.com)

Schenck, CH. (2007) Sleep Runners: the stories behind everyday parasomnias. DVD. www.sleeprunners.com

Simon, C., Gronfier, C., Schlienger, J.L., Brandenberger, G. (1998) Circadian and ultradian variations of leptin in normal man under continuous enteral nutrition: relationship to sleep and body temperature. *J.Clin.Endocrinol.Metab. 83,* 1893-1899.

Spaggiari, M.C., Granella, F., Parrino, L., Marchesi, C., Melli, I., Terzano, M.G. (1994) Nocturnal eating syndrome in adults. *Sleep, 17,* 339-344.

Spiegel, K., Leproult, R., Van Cauter, E. (1999) Impact of sleep debt on metabolic and endocrine function. *Lancet, 354,* 1435-1439.

Tsai, M.J., Tsai, Y.H., Huang, Y.B. (2007). Compulsive activity and anterograde amnesia after zolpidem use. *Clin. Toxicol. 45,* 179-181.

Van Cauter, E., Blackman, J.D., Roland, D., Spire, J.P., Refetoff, S., Polonsky, K.S. (1991) Modulation of glucose regulation and insulin secretion by circadian rhythmicity and sleep. *J.Clin.Invest.*, 88, 934-942.

Van Cauter, E., Leproult, R., Plat, L. (2000) Age-related changes in slow wave sleep and REM sleep and relationship with growth hormone and cortisol levels in healthy men. *JAMA, 284,* 861-868.

Vetrugno, R., Manconi, M., Ferini-Strambi, L., Provini, F., Plazzi, G., Montagna, P. (2006) Nocturnal eating: sleep-related eating disorder or night eating syndrome? A videopolysomnographic study. *Sleep, 29,* 949-954.

Whyte J.K.N. 1990. Somnambulistic eating: A report of three cases. *Int J Eat Disord., 9,* 577-581.

Winkelman, J.W. (1998) Clinical and polysomnographic features of sleep-related eating disorder. *J. Clin. Psychiatry, 59,* 14-19.

Winkelman, J.W. (2003) Treatment of nocturnal eating syndrome and sleep-related eating disorder with topiramate. *Sleep Med., 4,* 243-246.

Winkelman, J.W. (2006) Efficacy and tolerability of open-label topiramate in the treatment of sleep-related eating disorder: a retrospective case series. *J. Clin. Psychiatry, 67,* 1729-1734.

Winkelman, J.W. (2006) Sleep-related eating disorder and night eating syndrome: sleep disorders, eating disorders, or both? *Sleep, 29,* 876-877.

In: Pathways to Obesity and Main Roads to Recovery
Editor: Piergiuseppe Vinai

ISBN: 978-1-61122-740-6

Chapter XX

Obesity and its Treatment in Persons with Mental Illness

Jennifer D. Lundgren and Melisa V. Rempfer
Department of Psychology University of Missouri-Kansas City, MO, USA

Abstract

Persons with serious mental illness and individuals taking atypical antipsychotic medications have elevated risk for obesity compared to the general population. Several factors have been hypothesized to contribute to this problem, including abnormal eating behavior and energy consumption, economic and social factors. Further, individuals with mental illness and those prescribed atypical antipsychotic medications are at significantly greater risk of obesity-related health co-morbidities than is the general public. In response to this serious public health issue, there has been a burgeoning interest in developing lifestyle weight-management approaches targeted for people with serious mental illness. While studies have generally shown success in achieving modest weight loss for this population, mean weigh loss compares unfavorably to weight-loss interventions in non-psychiatric samples. Successful weight-management strategies for persons with serious mental illness require attention to various factors that can interfere with behavioral skill learning generally and with weight-loss behaviors specifically. Future treatment development and research will benefit from additional attention to the cognitive limitations often experienced by persons with serious mental illness.

Introduction

The Obesity Problem in Psychiatric Populations

Obesity is a well-known public health concern, with 65% of U.S. adults meeting criteria for overweight (BMI = 25.0 to 29.9 kg/m^2) or obesity (BMI >30.0 kg/m^2) (Flegal, Carroll,

Ogden, & Johnson, 2002). Persons with serious mental illness and individuals taking atypical antipsychotic medications are even more likely to be obese than is the general public (Dickerson et al., 2006a; Dickerson, Brown, Kreyenbuhl, Fang, Goldberg, Wohlheiter, et al., 2006b; Allison, Fontaine, Heo, Mentor, Capperlleri, Chandler, et al., 1999a; Theisen, Linden, Geller, Schafer, Martin, Remschmidt et al., 2001).

Allison and colleagues (1999a) compared the age adjusted BMIs of community dwelling individuals with schizophrenia to non-psychiatric controls enrolled in the Third National Health and Nutrition Examination Survey (NHANES-III). Women with schizophrenia had a significantly higher age-adjusted BMI (27.36 kg/m^2) compared to the female control group (BMI = 24.50 kg/m^2). The difference between males with schizophrenia and controls did not differ significantly; both, however, had age-adjusted BMIs in the overweight range (BMI between 25.0 and 29.9 kg/m^2). Dickerson and colleagues (2006a) found that both males and females diagnosed with serious mental illness (operationalized as schizophrenia, schzioaffective disorder, and mood disorders) were significantly more likely than a matched, non-psychiatric comparison group to meet criteria for obesity.

Why Is there a Problem?

Several factors have been hypothesized to contribute to excess weight among persons with SMI, including abnormal eating behavior and energy consumption (Strasnig, Brar, & Ganguli, 2003; Lundgren, Rempfer, Brown, Joetz, Hamera, 2010; Ramacciotti, Paoli, Catena, Ciapparelli, Dell'Osso, Schulte et al., 2004), decreased physical activity (Daumit, Goldberg, Anthony, Dickerson, Brown, Kreyenbuhl et al., 2005), and medication use (Allison, Mentore, Heo, Chandler, Cappelleri, Infante et al., 1999b).

With regard to energy consumption and eating behavior, Strasnig and colleagues (2003) found that persons with schizophrenia consumed more calories than did a reference group, consuming an average of 3,057 kcal/day. McCreadie and colleagues (1998) found that persons with schizophrenia, compared to matched controls, consumed fewer fruits (2.3 vs. 7.0) and fewer vegetables (10.0 vs. 19.0) per week. Ramaccotti and colleagues (2004) found that among individuals taking antipsychotic medication, binge eating disorder (BED) developed after the onset of antipsychotic treatment for 10% of individuals; an additional six percent reported BED before antipsychotic treatment. Our group has found that night eating syndrome (i.e., evening hyperphagia and nocturnal awakening and ingestion of food) is prevalent among obese individuals with SMI (both schizophrenia and mood disorders), with 26.8% reporting either evening hyperphagia or ≥ 3 nocturnal ingestions of food per week (Lundgren et al., 2010).

Physical activity patterns of persons with SMI are different from the general population (Daumit et al., 2005). Daumit and colleagues (2005) found that compared to the NHANES control sample, individuals with schizophrenia or mood disorders were more likely to report *no* physical activity during the month previous to assessment (patient = 25.7% vs. control = 17.5%). Persons with schizophrenia were less likely to jog (4.9%) and garden (17.8%) compared to controls (jog = 11.9%, garden = 50.8%). The most common type of physical activity reported among both groups was walking. Greater frequency of physical activity was associated with higher education and a diagnosis of depression; individuals with depression were 3.1 times more likely to engage in physical activity than were individuals diagnosed with schizophrenia and schizoaffective disorder. Inactivity was associated with less social contact and male gender.

The use of second generation (atypical) antipsychotics (SGAs) is a well-documented cause of excess weight and metabolic abnormalities among individuals with psychotic spectrum disorders (Allison et al., 1999b; Allison & Casey, 2001; Ganguli, 1999). Clozapine and Olanzapine are associated with the most weight gain (3.99 kg and 3.51kg weight gain at ten weeks respectively) (Allison et al., 1999b). The precise mechanism of weight gain due to SGAs remains unknown; regardless, obesity occurs when energy intake (calories) exceeds energy expenditure (Consensus Development Conference on Antipsychotic Drugs and Obesity and Diabetes). This is significant because it means that weight can be modified through lifestyle-behavior-change strategies aimed at regulating energy consumption and energy expenditure, even if the pathophysiology of obesity in this population is not fully understood.

Health Consequences and Mortality Associated with Obesity and Medication Use in Psychiatric Populations

In addition to excess weight, persons with SMI and those prescribed atypical antipsychotic medications are at significantly greater risk of obesity-related health co-morbidities, such as the Metabolic Syndrome (Met Syn), than is the general public (Newcomer & Haupt, 2006; McEvoy et al., 2005). Met Syn, as defined by the Third Report of the National Cholesterol Education Program Expert Panel on Detection, Evaluation, and Treatment of High Blood Cholesterol in Adults (NCEP-ATP III), is a cluster of conditions including abdominal obesity (waist circumference > 102 cm for men or > 88 cm for women), elevated triglycerides (≥ 150 mg/dl), low HDL cholesterol (< 40 mg/dl for men or < 50 mg/dl for women), elevated blood pressure (≥ 130/ ≥ 85 mm Hg), and elevated fasting glucose (≥ 110 mg/dl) (Expert Panel). Met Syn affects approximately 22% of adults in the general United States population (Ford, Giles, & Dietz, 2002). Met Syn increases the risks of coronary heart disease, myocardial infarction, stroke, and diabetes (Isomaa, Almgren, Tuomi, Forsen, Lahti, Nissen et al., 2001). The syndrome is associated with increased mortality, both all-cause and that associated with cardiovascular disease (Isomaa et al., 2001).

McEvoy and colleagues (2005) compared the prevalence of Met Syn between persons with schizophrenia enrolled in the Clinical Antipsychotic Trials of Intervention Effectiveness (CATIE) study and general public estimates from NHANES III. Forty percent (40%) of the CATIE participants met NCEP-ATP III criteria for Met Syn, which is significantly higher than the prevalence found among randomly selected matched participants from the NHANES III sample (19.7%). Nasrallah and colleagues (2006) reported on the pharmacologic treatment rates of CATIE participants meeting criteria for hypertension, dyslipidemia, and diabetes. Among the entire sample, 69.8% of persons with diabetes were receiving treatment, 37.6% of persons with hypertension were receiving treatment, and only 12% of persons with dyslipidemia were receiving treatment.

Paralleling the prevalence trends of obesity and Met Syn among individuals with serious mental illness, the mortality data provide even more cause for concern. Colton and Manderscheid (2006) studied the mortality rate and its causes in psychiatric samples in eight

U.S. states; they found that psychiatric patients, compared to nationwide life expectancies, had lost an average of 13 to 30 years of life (varying by state). The leading cause of death was heart disease, similar to non-psychiatric individuals' leading cause of death. Although the percent of patients who died of heart disease varied among the states, approximately 30% of deaths were attributable to this cause.

Despite the weight and metabolic abnormalities associated with atypical antipsychotic medications, they are considered the first line treatment for psychoses (American Psychiatric Association, 2004). It is not surprising, then, that increasingly more psychiatric patients are prescribed these medications. Data from the National Ambulatory Medical Care Survey and the National Hospital Ambulatory Medical Care Survey show a staggering increase in SGA use from 1996 to 2003: the number of healthcare visits associated with an atypical antipsychotic prescription increased by 195% and combination antipsychotic use (typical and atypical) increased by 149% (Sankaranarayanan & Puumala, 2007).

Given the negative health consequences associated with these medications, there is a clear need for improved treatment of both obesity and obesity related health co-morbidities in psychiatric populations prescribe these medications. Below, the weight-management options for psychiatric populations are reviewed.

Weight Management Programs Developed for Psychiatric Populations

Review of the Outcome Literature

Weight-management interventions for psychiatric populations are similar to those used in non-psychiatric populations, with a focus on behavior change, nutrition, and physical activity (Álvarez-Jiménez, Hetrick, Gonzáles-Blanch, Gleeson, McGorry, 2008; Ganguli, 2007; Brar, Ganguli, Pandina, Turkoz, Berry, Mahmoud, 2005). As with general weight management guidelines (see the National Institutes of Health Practical Guide: Identification, Evaluation, and Treatment of Overweight and Obesity in Adults for a review of current guidelines), pharmacotherapy (e.g., orlistat, sibutramine) is *not* considered the first-line intervention for psychiatric populations (Ganguli, 2007).

The outcome data on behavioral weight management among persons with SMI is limited compared to obesity treatment outcome in the general population. Álvarez-Jiménez and colleagues (2008) conducted a rigorous meta-analysis of controlled, non-pharmacologic interventions (i.e., cognitive-behavioral and nutritional counseling) for weight loss and weight-gain prevention in persons diagnosed with schizophrenia who were prescribed antipsychotic medications. Of the ten studies included in the analysis, five examined group programs and five examined individual programs; all programs were compared to treatment as usual. The treatments ranged in length from eight weeks to six months, and all but one intervention were conducted in *outpatient settings*. Four of the ten studies were aimed at weight-gain prevention, and one study (Álvarez-Jiménez, Gonzáles-Blanch, Vázquez-Barquero, Pérez-Iglesias, Martínez-García, Pérez-Pardal et al., 2006) included individuals with first-episode psychosis.

On average, the studies produced significant weight loss (M weighted change = -2.56kg), compared to the treatment as usual control conditions; there was some evidence that weight-gain prevention programs might have larger effects than weight-loss programs, although there was no statistically significant difference in weight change between studies aimed and prevention vs. loss. Similarly, individual programs appeared to be more beneficial, but the difference in weight gain between individual and group programs did not reach statistical significance. Finally, although only Álvarez-Jiménez and colleagues (2006) examined individuals with a first-onset psychosis, there was no statistically significant difference in weight change between this study (M weighted change = -2.8kg) and the studies examining persons with chronic schizophrenia (M weighted change = -2.4kg).

Clinical Management of Obesity in Persons with Mental Illness

As can be seen from the Álvarez-Jiménez (2008) comprehensive review of weight management interventions for persons with serious mental illness, treatment can be challenging. Researchers and clinicians might be left wondering if a) interventions for this population need to be enhanced to increase weight loss, b) prevention of weight gain, rather than weight loss, is a more realistic outcome variable, or c) treatments need to be enhanced, and expectations should be modified. Regardless, research has suggested that certain techniques are a helpful starting place for weight management in this population. These are reviewed below.

Self-monitoring of Food Intake and Physical Activity

A key aspect of weight-management programs, whether for psychiatric or non-psychiatric populations, is self-monitoring of caloric intake and caloric expenditure. This is enhanced by teaching the skill of self-monitoring through the use of food models and in-session practice with feedback from the clinician (Brar, Ganguli, Pandina, Turkoz, Berry, & Mahmoud, 2005). Making materials, such as food and exercise records, simple and repeated training in their use can also be helpful (Brown, Goetz, Van Sciver, Sullivan, & Hamera, 2006). Jean-Baptiste and colleagues (2007) used a novel food provision program to provide clients with schizophrenia a list of approved foods for which they could be reimbursed up to $25/week. Receipts were reviewed and used to provide feedback to clients about their food choices. This non-traditional method could be very useful in providing direct feedback to clients on food choice.

Cognitive and Behavioral Strategies to Modify Eating Behavior

Several methods can be used to help clients deal with urges to eat. Cognitive strategies, such as self-talk to delay or prevent snacking can be helpful (Brar et al., 2005). Eliminating cues in the environment that prompt eating, such as removing snacks from countertops, can be useful. These traditional cognitive and behavioral strategies have been supplemented for persons with serious mental illness in several ways. For instance, Brown and colleagues (2006) found that meal replacements can be beneficial in the beginning of treatment, before clients have the menu planning and cooking skills to reduce calories on their own.

Brownell's LEARN Program (2004) describes several behavioral techniques to slow eating, reduce portion size, and set behavioral goals so that caloric reduction can be achieved. The LEARN Program also provides education about nutrition and physical activity, and it can be used in both group and individual treatment contexts. This program has been adapted successfully for a psychiatric population, including additional strategies to facilitate learning such as simplified presentation of information, repetition of content, monetary incentive and in vivo skills training (Jean-Baptiste, Tek, Liskov, Chakunta, Nicholls, Hassan, Brownell, Wexler, 2007).

Promoting Physical Activity

Encouraging clients to increase physical activity is a key component of weight management, for both psychiatric and non-psychiatric populations. Donnelly, Blair, Jakicic, Manore, Rankin, & Smith (2009) reported in the recent American College of Sports Medicine Position Stand that engaging in between 150 minutes to 250 minutes of moderate physical activity per week will only lead to modest weight loss, and that clinically significant weight loss is associated with > 250 minutes/week of moderate physical activity. This translates to a minimum of 35 minutes/day of moderate physical activity to effect clinically significant weight loss. These recommendations suggest that physical activity should be structured into weight-management programs. In their weight-loss program for persons with serious mental illness, Brown and colleagues (2006) provide a model for this by devoting the first hour of each session to group physical activity and instruction.

Limitations of Current Weight-management Interventions for Psychiatric Populations

Despite the strong efforts by researchers to develop and test efficacious weight-management interventions adapted for psychiatric populations, the treatment outcome is less positive in comparison to non-psychiatric populations. For example, Loh and colleagues (2006) reported a mean 26-week weight loss of 10.31 lbs., which compares unfavorably to weight loss among non-psychiatric samples (mean 22 week loss = 18.74 lbs; Wadden & Butryn, 2003).

There are several potential reasons for the discrepancies in treatment outcomes between psychiatric and non-psychiatric populations, two of which are notably medication use and economic barriers to nutritious foods and physical activity. These are challenging barriers to overcome and not always amenable to behavioral intervention, short of unrealistic measures such taking someone off his/her medication. Even if economic challenges were reduced, cognitive deficits that impede behavioral performance would remain (Rempfer, Hamera, Brown, & Cromwell, 2003).

Table 20.1. Examples of cognitive adaptations for weight management

Cognitive difficulty	Potential Weight loss-related challenges	Examples of adapted intervention strategies
Difficulties with attention span	Distracted during treatment sessions Attention lapses during shopping, purchases high calorie foods	Additional repetition, monetary and other incentives, frequent breaks Assistance in preparing shopping lists, in vivo practice and reinforcement of shopping skills
Memory problems	Forgets what was consumed or forgets to use food record	Enhanced prompting to record eating behavior (e.g., use of reminder phone calls, alarms, etc.)
Executive functioning problems (e.g., problem solving, planning, reasoning, sequencing behavior)	Unable to execute multiple steps for food preparation, tends to eat high calorie prepared foods	Assistance in identifying and practicing simple food preparation recipes

We argue that a primary limitation of current weight-management programs for adults with schizophrenia is that they do not adequately address the *known cognitive impairments and consequent behavioral skill deficits* in this population. It is widely accepted that schizophrenia and other serious mental illnesses are associated with cognitive impairments in areas such as executive functioning, attention and memory. Further, cognition has been associated with various outcomes among people with serious mental illness, including social functioning (Vaskinn et al., 2008), activities of daily living (Rempfer, Hamera, Brown, and Cromwell, 2003; Semkovska et al., 2004), community independence (Heinrichs et al., 2010) and rehabilitation outcomes (Watzke et al., 2008). Thus, it is reasonable to assume that cognitive functioning may also impact outcomes associated with weight loss interventions.

To date, only one weight-management study in a psychiatric population has assessed cognitive functioning. Specifically, Jean-Baptiste and colleagues (2007) compared California Verbal Learning Test (CVLT) scores of successful and unsuccessful weight-loss participants. There was no difference in scores, leading the authors to conclude that "the results of this pilot study demonstrate that it is possible for patients with severe mental illness to lose weight while taking antipsychotic medications, regardless of the level of cognitive functioning" (Jean-Baptiste and colleagues, 2007 p. 202). However, given the small sample size in this pilot study (N=14), the findings require replication before definitive conclusions can be made about the potential influence of memory on behavioral weight management. Further, although a verbal memory deficit (as measured by the CVLT) may not be the limiting factor for weight loss in this population, it is well documented that other cognitive deficits in schizophrenia (e.g., executive functioning) predict the ability to perform basic activities of daily living. Promising environment interventions that bypass these cognitive problems have been shown to improve functional outcomes in persons with schizophrenia (Velligan, Diamond, Maples, Mintz, Glahn, & Miller, 2008a; Velligan, Diamond, Mintz, Maples, Li, Zeber et al., 2008b) and may similarly improve weight-loss outcomes.

Developing weight-management interventions that address the relationship between known cognitive impairments, behavioral skill, and functioning in the real world could reduce problems with transfer of skills and knowledge from the clinic to one's daily life and improve weight management efforts (Table 20.1).

Conclusion

In conclusion, obesity and its sequelae are a significant health concern for persons with serious mental illness. Weight gain in this population is promoted through a variety of intersecting factors such as economic difficulties that reduce access to nutritious foods and safe physical activity and medication use. Researchers are beginning to test behavioral weight-management interventions in this population, and thus far, results are not as promising as for non-psychiatric populations. Future treatment development work in this area should address known cognitive impairments and their relationship to functional behaviors necessary for weight management.

References

Allison, D.B., Casey, D.E. (2001). Antipsychotic-induced weight gain: a review of the literature. *Journal of Clinical Psychiatry, 62* (Suppl 7), 22-31.

Allison, D.B., Fontaine, K.R., Heo, M., Mentore, J.L., Cappelleri, J.C., Chandler, L.P., Weiden, P.J., Cheskin, L.J. (1999a). The distribution of body mass index among individuals with and without schizophrenia. *Journal of Clinical Psychiatry, 60*(4), 215-220.

Allison, D.B., Mentore, J.L., Heo, M., Chandler, L.P., Cappelleri, J.C., Infante, M.C., Weiden, P.J. (1999b). Antipsychotic-induced weight gain: a comprehensive research synthesis. *American Journal of Psychiatry, 156*, 1686-1696.

Álvarez-Jiménez, M., Gonzáles-Blanch, C., Vázquez-Barquero, J.L., Pérez-Iglesias, R., Martinez-Garcia, O., Pérez-Pardal, T., Ramirez-Bonilla, M.L., Crespo-Facorro, B. (2006). Attenuation of antipsychotic-induced weight gain with early behavioral intervention in drug-naïve first episode psychosis patients. A randomized controlled trial. *Journal of Clinical Psychiatry, 67,* 1253-1260.

Álvarez-Jiménez, M., Hetrick, S.E., Gonzáles-Blanch, C., Gleeson, J.F., & McGorry, P.D. (2008). Non-pharmacological management of antipsychotic-induced weight gain: systematic review and meta-analysis of randomized controlled trials. *The British Journal of Psychiatry, 193*, 101-107.

American Psychiatric Association. (April, 2004). *Practice guideline: treatment of patients with schizophrenia, 2nd ed.* http://www.psychiatryonline.com/pracGuide/pracGuideTopic_6.aspx.

Brar, J., Ganguli, R., Pandina, G., Turkoz, I., Berry, S., & Mahmoud, R. (2005). Effects of behavioral therapy on weight loss in overweight and obese patients with schizophrenia or schizoaffective disorder. *Journal of Clinical Psychiatry, 66*, 205-212.

Brown, C., Goetz, J., Van Sciver, A., Sullivan, D., & Hamera, E. (2006). A psychiatric rehabilitation approach to weight loss. *Psychiatric Rehabilitation Journal. 29(4),* 267-273.

Brownell, K.D. (2004). *The Learn Program for Weight Management,* 10th edition. American Health Publishing Company, Dallas, TX.

Colton, C.W., Manderscheid, R.W. (2006 Apr). Congruencies in increased mortality rates, years of potential life lost, and causes of death among public mental health clients in eight states; *Preventing Chronic Disease* [serial online], Available from: http://www.cdc.gov/ped/issues/2006/apr/05_0180.htm.

Daumit GL, Goldberg RW, Anthony C, Dickerson F, Brown CH, Kreyenbuhl J, Wohlheiter K, Dixon LB. (2005). Physical activity patterns in adults with severe mental illness. *Journal of Nervous Disease, 193* (10), 641-646.

Dickerson, F.B., Brown, C.H., Daumit, G.L., Li Juan, F., Goldberg, R.W., Wohlheiter, K., Dixon, L.B. (2006a). Health status of individuals with serious mental illness. *Schizophrenia Bulletin, 32*, 584-589.

Dickerson, F.B., Brown, C.H., Kreyenbuhl, J.A., Fang, L., Goldberg, R.W., Wohlheiter, K., Dixon, L.B. (2006b). Obesity among individuals with serious mental illness. *Acta Psychiatr Scand, 113,* 306-313.

Donnelly, J.E., Blair, S.N., Jakicic, J.M., Manore, M.M , Rankin, J.W., & Smith, B.K. (2009). American College of Sports Medicine Position Stand. Appropriate Physical Activity Intervention Strategies for Weight Loss and Prevention of Weight Regain for Adults. *Medicine and Science in Sports and Exercise, 41* (2), 459–471.

Flegal, K.M., Carroll, M.D., Ogden, C.L., Johnson C.L. (2002). Prevalencc and trends in obesity among U.S. adults, 1999--2000. *Journal of the American Medical Association, 288*, 1723-7.

Ford, E.S., Giles, W.H., Dietz, W.H. (2002). Prevalence of the metabolic syndrome among U.S. adults: findings from the third National Health and Nutrition Examination Survey. *Journal of the American Medical Association, 287(3),* 356-359.

Ganguli, R. (1999). Weight gain associated with antipsychotic drugs. *Journal of Clinical Psychiatry, 60,* 20-24.

Ganguli, R. (2007). Behavioral therapy for weight loss in patients with schizophrenia. *Journal of Clinical Psychiatry, 68*, 19-25.

Heinrichs, R.W., Ammari, N., Miles, A.A., Vaz, S.M. (2010). Cognitive performance and functional competence as predictors of community independence in schizophrenia. *Schizophrenia Bulletin, 36,* 381-387.

Isomaa, B., Almgren, P., Tuomi, T., Forsen, B., Lahti, K., Nissen, M., Taskinen, M., Groop, L. (2001). Cardiovascular Morbidity and Mortality Associated with the Metabolic Syndrome. *Diabetes Care, 2,* 683-689.

Jean-Baptiste, M., Tek, C., Liskov, E.,. Chakunta, U.R., Nicholls, S., Hassan, A.Q., Brownell, K.D., Wexler, B.E. (2007). A pilot study of a weight management program with food provisions in schizophrenia. *Schizophrenia Research, 96,* 198-205.

Loh, C., Meyer, J.M., & Leckband, S.G. (2006). A comprehensive review of behavioral interventions for weight management in schizophrenia. *Annals of Clinical Psychiatry, 18*, 23-31.

Lundgren, J.D., Rempfer, M.V., Brown, C.E., Goetz, J., Hamera, E. (2010). The prevalence of night eating syndrome and binge eating disorder among overweight and obese individuals with serious mental illness. *Psychiatry Research, 175,* 233-236.

McCreadie, R., Macdonald, E., Blacklock, C., Tilak-Singh, D., Wiles, D., Halliday, J., & Patterson, J. (1998). Dietary intake of schizophrenia patients in Nithsdale, Scotland: case-control study. *British Medical Journal, 317*, 784-785.

McEvoy, J.P., Meyer, J.M., Goff, D., Nasrallah, H.A., Davis, S.M., Sullivan, L., Meltzer, H.Y., Hsiao, J., Stroup, T.S., & Lieberman, J.A. (2005). Prevalence of the metabolic syndrome in patients with schizophrenia: baseline results from the CATIE schizophrenia trial and comparison with national estimates from NHANES III. *Schizophrenia Research, 80*,19-32.

Nasrallah, H.A., Meyer, J.M., Goff, D.C., McEvoy, J.P., Davis, S.M., Stroup, T.S., Lieberman, J.A. (2006). Low rates of treatment for hypertension, dyslipidemia and diabetes in schizophrenia: data from the CATIE schizophrenia trial sample at baseline. *Schizophrenia Research, 86*, 15-22.

Newcomer, J.W., Haupt, D.W. (2006). The metabolic effects of antipsychotic medications. *Canadian Journal of Psychiatry, 51 (8),* 480-491.

Ramacciotti, C.A., Paoli, R.A., Catena, M., Ciapparelli, A., Dell'Osso, L., Schulte, F., Garfinkel, P.E. (2004). Schizophrenia and binge-eating disorders. *Journal of Clinical Psychiatry, 65*, 1016-1017.

Rempfer, M.V., Hamera, E.K., Brown, C.E., Cromwell, R.L. (2003). The relation between cognition and the independent living skill of shopping in people with schizophrenia. *Psychiatry Research, 117*, 103-112.

Sankaranarayanan, J. & Puumala, S.E. (2007). Antipsychotic use at adult ambulatory care visits by patients with mental health disorders in the United States, 1996-2003: national estimates and associated factors. *Clinical Therapeutics, 29 (4),* 723-741.

Semkovska, M., Bedard, M., Godbout, L., Limoge, F., & Stip, E. (2004). Assessment of executive dysfunction during activities of daily living in schizophrenia. *Schizophrenia Research*, *69*, 289-300.

Strasnig, M., Brar, J.S., Ganguli, R. (2003). Nutrition assessment of patients with schizophrenia: a preliminary study. *Schizophrenia Bulletin, 29*, 393-397.

Theisen, F.M., Linden A., Geller, F., Schafer, H., Martin, M., Remschmidt, H.,. Hebebrand, J. (2001). Prevalence of obesity in adolescent and young adult patients with and without schizophrenia and in relationship to antipsychotic medication. *Journal of Psychiatric Research, 35,* 339-345.

Vaskinn, A., Sundet, K., Friis, S., Simonson, C., Birkenaes, A.B., Jonsdottir, H., Ringen, P.A., Andreassen, O.A. (2008). Emotion perception and learning potential: mediators between neurocognition and social problem-solving in schizophrenia? *Journal of the International Neuropsychological Society, 14,* 279-288.

Velligan, D.I., Diamond, P.M., Maples, N.J., Mintz, J., Li, X., Glahn, D.C., Miller, A.L. (2008a). Comparing the efficacy of interventions that use environmental supports to improve outcomes in patients with schizophrenia. *Schizophrenia Research, 102*, 312-319.

Velligan, D.I., Diamond, P.M., Mintz, J., Maples, N., Li, X., Zeber, J., Ereshefsky, L., Lam, Y.F., Castillo, D., & Miller, A.L. (2008b). The use of individually tailored supports to improve medication adherence and outcomes in schizophrenia. *Schizophrenia Bulleting, 34(3),* 483-493.

Wadden, T.A., Berkowitz, R.I., Sarwer, D.B., Purs-Wisniewski, R., & Steinberg, C. (2001). Benefits of lifestyle modification in the pharmacologic treatment of obesity. *Archives of Internal Medicine, 161*, 218-227.

Watzke, S., Brieger, P., Kuss, O., Schoettke, H., & Wiedl, K., (2008). A longitudinal study of learning potential and rehabilitation outcomes in schizophrenia. *Psychiatric Services 59,* 248-255.

In: Pathways to Obesity and Main Roads to Recovery
Editor: Piergiuseppe Vinai
ISBN: 978-1-61122-740-6

Chapter XXI

Neurosurgery in the Treatment of Obesity

Casey H. Halpern[1], Ephraim Church[1], John A. Wolf[2], Tracy L. Bale[3], Albert J. Stunkard[4], Jurg L. Jaggi[1], M. Sean Grady[1], Thomas Wadden[4] and Gordon H. Baltuch[1]

[1]Ephraim Church, B.A. Departments of Neurosurgery University of Pennsylvania School of Medicine Philadelphia, PA, USA

[2]Departments of Psychiatry, University of Pennsylvania School of Medicine Philadelphia, PA, USA

[3]Departments of Neuroscience University of Pennsylvania School of Medicine Philadelphia, PA, USA

[4]Departments of Psychiatry, Center for Weight and Eating Disorders University of Pennsylvania School of Medicine Philadelphia, PA, USA

Abstract

Current pharmacological and behavioral approaches to obesity face high dietary relapse rates. Suboptimal outcomes have also been reported following bariatric surgery. Neuropsychiatric components of obesity may be responsible for such relapse, and neuromodulation of brain regions associated with appetite, satiety, and reward may be useful for patients who have failed bariatric surgery. Deep brain stimulation (DBS) surgery has been shown to be safe and effective in the treatment of movement disorders, and it is increasingly used for the treatment of neuropsychiatric disorders. In DBS, an electrode is lowered to a specific neural target and adjustable electrical stimulation is administered. We propose DBS as a potential approach in the treatment of refractory obesity. In this chapter, we discuss potential indications, the DBS procedure, candidate neural targets, and challenges inherent in surgically targeting specific brain regions.

Introduction

Obesity is a worldwide epidemic affecting more than 300 million people (Deitel, 2002). A greater than ten-fold increase in bariatric surgeries performed over the past eight years (Sturm, 2007) may be explained by the limitations of pharmacological therapies and behavioral techniques (Jeffery et al., 2004; Li et al., 2005) Although mean weight loss after bariatric surgery ranges from about 20 to 60%, with concomitant improvement in morbidity (Maggard et al., 2005), adverse events occur in up to 20% of patients. However, major complications of bariatric surgery are typically seen in less than 9%, and the perisurgical mortality is below 0.8% (Flum et al., 2009; Hauser et al., 2010; Marsk et al., 2009). Unfortunately, patients undergoing bariatric surgery are not free from relapse, and significant weight gain can occur within two years of surgery after the nadir weight is reached (Kalarchian et al., 2002). The failure rate due to noncompliant eating patterns in patients followed for ten years has been reported to be as high as 20% for obese and 40% for super-obese (BMI > 50 kg/m2) patients (Christou et al., 2006).

Neuropsychiatric components of obesity may explain the refractory nature of this condition. Based on evidence from our experience in treating movement disorders and, more recently, neuropsychiatric disease with deep brain stimulation (DBS) (Halpern et al., 2007), there is a potential role for this approach in obesity treatment. DBS may aid in addressing treatment-resistant components of refractory obesity by modulating specific neural centers implicated in the pathophysiology of obesity. Appetite and satiety centers in the brain are well documented (Rolls, 1984) and represent primary areas for investigation (Covalin et al., 2005; Sani et al., 2007; Halpern et al., 2008). On the other hand, studies indicate that the reward sensation associated with food intake is important in the pathophysiology of obesity (Wise and Rompre, 1989; Halpern et al., 2008). Thus, neural modulation may be accomplished by targeting appetite, satiety, or reward circuitry using DBS, a well-established technique of stereotactic functional neurosurgery. Below, we review three potential neural targets for DBS believed to be involved in the excessive consumption of food in obesity, the lateral hypothalamus (LH), ventromedial hypothalamus (VMH) and nucleus accumbens (NAc).

Indications and Potential Complications of DBS for Obesity

DBS for obesity may be an appropriate treatment option for patients who have failed bariatric surgery. Reward sensation associated with food intake is important in the pathophysiology of obesity, and failed surgical patients may well suffer from obesity driven by dysregulation of reward circuitry. By addressing an underlying contributor to their obesity, neurosurgical treatment may be most effective for patients with obesity poorly controlled by bariatric surgery.

DBS, though undoubtedly an invasive procedure, is remarkably safe. Side effects are generally transient and most commonly include eyelid-opening apraxia, dyskinesia and paresthesias. These often occur when stimulators are adjusted during the procedure or after surgery in the follow-up period. However, rare deaths have been reported from pulmonary emboli, myocardial infarction, stroke, intracerebral hermorrhage, and suicide. The majority of intracranial hemorrhages associated with DBS, however, are asymptomatic.

It is important to consider adverse effects and complications of DBS on a target-specific level. The LH is a relatively large region of the hypothalamus (Figure 1) with many nuclei that have diverse physiologic functions in addition to appetite control, including body temperature regulation, sexual activity, reproductive endocrinology, and the fight-or-flight response (Purves et al., 2001). There are other important structures nearby including the fornix and the optic nerve. Indeed, targeting of LH has been associated with risk of stimulation spread to the various nuclei and targeting efforts may be complicated by the proximity of critical structures.

There are a number of challenges to surgically targeting the VMH. This region is bilobed and somewhat smaller than LH (Figure 2). Its proximity to the anterior commissure, a structure that is easily visualized on MRI, may aid in localization. However, it is medially positioned and an intraventricular trajectory, an approach that is considered sub-optimal due to potential complications, may be required. Moreover, the optic nerve is directly anterior, and the mammillary body is posterior, to VMH. The mammillary bodies form a portion of the Circuit of Papez, which is believed to play a role in seizure propagation and expression, and stimulation spread may induce seizures (Mirski and Ferrendelli, 1984). Finally, the position of the VMH just inferior and medial to LH, and the interconnectedness of hypothalamic nuclei, raise the possibility of inducing an antagonisitic effect in LH due to the spread of low-frequency stimulation.

Like the STN, which is targeted in Parkinson's disease (PD), the NAc may be localized in relation to the anterior commissure (3 mm anterior) and midline (6 mm lateral). The electrode trajectory to the NAc would be just lateral to the ventricle through caudate, an approach that has been well tolerated in DBS for OCD and depression and DBS of the globus pallidus for PD. Although microtrauma to the caudate may result in memory deficits, this is less likely in the absence of preoperative dementia (Broggi et al., 2003). Nearby structures that could complicate this approach are the anterior cerebral artery located inferiorly and the optic nerve located inferomedially.

DBS Surgery: The Procedure

DBS employs a stereotactic approach to introduce electrodes through a frontal burr hole to a neural target associated with the pathophysiology of the disease (Halpern et al., 2007; Jaggi et al., 2004). The clinical efficacy of DBS depends on highly accurate, MRI-directed targeting (Schrader et al., 2002). A stereotactic frame is positioned on the patient's head, and imaging is obtained and imported into targeting software. The electrode trajectory is determined using statistical data from atlases (Schaltenbrand and Warren, 1977), which provides neurosurgeons with target coordinates chosen empirically for their effect on symptoms. Trajectory planning ensures that critical structures can be avoided, including deep sulci, ventricles and superficial large veins if contrast is used. During electrode insertion, electrophysiologic recordings identify anatomic boundaries of the target. In the treatment of some conditions such as PD and essential tremor, clinical effects of stimulation may be evaluated with the patient awake to assess for symptom relief and adverse effects of stimulation prior to closure. Thus, preoperative targeting, intraoperative electrophysiologic recordings, and symptom response with stimulation may be used to achieve remarkable accuracy in electrode placement. Once the electrode is in its fixed, correct position, the surgeon inserts the internal pulse generator (IPG) into a subcutaneous pocket adjacent to the clavicle. The IPG is attached to the DBS lead by a subcutaneously tunneled wire, the top end of which is anchored to the burr hole site at the top of the skull.

DBS of the Hypothalamus for Obesity

The relative balance between food intake and energy expenditure is an important determinant of body weight. Imbalance between energy input and output leads to obesity, and overconsumption of calorically dense foods is likely an important element of the obesity epidemic. The hypothalamus is the region of the brain that has been shown to be important in maintaining energy homeostasis. This region contains a feeding center in the LH and a satiety center in the VMH. These areas play an important role in food intake (Rolls, 1984; Rolls et al., 1980). Therefore, LH and VMH represent potential targets of DBS.

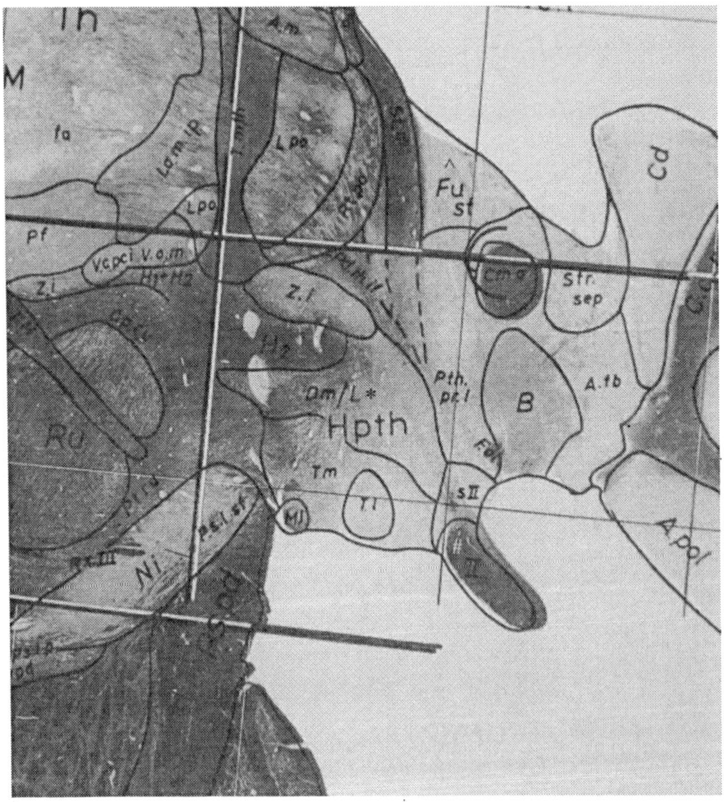

Figure 21.1. A sagittal section of the lateral hypothalamus. *lateral hypothalamus (L); #optic nerve (II); ^nucleus accumbens (Fu.st). From Schaltenbrand G, Warren W: Atlas for Stereotaxy of the Human Brain. Stuttgart: Thieme, 1977. Reprinted, with the addition of *, #, and ^, with permission.

In numerous studies over the past 50 years, the LH has been implicated in feeding behavior and energy expenditure (Bernardis and Bellinger, 1996). Lesioning of this region in rats induced leanness (Anand and Brobeck, 1951) and appeared to impact appetite regulation, an effect that can be partially explained by stimulatory peptides and their receptors expressed in the LH (Sakurai et al., 1998). These peptides, which include MCH and orexins (hypocretins), have been well studied in rodent models and are implicated in eating behavior and obesity (Ludwig et al., 2001). Other important regulators of feeding behavior and body weight include neuropeptide Y and agouti-related protein, which densely project to the LH (Stanley et al., 1993; Elmquist et al., 1999).

Targeting the hypothalamus for cluster headaches has been shown to be safe and potentially effective (Leone et al., 2005). Additionally, electrocoagulation of the LH in obese humans more than 30 years ago resulted in significant, though transient, appetite suppression with weight reduction (Quaade et al., 1974). Thus, it has been proposed that bilateral, high-frequency DBS of the LH could mimic results of lesion studies (Sani et al., 2005). This hypothesis was recently tested by Sani et al. (Sani et al., 2007) by implanting electrodes bilaterally in the rat LH. Although high-frequency stimulation (180-200 Hz) was associated with significant weight loss in the experimental group, there was no change in eating behavior. The authors surmised that the effect might have been due to changes in metabolic profile. Low-frequency stimulation (50 to 100 Hz) has been associated before with increased consumptive or hoarding behaviors in various animal models (Mendelson and Chorover, 1965; Berridge and Valenstein, 1991; Delgado and Anand, 1952).

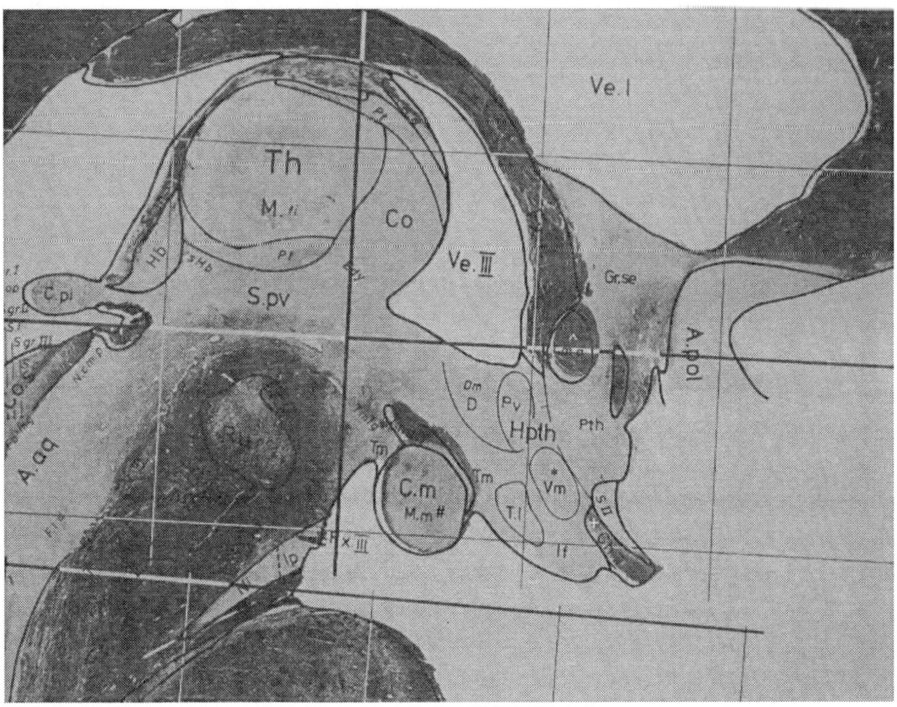

* ventromedial hypothalamus (Vm); #mammillary body (M.m); +optic chiasm (Ch. II); ^anterior commissure (Cm.a). From Schaltenbrand G, Warren W: Atlas for Stereotaxy of the Human Brain. Stuttgart: Thieme, 1977. Reprinted, with the addition of *, #, +, and ^, with permission.

Figure 21.2. A sagittal section of the ventromedial hypothalamus.

Similar to the LH, the VMH is implicated in appetite regulation and energy homeostasis (Hetherington and Ranson, 1942). Lesions of the VMH induced weight gain in obese animals

(Brobeck, 1946), and this effect appeared to be due to metabolic changes (Cox and Powley, 1981). Low-frequency stimulation of the VMH (60-100 Hz) inhibited feeding in hungry rats and goats, an effect that was reversible (Krasne, 1962; Andersson, 1951). Stimulation caused additional results that may have been due to autonomic activation, including fear, aversion, restlessness, and attempts to escape. Stimulation of the VMH has been shown to increase metabolic rate and is associated with utilization of fat stores as revealed by a drop in respiratory quotient (Ruffin and Nicolaidis, 1999). Using indirect calorimetry, a recent study assessed metabolic activity during VMH DBS at 25, 50, 75, and 100 Hz and revealed a trend toward an indirect relationship between energy expenditure and increasing frequencies (Covalin et al., 2005). Hence, the effect of stimulation in VMH appears to be frequency dependent with lower frequencies driving VMH activity and higher frequencies causing lesional effects (A.L. Benabid, 2006, personal communication).

DBS of the Nucleus Accumbens for Obesity

Evidence presented above indicates that DBS of LH or VMH may alter energy homeostasis. These may prove to be useful neurosurgical approaches in the treatment of obesity. However, the assumption that modulation of appetite or satiety will significantly affect feeding behavior associated with obesity may be false. This notion is supported by studies in which mice fed a highly palatable (high-fat) diet consumed 90% more than those fed standard house chow (Teegarden and Bale, 2007) Such an effect is due to reinforcing properties of palatable food, which appear to be modulated by a region of the brain that is essential in reward and reinforcement, the NAc (Smith et al., 1998). DBS of NAc offers the possibility of modulating reinforcing properties of high-fat foods and altering behaviors associated with obesity.

The NAc is similar to the principal target in DBS for PD, the subthalamic nucleus (STN). Both are located in the basal ganglia, although the NAc is slightly larger than the STN (Figs. 1 and 3). It is important to recognize that the NAc, though well circumscribed on myelin-stained sections, is composed of core and shell subregions that differ in their cytoarchitecture, neurostransmitter characteristics, and connections (Zaborszky et al., 1985). The core region connects to extrapyramidal motor structures such as the ventral pallidum (VP), STN, and the substantia nigra (Deutch and Cameron, 1992) The shell region, on the other hand, is embedded in a complex mesocorticolimbic circuit providing control of reward sensitivity. In addition to dopaminergic input from the ventral tegmental area in the midbrain, the shell receives afferents from the amygdala, hippocampus, prefrontal cortex, and thalamus, and its efferents project largely to the VP and thalamus (Zahm, 2000; Zahm and Brog, 1992). Notably, there is evidence that some output from the NAc shell may bypass the VP and project directly to the LH (Zahm, 2000), which suggests that there exists communication between reward processing and feeding centers in the brain.

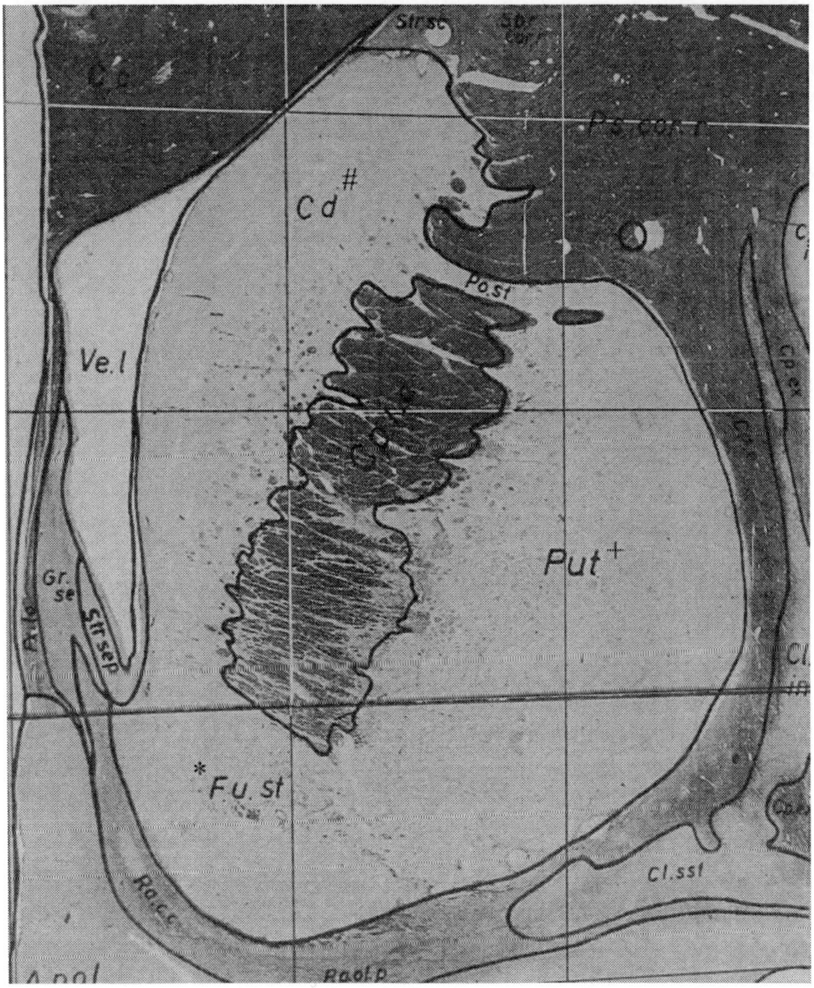

* Nucleus accumbens (Fu.st); #caudate nucleus (Cd); +putamen (Put). From Schaltenbrand G, Warren W: Atlas for Stereotaxy of the Human Brain. Stuttgart: Thieme, 1977. Reprinted, with the addition of *, #, and ^, with permission.

Figure 21.3. A coronal section of the nucleus accumbens located in the ventral striatum.

The NAc plays a central role in the modulation of reward sensation shown to be associated with palatability of foods. For example, rodents preferred chow with high-fat content (45 kcal % fat) to standard house chow because of its reinforcing properties, and this effect was believed to be mediated in part by dopamine neurotransmission in the NAc (Wise and Rompre, 1989). Indeed, there is evidence that dopamine is integral in the modulation of reward sensation in the NAc, for example, injections of dopamine antagonists in NAc suppressed feeding (Bendotti et al., 1986). In another study, levels of dopamine release were proportional to the amount ingested (Martel and Fantino, 1996), and when comparing obese and lean rats, there was a significantly greater amount of dopamine released in response to food stimuli in the obese rats (Wise and Rompre, 1989; Meguid et al., 2000). Neurotransmitters other than dopamine likely play an important role in NAc reward processing (Maldonado-Irizarry et al., 1995), and further studies including computational modeling will help delineate the precise effects of DBS on these systems (Moyer et al., 2007).

Although there is much variability between individuals, those with more frequent and intense food cravings are more likely to be obese (Beaver et al., 2006). Mice will endure significant levels of stress to obtain preferred foods (Teegarden and Bale, 2007). Thus, evidence supports the notion that one important feature of obesity is dysregulation of the reward system. This line of thinking has culminated in the recent suggestion that at least some forms of obesity may be characterized by an excessive motivational drive for food intake that overrides the hypothalamic circuitry normally involved in food consumption (Morton et al., 2006). There is evidence of altered expression of peptides related to feeding behavior in the LH with concomitant hunger for highly palatable food (Huang et al., 2003), and the presence of anatomical projections from LH to NAc suggest a modulatory role of hypothalamus on food reward (Peyron et al., 1998). Hypothalamic control of intake may be impaired in obesity (Wortley et al., 2003). It is a dysregulated reward system that may underlie significant rates of relapse and common failure of many current treatments.

Evidence from lesion studies, neurofunctional imaging, and stimulation studies indicate that DBS of NAc is a highly promising approach. Chemical lesion of dopaminergic neuron terminals in NAc resulted in attenuation of food hoarding and weight loss in rats, and levodopa reversed this effect (Kelley and Stinus, 1985). It is well known that DBS has lesioning effects at high frequencies; it could mimic chemical lesioning. However, it is difficult to predict the sum effect of electrical stimulation of various neurotransmitter systems in the NAc. Additionally, stimulation may have differential effects on NAc core and shell subregions. For example, N-methyl-D-aspartate lesions of the NAc core induced weight loss in rats, whereas the shell-lesion group gained weight (Maldonado-Irizarry and Kelley, 1995). Given that large excitotoxic lesions of both core and shell did not affect weight, it is possible that these subregions have opposing effects. Further study and rigorous stereotactic techniques will be necessary to ensure precise, efficacious placement of the electrode.

Evidence from functional neuroimaging points to the NAc as a promising DBS target for obesity. Striatal reward areas, which encompass NAc, are activated during exposure to a high-fat stimulus, and this is particularly true of patients with enhanced reward sensitivity (Beaver et al., 2006). Our experience treating PD with high-frequency stimulation of the over-active STN suggests that a hyperfunctioning region within the brain may be susceptible to DBS. Interestingly, positron emission tomography and autoradiographic studies have revealed reduced D2 receptors and increased dopamine transporters (Wang et al., 2004), and although obese patients show increased accumbal dopamine release in response to food stimuli, clearance may also be increased. It is conceivable that an abnormally short-lived dopaminergic signal may result in the need to compensate with food reinforcers. This, along with an increased stress response to palatable food restriction, may underlie the reported high rates of recurrent binge eating and long-term failures in patients undergoing bariatric surgery.

Electrical stimulation of the NAc in rats at 60 Hz resulted in increased sniffing, excitement, and aggression (Predy and Kokkindis, 1984; McCracken and Grace, 2007). These findings were replicated in cats (Goldstein and Siegel, 1980). Although no consistent effect on feeding behavior has been reported, none of these studies was conducted in overweight or obese animals. Moreover, reward circuitry DBS has shown great promise in addressing treatment-resistant OCD and depression. High-frequency stimulation appears to diminish symptoms in rat models of OCD (van Kuyck et al., 2003). In humans suffering from OCD, DBS of the ventral capsule/ventral striatum, a region that encompasses the NAc, resulted in a significant decrease in disease severity and improvement in global functioning (Greenberg et al., 2006). Additionally, an abnormal response to pleasurable stimuli in the ventral striatum, and particularly the NAc, has been implicated in depression (Tremblay et al., 2005). One study demonstrated an improvement in the severity of depression with stimulation of the NAc (Schlaepfer et al., 2007). Furthermore, DBS of the NAc has been shown to be effective in attenuating the reinstatement of drug-seeking behavior in rats (Vassoler et al., 2008). Such relapse behavior has been demonstrated in mice withdrawn from a highly palatable diet (Teegarden and Bale, 2007). These results provide evidence for the safety of NAc DBS, as well as its capacity to modulate neural transmission in an area of the brain that is integral in reward sensation associated with treatment-resistant obesity.

Conclusion

Hypothalamic DBS is an appealing option for obesity treatment. Hypothalamic lesions produce appetite modulation as well as enhancement of metabolic rate in both animal models and humans. These effects appear to be reproduced by DBS with the added benefits of titratability and reversibility. In the long term, however, suppressing appetite and increasing energy expenditure may be inadequate. For example, palatability significantly increases food intake. Electrocoagulation of LH in humans only transiently suppressed appetite and provided minimal weight loss. Thus, other potential anatomic targets such as NAc may be considered. By modulating reward sensation, NAc DBS may provide weight reduction over time and lessen relapse rates associated with conservative and surgical treatments. Nucleus accumbens DBS may interact with systems known to be involved in the reinforcing properties of food, and stimulation frequency may be titratable to adequate inhibition of food preference. This approach may be particularly useful for those forms of obesity caused by excessive motivational drive for food and may be a helpful option for patients who have failed bariatric surgery.

The worldwide epidemic of obesity likely has several contributing factors. Among these is the abundance of highly palatable, calorie-rich food and its effect on reward systems in the human brain. Disordered reward circuitry involving the NAc may contribute to obesity in some patients and may be addressed with neurosurgical management. DBS of NAc has been established as safe in the treatment of patients with refractory OCD and depression. Moreover, animal models of obesity exist and should be used to explore the effects of NAc DBS on weight loss.

References

Anand B.K., Brobeck J.R. (1951) Localization of a "feeding center" in the hypothalamus of the rat. *Proc Soc Exp Biol Med, 77,* 323-4.

Andersson B. (1951) The effect and localization of electrical stimulation of certain parts of the brain stem in sheep and goats. *Acta Physiol Scand., 23*, 8-23.

Beaver J.D., Lawrence A.D., van Ditzhuijzen J., Davis M.H., Woods A., Calder A.J. (2006) Individual differences in reward drive predict neural responses to images of food. *J Neurosci., 26*, 5160-6.

Bendotti C., Berettera C., Invernizzi R., Samanin R. (1986) Selective involvement of dopamine in the nucleus accumbens in the feeding response elicited by muscimol injection in the nucleus raphe dorsalis of sated rats. *Pharmacol Biochem Behav., 24,* 1189-93.

Bernardis L.L., Bellinger L.L. (1996) The lateral hypothalamic area revisited: ingestive behavior. *Neurosci Biobehav Rev., 20,* 189-287.

Berridge K.C., Valenstein E.S. (1991) What psychological process mediates feeding evoked by electrical stimulation of the lateral hypothalamus? *Behav Neurosci., 105,* 3-14.

Brobeck J.R. (1946) Mechanism of the development of obesity in animals with hypothalamic lesions. *Physiol Rev., 26,*:541–559.

Broggi G., Franzini A., Marras C., Romito L., Albanese A. (2003) Surgery of Parkinson's disease: inclusion criteria and follow-up. *Neurol Sci., 24 Suppl 1,* S38-40.

Christou N.V., Look D., Maclean L.D. (2006) Weight gain after short- and long-limb gastric bypass in patients followed for longer than 10 years. *Ann Surg., 244,* 734-40.

Covalin A., Feshali A., Judy J. (2005) Deep brain stimulation for obesity control: Analyzing stimulation parameters to modulate energy expenditure, Proceedings of the 2nd International IEEE EMBS, Arlington, VA. pp. v-viii.

Cox J.E., Powley T.L. (1981) Intragastric pair feeding fails to prevent VMH obesity or hyperinsulinemia. *Am J Physiol., 240,* E566-72.

Deitel M. (2002) The International Obesity Task Force and "globesity." Obes Surg 12:613-4.

Delgado J.M.R., Anand B.K. (1952) Increase of food intake induced by electrical stimulation of the lateral hypothalamus. *Am J Physiol., 172,* 162-8.

Deutch A.Y., Cameron D.S. (1992) Pharmacological characterization of dopamine systems in the nucleus accumbens core and shell. *Neuroscience, 46,* 49-56.

Elmquist J.K., Elias C.F., Saper C.B. (1999) From lesions to leptin: hypothalamic control of food intake and body weight. *Neuron., 22,* 221-32.

Flum D.R., Belle S.H., King W.C., Wahed A.S., Berk P., Chapman W., Pories W., Courcoulas A., McCloskey C., Mitchell J., Patterson E., Pomp A., Staten M.A., Yanovski S.Z., Thirlby R., Wolfe B. (2009) Perioperative safety in the longitudinal assessment of bariatric surgery. *N Engl J Med., 361,* 445-54.

Goldstein J.M., Siegel J. (1980) Suppression of attack behavior in cats by stimulation of ventral tegmental area and nucleus accumbens. *Brain Res., 183,* 81-92.

Greenberg B.D., Malone D.A., Friehs G.M., Rezai A.R., Kubu C.S., Malloy P.F., Salloway S.P., Okun M.S., Goodman W.K., Rasmussen S.A. (2006) Three-year outcomes in deep brain stimulation for highly resistant obsessive-compulsive disorder. *Neuropsychopharmacology, 31,* 2384-93.

Halpern C., Hurtig H., Jaggi J., Grossman M., Won M., Baltuch G. (2007) Deep brain stimulation in neurologic disorders. *Parkinsonism Relat Disord., 13,* 1-16.

Halpern C.H., Wolf J.A., Bale T.L., Stunkard A.J., Danish S.F., Grossman M., Jaggi J.L., Grady M.S., Baltuch G.H. (2008) Deep brain stimulation in the treatment of obesity. *J Neurosurg., 109,* 625-34.

Hauser D.L., Titchner R.L., Wilson M.A., Eid G.M. (2010) Long-term outcomes of laparoscopic Roux-en-Y gastric bypass in U.S. veterans. *Obes Surg., 20,* 283-9.

Hetherington, A.W., Ranson, S.W. (1942) The spontaneous activity and food intake in rats with hypothalamic lesions. *Am. J. Physiol., 36,* 609–616.

Huang, X.F., Han, M., South, T., Storlien, L. (2003) Altered levels of POMC, AgRP and MC4-R mRNA expression in the hypothalamus and other parts of the limbic system of mice prone or resistant to chronic high-energy diet-induced obesity. *Brain Res., 992,* 9-19.

Jaggi, J.L., Umemura, A., Hurtig, H.I., Siderowf, A.D., Colcher, A., Stern, M.B., Baltuch, G.H. (2004) Bilateral stimulation of the subthalamic nucleus in Parkinson's disease: surgical efficacy and prediction of outcome. *Stereotact Funct Neurosurg, 82,* 104-14.

Jeffery, R.W., Kelly, K.M., Rothman, A.J., Sherwood, N.E., Boutelle, K.N. (2004) The weight loss experience: a descriptive analysis. *Ann Behav Med., 27,* 100-6.

Kalarchian, M.A., Marcus, M.D., Wilson, G.T., Labouvie, E.W., Brolin, R.E., LaMarca, L.B. (2002) Binge eating among gastric bypass patients at long-term follow-up. *Obes Surg 12*:270-5.

Kelley, A.E., Stinus, L. (1985) Disappearance of hoarding behavior after 6-hydroxydopamine lesions of the mesolimbic dopamine neurons and its reinstatement with L-dopa. *Behav Neurosci., 99,* 531-45.

Krasne, F.B. (1962) General Disruption Resulting from Electrical Stimulus of Ventromedial Hypothalamus. *Science, 138,* 822-823.

Leone, M., Franzini, A., Felisati, G., Mea, E., Curone, M., Tullo, V., Broggi, G., Bussone, G. (2005) Deep brain stimulation and cluster headache. *Neurol Sci., 26, Suppl 2*:s138-9.

Li, Z., Maglione, M., Tu, W., Mojica, W., Arterburn, D., Shugarman, L.R., Hilton, L., Suttorp, M., Solomon, V., Shekelle, P.G., Morton, S.C. (2005) Meta-analysis: pharmacologic treatment of obesity. *Ann Intern Med., 142,* 532-46.

Ludwig, D.S., Tritos, N.A., Mastaitis, J.W., Kulkarni, R., Kokkotou, E., Elmquist, J., Lowell, B., Flier, J.S., Maratos-Flier, E. (2001) Melanin-concentrating hormone overexpression in transgenic mice leads to obesity and insulin resistance. *J Clin Invest., 107,* 379-86.

Maggard, M.A., Shugarman, L.R., Suttorp, M., Maglione, M., Sugerman, H.J., Livingston, E.H., Nguyen, N.T., Li Z., Mojica, W.A., Hilton, L., Rhodes, S., Morton, S.C., Shekelle, P.G. (2005) Meta-analysis: surgical treatment of obesity. *Ann Intern Med., 142,* 547-59.

Maldonado-Irizarry, C.S., Kelley, A.E. (1995) Excitotoxic lesions of the core and shell subregions of the nucleus accumbens differentially disrupt body weight regulation and motor activity in rat. *Brain Res Bull., 38,* 551-9.

Maldonado-Irizarry, C.S., Swanson, C.J., Kelley, A.E. (1995) Glutamate receptors in the nucleus accumbens shell control feeding behavior via the lateral hypothalamus. *J Neurosci., 15,* 6779-88.

Marsk, R., Tynelius, P., Rasmussen, F., Freedman, J. (2009) Short-term morbidity and mortality after open versus laparoscopic gastric bypass surgery. A population-based study from Sweden. *Obes Surg. ,19,* 1485-90.

Martel, P., Fantino, M. (1996) Mesolimbic dopaminergic system activity as a function of food reward: a microdialysis study. *Pharmacol Biochem Behav., 53,* 221-6.

McCracken, C.B., Grace, A.A. (2007) High-frequency deep brain stimulation of the nucleus accumbens region suppresses neuronal activity and selectively modulates afferent drive in rat orbitofrontal cortex in vivo. *J Neurosci., 27,* 12601-10.

Meguid, M.M., Fetissov, S.O., Varma, M., Sato, T., Zhang, L., Laviano, A., Rossi-Fanelli, F. (2000) Hypothalamic dopamine and serotonin in the regulation of food intake. *Nutrition, 16,* 843-57.

Mendelson, J., Chorover, S.L. (1965) Lateral hypothalamic stimulation in satiated rats: T-maze learning for food. *Science, 149,* 559-561.

Mirski, M.A., Ferrendelli, J.A. (1984) Interruption of the mammillothalamic tract prevents seizures in guinea pigs. *Science, 226,* 72-4.

Morton, G.J., Cummings, D.E., Baskin, D.G., Barsh, G.S., Schwartz, M.W. (2006) Central nervous system control of food intake and body weight. *Nature, 443,* 289-95.

Moyer, J.T., Wolf, J.A., Finkel, L.H. (2007) Effects of dopaminergic modulation on the integrative properties of the ventral striatal medium spiny neuron. *J Neurophysiol., 98,* 3731-48.

Peyron, C., Tighe, D.K., van den Pol, A.N., de Lecea, L., Heller, H.C., Sutcliffe, J.G., Kilduff, T.S. (1998) Neurons containing hypocretin (orexin) project to multiple neuronal systems. *J Neurosci., 18,* 9996-10015.

Predy, P.A., Kokkindis, L. (1984) Sensitization to the effects of repeated amphetamine administration on intracranial self-stimulation: evidence for changes in reward processes. *Behav Brain Res.,13,* 251-9.

Purves, D., Augustine, G.J., Fitzpatrick, D., Katz, L., LaMantia, A., McNamara, J.O., Williams, S.M. (2001) (Eds.) *Neuroscience*, Sinauer Associated, Inc., Sunderland, MA.

Quaade, F., Vaernet, K., Larsson, S. (1974) Stereotaxic stimulation and electrocoagulation of the lateral hypothalamus in obese humans. *Acta Neurochir (Wien), 30,* 111-7.

Rolls, E.T. (1984) The neurophysiology of feeding. *Int J Obes 8* Suppl 1:139-50.

Rolls, E.T., Burton, M.J., Mora F. (1980) Neurophysiological analysis of brain-stimulation reward in the monkey. Brain Res., 194, 339-57.

Ruffin, M., Nicolaidis, S. (1999) Electrical stimulation of the ventromedial hypothalamus enhances both fat utilization and metabolic rate that precede and parallel the inhibition of feeding behavior. *Brain Res., 846,* 23-9.

Sakurai, T., Amemiya, A., Ishii, M., Matsuzaki, I., Chemelli, R.M., Tanaka, H., Williams, S.C., Richardson, J.A., Kozlowski, G.P., Wilson, S., Arch, J.R., Buckingham, R.E., Haynes, A.C., Carr, S.A., Annan, R.S., McNulty, D.E., Liu, W.S., Terrett, J.A., Elshourbagy, N.A., Bergsma, D.J., Yanagisawa, M. (1998) Orexins and orexin receptors: a family of hypothalamic neuropeptides and G protein-coupled receptors that regulate feeding behavior. *Cell, 92,* 573-85.

Sani, S., Jobe, K., Smith, A., Kordower, J.H., Bakay, R.A. (2007) Deep brain stimulation for treatment of obesity in rats. *J Neurosurg., 107,* 809-13.

Sani, S.B., Jobe, K.W., Kordower, J., Bakay, R.A. (2005) *Deep Brain Stimulation for the Treatment of Obesity in the Rat*, 73rd Annual Meeting, American Association of Neurological Surgeons, New Orleans, Louisiana.

Schaltenbrand, G., Warren, W. (1977) *Atlas for Stereotaxy of the Human Brain*, Thieme, Stuttgart.

Schlaepfer, T.E., Cohen, M.X., Frick, C., Kosel, M., Brodesser, D., Axmacher, N., Joe, A.Y., Kreft, M., Lenartz, D., Sturm, V. (2008) Deep Brain Stimulation to Reward Circuitry Alleviates Anhedonia in Refractory Major Depression. *Neuropsychopharmacology, 33(2),* 368-77.

Schrader, B., Hamel, W., Weinert, D., Mehdorn, H.M. (2002) Documentation of electrode localization. *Mov Disord, 17 Suppl 3,* S167-74.

Smith, Y., Shink, E., Sidibe, M. (1998) Neuronal circuitry and synaptic connectivity of the basal ganglia. *Neurosurg Clin N Am., 9,* 203-22.

Stanley, B.G., Magdalin, W., Seirafi, A., Thomas, W.J., Leibowitz, S.F. (1993) The perifornical area: the major focus of (a) patchily distributed hypothalamic neuropeptide Y-sensitive feeding system(s). *Brain Res., 604,* 304-17.

Sturm, R. (2007) Increases in morbid obesity in the USA: 2000-2005. *Public Health 121*(7):492-6.

Teegarden, S.L., Bale, T.L. (2007) Decreases in Dietary Preference Produce Increased Emotionality and Risk for Dietary Relapse. *Biol Psychiatry, 61(9),* 1021-9.

Tremblay, L.K., Naranjo, C.A., Graham, S.J., Herrmann, N., Mayberg, H.S., Hevenor S., Busto, U.E. (2005) Functional neuroanatomical substrates of altered reward processing in major depressive disorder revealed by a dopaminergic probe. *Arch Gen Psychiatry, 62,* 1228-36.

van Kuyck, K., Demeulemeester, H., Feys, H., De Weerdt, W., Dewil, M., Tousseyn, T., De Sutter, P., Gybels, J., Bogaerts, K., Dom, R., Nuttin, B. (2003) Effects of electrical stimulation or lesion in nucleus accumbens on the behaviour of rats in a T-maze after administration of 8-OH-DPAT or vehicle. *Behav Brain Res., 140,* 165-73.

Vassoler, F.M., Schmidt, H.D., Gerard, M.E., Famous, K.R., Ciraulo, D.A., Kornetsky, C., Knapp, C.M., Pierce, R.C. (2008) Deep brain stimulation of the nucleus accumbens shell attenuates cocaine priming-induced reinstatement of drug seeking in rats. *J Neurosci., 28,* 8735-9.

Wang, G.J., Volkow, N.D., Thanos, P.K., Fowler, J.S. (2004) Similarity between obesity and drug addiction as assessed by neurofunctional imaging: a concept review. *J Addict Dis., 23,* 39-53.

Wise, R.A., Rompre, P.P. (1989) Brain dopamine and reward. *Annu Rev Psychol., 40,* 191-225.

Wortley, K.E., Chang, G.Q., Davydova, Z., Leibowitz, S.F. (2003) Peptides that regulate food intake: orexin gene expression is increased during states of hypertriglyceridemia. *Am J Physiol Regul Integr Comp Physiol., 284,* R1454-65.

Zaborszky, L., Alheid, G.F., Beinfeld, M.C., Eiden, L.E., Heimer, L., Palkovits, M. (1985) Cholecystokinin innervation of the ventral striatum: a morphological and radioimmunological study. *Neuroscience, 14,* 427-53.

Zahm, D.S. (2000) An integrative neuroanatomical perspective on some subcortical substrates of adaptive responding with emphasis on the nucleus accumbens. *Neurosci Biobehav Rev., 24,* 85-105.

Zahm, D.S., Brog, J.S. (1992) On the significance of subterritories in the "accumbens" part of the rat ventral striatum. *Neuroscience, 50,*:751-67.

Index

A

abstraction, 142
abuse, 131, 179, 255, 269
academic performance, 65, 76
academic success, 66
access, 178, 187, 227, 229, 269, 271, 291, 316
accessibility, 179, 188, 195, 293
acid, 14, 19, 23, 26, 32, 51, 206, 209, 254, 257, 259
activity level, 186, 190, 208, 218
acute stress, 168
adaptation, 30, 220
adaptations, 315
ADHD, 68, 281
adipocytc, 12, 254, 259
adiponectin, 51, 54, 57
adipose, 12, 22, 27, 147, 153, 207, 208, 210, 211
adipose tissue, 12, 22, 27, 147, 153, 207, 208, 210, 211
adiposity, 1, 3, 14, 16, 18, 19, 23, 26, 43, 44, 51, 56, 63, 72, 77, 153, 181, 209, 262
adjustment, 79, 165, 168, 207, 208, 209
adolescent female, 37
adolescents, 36, 37, 40, 43, 49, 55, 60, 61, 62, 63, 64, 65, 66, 67, 69, 70, 71, 72, 73, 74, 75, 76, 77, 78, 79, 80, 119, 136, 153, 178, 179, 185, 188, 189, 190, 191, 193, 194, 195, 197, 198, 199, 201, 208, 213, 255, 256, 257, 258, 260, 261, 263, 264, 269
adrenal gland, 22, 28
adrenocorticotropic hormone, 7, 28
adult obesity, 4, 14, 17, 19, 64, 79, 194, 195, 201
adult onset diabetes, 278
adulthood, xi, 14, 29, 68, 69, 72, 73, 75, 76, 80, 92, 155, 175, 179, 195, 197, 198
adults, xiii, 2, 4, 11, 12, 18, 23, 29, 30, 32, 33, 36, 40, 42, 43, 48, 60, 65, 69, 70, 85, 104, 106, 120, 135, 148, 149, 153, 162, 173, 174, 178, 209, 210, 211, 212, 222, 232, 234, 235, 237, 247, 249, 250, 255, 257, 260, 262, 263, 267, 308, 309, 311, 315, 317
advancement, xiii, 237
adverse effects, 106, 253, 323
adverse event, 281, 304, 322
advertisements, 180, 181, 189, 191, 195, 199, 241
aerobic exercise, 208, 211
aesthetic, 125
affective disorder, 104
African Americans, 2, 13
African-American, 62, 63, 65, 67, 69, 179, 235
age, 6, 8, 29, 36, 47, 48, 51, 60, 61, 63, 64, 65, 66, 67, 68, 69, 70, 71, 72, 74, 75, 76, 79, 80, 85, 86, 99, 162, 164, 167, 179, 188, 196, 199, 207, 209, 217, 219, 220, 256, 257, 269, 290, 310
aggressiveness, 284
albumin, 149
alcohol consumption, 205
alertness, 109, 110, 112, 302
alexithymia, 131, 139, 141
algorithm, 159, 247
alimentation, 135, 138
allele, 11, 15, 17, 35, 37, 43, 53, 55
almonds, 218
alpha activity, 115, 116
ALT, 149
alternative behaviors, 242, 243, 283
American Psychiatric Association, 72, 245, 248, 312, 316
amino, 259, 300
amino acid, 300
amino acids, 300
amnesia, 115, 299, 300, 302
amphetamines, 252
amygdala, 31, 32, 33, 34, 36, 38, 39, 40, 326
amylase, 204
anastomosis, 273, 275
anatomy, 158
anger, 53, 88, 131, 141, 240

anhydrase, 259
anorexia, 24, 44, 68, 84, 95, 97, 109, 110, 111, 113, 118, 130, 136, 137, 138, 139, 221, 257, 286, 289
anorexia nervosa, 44, 68, 84, 109, 110, 130, 136, 139, 221, 286
anterior cingulate cortex, 31
anterograde amnesia, 308
anticonvulsant, 281
antidepressant, 105, 257, 281
antidepressants, 104, 150, 253, 280
antioxidant, 205, 254
antipsychotic, xiii, 150, 256, 260, 261, 309, 310, 311, 312, 315, 316, 317, 318
antipsychotic drugs, 260, 261, 317
anxiety, 60, 64, 66, 67, 70, 71, 78, 87, 88, 89, 90, 97, 98, 99, 101, 102, 106, 127, 128, 130, 131, 139, 140, 141, 160, 164, 172, 239, 255, 293, 294, 295
anxiety disorder, 89, 131, 160, 164, 172
APA, 69, 70, 84, 129
apathy, 221
aplasia, 9
appetite, xi, 15, 21, 22, 23, 24, 25, 26, 27, 28, 29, 30, 32, 33, 37, 40, 41, 42, 43, 44, 46, 49, 50, 51, 53, 55, 57, 92, 102, 103, 150, 254, 255, 259, 262, 300, 305, 321, 322, 323, 325, 326, 329
apraxia, 322
aspartate, 149, 328
assertiveness, 125, 284
assessment, xii, 29, 56, 71, 85, 93, 94, 97, 100, 121, 123, 126, 127, 128, 129, 132, 139, 140, 141, 142, 143, 144, 145, 146, 149, 151, 152, 155, 166, 167, 168, 169, 170, 174, 176, 191, 211, 260, 276, 282, 285, 296, 310, 318, 330
assessment techniques, 71
assessment tools, 71
asymptomatic, 323
atmosphere, 185
ATP, 204, 213, 311
autosomal dominant, 7
aversion, 54, 326
avoidance, 283
awareness, 88, 96, 97, 99, 109, 111, 113, 115, 138, 182, 188, 191, 243, 290, 292, 294, 299, 302, 303

B

bariatric surgery, xiii, 25, 26, 45, 46, 47, 50, 52, 83, 85, 90, 96, 98, 104, 133, 157, 158, 159, 160, 163, 164, 165, 167, 168, 169, 170, 171, 172, 173, 174, 175, 176, 253, 267, 268, 269, 270, 275, 276, 278, 280, 321, 322, 328, 329, 330
barriers, 168, 171, 190, 198, 201, 293, 294, 295, 314
basal ganglia, 326, 332
base, 8, 123, 132, 140, 165
base pair, 8
BBB, 25, 26, 27
Beck Depression Inventory, 139, 151, 166, 167, 172
beef, 218
behavior modification, 215, 276
behavior therapy, 216, 233, 246, 250, 282, 285, 287, 289, 296
behavioral aspects, 175, 239
behavioral assessment, 167
behavioral change, 41, 151, 167, 179, 182, 238
behavioral disorders, 68
behavioral medicine, 232
behavioral problems, 68, 76
behavioral theory, 238
behaviorism, 238
Beijing, 75, 196
beneficial effect, 185, 267
benefits, xiii, 125, 141, 167, 170, 198, 207, 210, 212, 220, 237, 238, 251, 252, 260, 262, 267, 268, 276, 329
benzodiazepine, 118, 138, 299
beverages, 2, 178, 201, 202, 247
bias, 141
bicarbonate, 149
bingeing, 1, 69, 70, 84, 86, 87, 88, 89, 99, 102, 130, 131, 297
biological processes, 22
biomarkers, 210
bipolar disorder, 160
blood, 6, 22, 23, 24, 26, 30, 31, 42, 49, 51, 52, 55, 65, 149, 204, 209, 212, 253, 255, 256, 257, 281, 311
blood pressure, 55, 65, 204, 253, 255, 256, 257, 281, 311
blood urea nitrogen, 149
blood-brain barrier, 22, 42, 49, 52
bloodstream, 26
BMI, 3, 6, 11, 12, 13, 16, 18, 19, 29, 30, 35, 37, 44, 46, 53, 60, 61, 62, 63, 64, 65, 66, 67, 68, 71, 73, 76, 85, 89, 98, 99, 100, 101, 129, 146, 147, 148, 158, 159, 160, 162, 164, 174, 181, 186, 187, 190, 191, 203, 216, 217, 235, 237, 244, 245, 247, 252, 268, 269, 309, 310, 322
body composition, 54, 186
body dissatisfaction, 64, 65, 66, 67, 68, 76
body fat, 1, 3, 27, 49, 51, 68, 79, 146, 147, 197, 207, 208, 209, 216
body image, xi, 65, 77, 87, 92, 126, 128, 139, 142, 160, 168, 221, 284
body mass, 12, 17, 19, 20, 45, 47, 48, 55, 60, 77, 80, 147, 158, 172, 176, 192, 197, 199, 210, 237, 316
body mass index, 17, 19, 20, 45, 47, 48, 60, 77, 80, 158, 172, 176, 192, 197, 199, 210, 237, 316

body shape, 3, 139
body size, 63
body weight, xi, 3, 11, 12, 15, 19, 20, 22, 25, 26, 27, 30, 37, 41, 43, 49, 51, 52, 53, 76, 78, 79, 98, 105, 127, 133, 158, 160, 170, 199, 201, 203, 204, 209, 215, 216, 220, 221, 222, 223, 226, 229, 244, 247, 252, 268, 271, 275, 280, 306, 324, 325, 330, 331, 332
bone, 147, 208, 275
bone mass, 208, 275
bone mineral content, 147
borborygmi, 258
boredom, 88, 89, 127, 136, 240, 294
brain, 7, 11, 12, 14, 15, 17, 19, 22, 23, 24, 26, 27, 29, 31, 32, 33, 34, 36, 37, 38, 39, 40, 41, 42, 43, 44, 46, 47, 48, 51, 52, 53, 54, 56, 92, 104, 300, 306, 321, 322, 324, 326, 328, 329, 330, 331, 332, 333
brain activity, 31, 51, 53, 54, 92
brain stem, 329
brainstem, 23, 25, 29, 36
Brazil, 5, 199
breakdown, 27
breastfeeding, 258
breathing, 113, 115, 203, 207, 295, 305
breathing rate, 115
Britain, 3
bulimia, 44, 68, 84, 88, 91, 92, 93, 99, 105, 107, 109, 110, 118, 119, 130, 131, 136, 139, 221, 257, 259, 280, 285, 286, 287, 296, 297
bulimia nervosa, 68, 84, 88, 91, 92, 93, 107, 118, 130, 136, 139, 221, 257, 259, 280, 285, 286, 296, 297

C

Ca^{2+}, 13
calcium, 149, 242, 275
caloric intake, 24, 28, 96, 97, 102, 104, 143, 145, 180, 206, 208, 219, 220, 243, 284, 292, 293, 295, 306, 313
caloric restriction, 145, 215, 221, 232
calorie, 2, 32, 34, 50, 53, 55, 168, 178, 180, 181, 207, 208, 215, 216, 217, 218, 219, 220, 231, 245, 256, 257, 260, 282, 291, 315, 329
calorimetry, 326
campaigns, 189
cancer, 24, 158, 237, 268, 278, 282
cancer death, 268
candidates, xii, 15, 98, 133, 157, 159, 160, 163, 164, 167, 168, 169, 172, 173, 174, 175, 176, 234
capsule, 328
carbamazepine, 259
carbohydrate, 2, 29, 51, 93, 102, 204, 205, 206, 212, 219, 220, 221, 232
carbohydrates, 2, 112, 206, 211, 213, 217, 219
carbonic anhydrase inhibitors, 259
cardiac arrest, 257
cardiac muscle, 13
cardiac risk, 257
cardiac risk factors, 257
cardiomyopathy, 9
cardiovascular disease, xiii, 148, 153, 158, 174, 203, 204, 205, 208, 210, 211, 213, 237, 257, 282, 311
cardiovascular morbidity, 260
cardiovascular risk, 147, 152, 175, 208, 209, 252, 255, 264
care model, 231, 234
caregivers, 72, 283
case studies, 292, 301
Caucasians, 11, 62, 67, 210
central nervous system, 15, 255, 306
central obesity, 48
cerebellum, 32, 33
cerebral blood flow, 49
challenges, 5, 16, 184, 314, 315, 321, 323
cheese, 145, 218
chemical, 87, 205, 328
chemical properties, 205
chicken, 32, 218
child maltreatment, 195
childhood, xi, 4, 7, 8, 17, 19, 43, 47, 52, 60, 61, 64, 68, 69, 70, 71, 72, 73, 74, 75, 76, 77, 78, 79, 80, 131, 143, 177, 178, 179, 180, 181, 182, 184, 185, 187, 188, 189, 190, 191, 192, 193, 194, 195, 196, 197, 198, 199, 200, 201, 202
childhood sexual abuse, 199
China, 2, 61, 75, 76, 196
cholestasis, 258
cholesterol, 149, 204, 205, 206, 207, 208, 209, 256, 257, 258, 263, 268, 311
chromosomal abnormalities, 7
chromosome, 13
chronic diseases, 146
chronic renal failure, 257
circadian rhythm, 102, 103, 296, 308
circadian rhythmicity, 308
circadian rhythms, 102, 103, 296
citalopram, 280
City, 186, 193, 277, 309
classes, 3, 85, 167, 305
classification, 6, 19, 76, 119
clavicle, 324
cleaning, 112
clients, 230, 231, 243, 313, 314, 317
clinical assessment, 142
clinical depression, 129
clinical presentation, 7, 123

clinical trials, 41, 220, 252, 262
close relationships, 39
cluster headache, 325, 331
clustering, 210
clusters, 139
CNS, 23, 104, 105, 254, 307
cocaine, 27, 48, 333
cognition, 31, 42, 172, 315, 318
cognitive abilities, 171
cognitive biases, 127, 140
cognitive deficit, 314, 315
cognitive deficits, 314, 315
cognitive development, 80
cognitive dysfunction, 306
cognitive function, 17, 76, 166, 315
cognitive impairment, 315, 316
cognitive models, 140
cognitive performance, 64
cognitive style, 165
cognitive tasks, 48
cognitive theory, 200
cognitive-behavioral therapy, 168, 237, 250, 285, 287
collaboration, 144, 196
commercial, 190, 197, 201, 227, 228, 232, 233, 235, 244
commercials, 181, 199
commissure, 323, 325
common symptoms, 99
communication, 43, 171, 198, 247, 261, 326
community, 60, 65, 66, 67, 68, 69, 70, 71, 78, 84, 85, 86, 91, 96, 98, 111, 129, 130, 135, 189, 200, 231, 267, 310, 315, 317
comorbidity, 72, 80, 139, 151
compensation, 3
complex behaviors, 307
complex carbohydrates, 205, 206, 275
complexity, xii, 157, 159
compliance, 80, 144, 145, 189, 251, 252
complications, 90, 91, 158, 164, 167, 170, 209, 251, 252, 257, 270, 271, 272, 275, 276, 322, 323
composition, 46, 86, 147, 167, 205, 207, 209, 213, 215, 216, 219, 220
compounds, 253, 259
compulsive behavior, 159
compulsive personality disorder, 163
computational modeling, 327
computed tomography, 103
computer, 224, 231, 234, 241
conception, 200
confounders, 184
confounding variables, 64
connectivity, 38, 43, 332
conscious awareness, 110
consciousness, 110, 111, 112, 115, 299, 302
consensus, 60, 95, 96, 171
consent, 167, 168, 188, 275
constipation, 216, 217
consumption, 2, 25, 26, 28, 32, 33, 37, 96, 100, 111, 112, 113, 130, 132, 134, 179, 181, 182, 183, 184, 185, 186, 195, 196, 201, 205, 206, 209, 243, 307, 322, 328
content analysis, 192
contingency, 239, 240
contraceptives, 259
control condition, 313
control group, 100, 128, 163, 248, 256, 268, 293, 310
controlled studies, 150, 184
controlled trials, 150, 165, 171, 292, 295, 305, 316
controversial, 89, 90, 103, 109, 110, 112, 115, 128, 256
convergence, 46, 51
conviction, 98, 143
cooking, 110, 111, 137, 184, 314
coping strategies, 64, 283
coronary heart disease, 52, 152, 153, 204, 212, 257, 311
correlation, 3, 98, 99, 102, 128, 178, 204, 205, 226
correlations, 54
cortex, 31, 32, 33, 34, 35, 36, 38, 50, 53, 56, 331
cortical pathway, 35
corticosteroids, 150
corticotropin, 27
cortisol, 22, 28, 45, 46, 48, 53, 101, 102, 300, 308
cost, 30, 147, 195, 244, 246
counsel, 171
counseling, 169, 171, 173, 193, 231, 234, 244, 247, 250, 256, 258, 312
craving, 48, 259
creatinine, 149, 253, 259
creativity, 171
critical analysis, 60, 177
criticism, 63, 71, 122
cross-sectional study, 77, 198, 199, 302, 307
cues, 32, 33, 34, 35, 36, 37, 38, 40, 41, 42, 45, 49, 54, 89, 103, 184, 242, 243, 283, 284, 313
cultural differences, 77
cultural influence, 197
cycles, 14, 79, 80, 107
cyclosporine, 258
cytoarchitecture, 326

D

data collection, 151
database, 176

deaths, 152, 312, 322
deep brain stimulation, xiii, 322, 330, 331
defects, 7, 9, 15
deficiencies, 275, 277
deficiency, 7, 25, 258
deficit, 68, 71, 72, 215, 216, 220, 251, 315
deflation, 273
degenerate, 1
degradation, 26, 207
dehiscence, 271, 273
dehydration, 216
dementia, 323
demographic characteristics, 200
denial, 169, 176
Department of Health and Human Services, 250
deposition, 28, 103
depression, 31, 60, 64, 66, 67, 68, 69, 70, 71, 75, 76, 78, 79, 90, 101, 105, 127, 129, 130, 131, 138, 139, 150, 159, 164, 179, 194, 195, 221, 239, 245, 253, 255, 259, 269, 290, 293, 310, 323, 328, 329
depressive symptoms, 78, 101, 131, 140, 262, 281, 290
deprivation, 17, 88, 179
depth, 125, 133, 229, 283
deregulation, 15
destiny, 142
detection, 209
developed countries, 3, 158, 289
developing countries, 61
developing nations, 158
developmental change, 36
dexamethasone suppression test, 105
diabetes, 4, 18, 20, 25, 27, 41, 45, 47, 48, 52, 106, 142, 143, 148, 150, 175, 206, 207, 208, 209, 210, 211, 212, 213, 235, 237, 247, 252, 256, 257, 260, 262, 263, 264, 268, 282, 311, 318
diabetic patients, 171, 204, 213, 261, 262, 263, 264, 268
diacylglycerol, 13
Diagnostic and Statistical Manual of Mental Disorders, 72, 96
diagnostic criteria, xii, 84, 85, 86, 90, 95, 96, 98, 100, 101, 104, 112, 121, 130, 136, 137, 138, 153, 154, 164, 204, 244, 283, 289
diarrhea, 253, 257, 260, 275
diastolic blood pressure, 204, 256, 260
diet, xiii, 3, 24, 36, 40, 45, 53, 62, 63, 64, 70, 71, 80, 87, 98, 101, 102, 123, 125, 128, 133, 134, 140, 141, 142, 143, 144, 145, 169, 170, 180, 190, 204, 205, 206, 208, 210, 211, 212, 213, 215, 216, 217, 218, 219, 221, 224, 226, 227, 228, 230, 231, 232, 242, 245, 251, 252, 255, 257, 260, 264, 282, 283, 284, 291, 326, 329, 331
dietary fat, 212, 213
dietary fiber, 211, 212
dietary habits, 182, 187, 220, 221
dietary intake, 178, 183
dieting, 1, 57, 65, 68, 69, 70, 71, 74, 79, 92, 93, 131, 143, 167, 183, 187, 216, 220, 221, 222, 262
differential diagnosis, 136
digestion, 22, 26, 204
digestive enzymes, 26
direct measure, 216
disability, 278
discomfort, 135, 188
discordance, 6
discrimination, 3, 175
discussion groups, 184
diseases, xii, 10, 15, 16, 18, 61, 89, 110, 148, 149, 205, 211, 252, 260, 276
disgust, 130, 131
disorders, xii, xiii, 15, 17, 67, 68, 72, 75, 77, 80, 85, 89, 90, 91, 92, 97, 98, 100, 101, 110, 111, 113, 117, 118, 128, 131, 135, 160, 162, 164, 165, 167, 168, 169, 170, 172, 174, 178, 188, 203, 204, 248, 258, 264, 269, 286, 303, 306, 307, 310, 311, 318, 321, 322, 330
dissatisfaction, 65, 79, 130, 160, 253, 290
dissociation, 110
distress, 64, 67, 75, 81, 84, 85, 87, 90, 95, 96, 97, 101, 137, 160, 168, 171, 183, 195, 221, 290
distribution, 6, 18, 49, 53, 86, 147, 152, 153, 210, 316
divergence, 111
dizygotic, 6
dizygotic twins, 6
dopamine, 23, 31, 33, 35, 36, 37, 39, 42, 43, 45, 46, 47, 49, 52, 53, 54, 55, 56, 303, 305, 307, 327, 328, 330, 331, 333
dopamine agonist, 305, 307
dopamine antagonists, 327
dopaminergic, 23, 38, 40, 48, 255, 305, 326, 328, 331, 332, 333
dorsolateral prefrontal cortex, 31, 32, 50, 51
dosage, 118, 292
double blind study, 49
double-blind trial, 286
dough, 290
down-regulation, 24, 30, 35
draft, 278
drawing, xv, 125
drug abuse, 257
drug addict, 31, 46, 333
drug addiction, 31, 46, 333
drug discovery, 41
drug side effects, 149

drug treatment, 154, 252
drugs, xiii, 24, 41, 117, 118, 149, 150, 153, 251, 252, 253, 254, 255, 257, 258, 259, 260, 264, 265
duodenum, 267, 270, 273, 275
dyslipidemia, 148, 203, 204, 216, 252, 257, 260, 311, 318

E

East Asia, 2, 11
eating disorders, 16, 18, 31, 44, 67, 68, 71, 75, 76, 78, 84, 85, 90, 91, 92, 93, 94, 98, 100, 109, 110, 119, 120, 121, 127, 128, 129, 130, 131, 132, 134, 139, 151, 152, 153, 164, 167, 168, 198, 199, 221, 222, 232, 233, 234, 239, 244, 249, 250, 252, 257, 286, 296, 307, 308, 318
eating disturbances, 76
economic consequences, 4, 75
economic status, 4, 62, 79, 177, 178, 189, 191, 197, 201
education, 62, 63, 64, 162, 178, 179, 184, 185, 186, 187, 196, 200, 209, 215, 223, 239, 246, 256, 283, 314
educational attainment, 64
educational materials, 181
educators, 66
EEG activity, 113, 115
egg, 143, 144
EKG, 113, 114, 115, 116, 117, 118
elderly population, 212
electrocardiogram, 149
electrodes, 117, 323, 325
electroencephalogram, 113
electrophoresis, 149
elementary school, 20, 74, 78, 197, 198
e-mail, 234, 246, 247
emotion, 31, 38, 42, 43, 87, 88, 140, 141, 151, 172
emotional conflict, 242
emotional disorder, 178
emotional distress, 70, 87, 89, 95, 100, 111
emotional problems, 67, 123
emotional state, 88, 131, 179
emotional well-being, 64
employment, 75, 195, 221
encephalopathy, 275
endocrine, 24, 28, 39, 41, 43, 61, 87, 308
endocrinology, 323
endorsements, 181
endothelial cells, 26
energy, 11, 12, 14, 15, 19, 22, 23, 24, 26, 40, 45, 49, 52, 53, 54, 55, 103, 104, 147, 154, 179, 180, 181, 182, 185, 207, 210, 215, 216, 217, 220, 221, 222, 226, 240, 248, 251, 252, 254, 262, 264, 300, 309, 310, 311, 324, 325, 326, 329, 330, 331
energy consumption, 185, 208, 309, 310, 311
energy density, 181
energy expenditure, 12, 14, 15, 26, 185, 207, 210, 220, 222, 251, 254, 262, 311, 324, 325, 326, 329, 330
energy input, 324
enrollment, 246
entorhinal cortex, 32
environment, 5, 6, 16, 73, 86, 91, 94, 170, 179, 183, 186, 188, 193, 201, 239, 245, 295, 313, 315
environment factors, 179
environmental change, 192
environmental factors, 6, 15, 16, 19, 22, 61, 86, 106
environmental influences, 6, 19, 73, 86, 93
environmental resources, 172
environmental stimuli, 186
enzyme, 11, 14, 19
epidemic, 2, 4, 57, 61, 80, 94, 150, 157, 176, 196, 213, 237, 246, 322, 324, 329
epidemiologic studies, 85
epidemiology, 91, 192, 193, 283
epilepsy, 9, 150
erosion, 273
error detection, 31
escitalopram, 280, 286
ESI, 136
essential tremor, 323
estrogen, 22, 29
ethical issues, 41
ethnic background, 63
ethnicity, 64, 67, 73, 162, 179, 189
Europe, 2, 12, 41, 252, 255, 271
European Union, 61
evidence, 4, 5, 6, 10, 12, 14, 15, 16, 21, 27, 28, 29, 34, 43, 44, 47, 53, 69, 70, 76, 85, 86, 87, 90, 102, 129, 159, 164, 165, 169, 174, 204, 206, 210, 219, 222, 223, 224, 225, 226, 227, 234, 239, 249, 276, 282, 290, 313, 322, 326, 327, 328, 329, 332
examinations, 149, 160
excess body weight, 24
exclusion, 267, 270
execution, 275
executive function, 31, 315
executive functioning, 315
executive functions, 31
exercise, 24, 49, 68, 80, 84, 126, 131, 136, 168, 170, 186, 189, 190, 196, 202, 207, 208, 210, 212, 215, 223, 224, 225, 226, 227, 230, 231, 241, 245, 249, 251, 252, 284, 295, 313
exocytosis, 47
experimental design, 165
expertise, 159, 167, 169, 172

exposure, 30, 35, 37, 38, 40, 49, 76, 178, 180, 181, 198, 305, 328
external locus of control, 131
extraction, 205
eye movement, 110

F

facial muscles, 117
facilitators, 187
false positive, 10
families, 6, 8, 10, 14, 62, 71, 86, 87, 179, 180, 182, 183, 184, 189, 190, 192, 201, 247
family characteristics, 198
family environment, 202
family functioning, 191
family history, 15, 69, 129, 167, 210, 235
family income, 182
family meals, 68, 183
family members, 189, 283
family relationships, 69
family studies, 6, 86
family support, 186, 231
fast food, 143, 144, 178, 179, 180, 190, 245
fasting, 7, 24, 25, 26, 27, 29, 32, 39, 46, 49, 50, 56, 130, 134, 136, 204, 208, 209, 211, 311
fasting glucose, 39, 204, 209, 311
fat, 2, 3, 6, 12, 18, 20, 22, 25, 26, 27, 28, 29, 35, 51, 53, 87, 93, 102, 126, 147, 152, 155, 178, 179, 180, 181, 184, 186, 188, 193, 197, 204, 205, 207, 208, 210, 213, 215, 217, 218, 220, 245, 254, 257, 258, 326, 327, 328, 332
fat intake, 102, 184, 205, 208, 213, 258
fat soluble, 258
fatty acids, 205, 207, 213, 262
FDA, 253, 255, 257, 261, 281
fear, 98, 141, 142, 326
feelings, 97, 101, 126, 141, 220, 221, 238, 239, 240, 241, 245, 283, 284
female rat, 44, 49
fertility, 1, 2, 7
fiber, 205, 209, 211, 213, 217
fibers, 205, 216
fibrosarcoma, 13, 14
financial, 229
first degree relative, 92
fitness, 186, 199, 203, 207, 208, 209, 210, 211, 249
flatulence, 258, 275
flavor, 31, 51
flavour, 46
flexibility, 73, 248
flight, 323
fluctuations, 29
fluoxetine, 280, 281, 282, 285, 286, 304, 306
fluvoxamine, 280, 281, 286, 287, 292, 304
focus groups, 73, 183
food habits, 181
food intake, xii, 7, 11, 12, 14, 22, 23, 24, 25, 26, 27, 28, 29, 33, 35, 42, 43, 44, 46, 48, 50, 52, 53, 54, 55, 56, 57, 70, 83, 87, 96, 100, 103, 105, 106, 109, 111, 113, 120, 130, 131, 133, 134, 137, 144, 158, 181, 182, 184, 197, 223, 251, 289, 293, 294, 296, 297, 300, 322, 324, 328, 329, 330, 331, 332, 333
food products, 181, 188
Ford, 41, 47, 203, 210, 212, 311, 317
formation, 26, 33, 75, 195, 271
formula, 36
fractures, 275
fragments, 254
France, 61
fraternal twins, 119
frontal cortex, 36
fructose, 204
fruits, 112, 183, 217, 310
functional MRI, 47, 48, 51

G

GABA, 118, 253, 259, 302
gallbladder, 51
gastrectomy, 49, 158, 174, 275
gastrin, 57
gastrointestinal tract, 9, 22
gender differences, 75, 196
gene expression, 20, 54, 333
gene pool, 61, 191
general practitioner, 190
generalized anxiety disorder, 129
Generalized Anxiety Disorder, 163
genes, 5, 6, 7, 8, 9, 10, 12, 14, 15, 50, 86, 106, 212
genetic alteration, 7, 40
genetic defect, 7
genetic factors, 5, 6, 8, 14, 37, 86, 102
genetic marker, 8, 9, 10, 15
genetic predisposition, 15, 112, 167
genetic syndromes, 30
genetics, 5, 6, 8, 15, 18, 20, 86
genome, 5, 6, 8, 9, 10, 12, 13, 14, 16, 17, 18, 19
genotype, 9, 10, 19
genotyping, 10
gestational age, 30
glasses, 37, 218
globalization, 3
globus, 39, 323
glucagon, 21, 22, 25, 38, 49, 51, 52, 57
glucocorticoid receptor, 14
gluconeogenesis, 22, 300

glucose, 7, 22, 23, 25, 26, 33, 35, 39, 48, 51, 54, 55, 56, 149, 203, 204, 205, 206, 207, 210, 211, 212, 213, 258, 259, 260, 273, 300, 301, 306, 308
glucose regulation, 308
glucose tolerance, 203, 210, 212, 258, 259, 260, 301
glue, 112
graduate students, 225
graph, 145, 146
grazing, 294
Great Britain, 4, 282
Greece, 61, 198
growth, 7, 8, 12, 13, 23, 25, 30, 46, 47, 52, 60, 61, 203, 254, 308
growth factor, 47
growth hormone, 7, 23, 46, 254, 308
guidance, 230, 286
guidelines, 2, 4, 129, 152, 159, 174, 186, 201, 216, 234, 237, 241, 244, 246, 248, 249, 252, 268, 276, 277, 312
guilt, 87, 88, 89, 97, 98, 101, 130, 131, 144, 167, 220, 241
guilty, 84, 102, 135
gynecomastia, 9

H

half-life, 118
hallucinations, 305
health care, 63, 71, 190, 191, 192, 193, 199, 216, 234
health care professionals, 63, 71, 190, 191, 192, 193, 216
health condition, 75
health effects, 262
health information, 247
health problems, 73, 279, 290
health promotion, 189, 191
health risks, 126, 147, 170, 237, 246
health status, 174, 186, 212
hearing loss, 9
heart attack, 257
heart disease, 232, 312
heart rate, 253, 255, 256, 281
height, 2, 3, 146, 147, 162, 187, 197, 217
helplessness, 101, 220
heritability, 6, 14, 18, 86
heterogeneity, 56, 115
high blood cholesterol, 209
high fat, 220
higher education, 185, 310
hippocampus, 31, 32, 34, 53, 326
Hispanics, 2
history, xiii, 1, 16, 77, 90, 91, 93, 122, 133, 145, 160, 164, 167, 168, 169, 199, 237, 257, 270, 282, 301, 302, 303, 305
homeostasis, 7, 12, 23, 52, 53, 55, 105, 205, 300, 301, 324, 326
homework, 127, 283, 294
Hong Kong, 65, 77
hormone, 22, 24, 25, 26, 27, 28, 29, 39, 40, 41, 43, 44, 49, 50, 54, 254, 300, 331
hormone levels, 39, 41, 44
hormones, xi, 9, 11, 21, 22, 29, 40, 41, 42, 43, 44, 47, 52, 55, 56, 57, 102, 103, 252, 270, 273
hospitalization, 275
host, 22, 64, 86, 177, 191
hotel, 291
HPA axis, 28, 42, 45
human, 1, 2, 7, 12, 16, 18, 19, 20, 24, 41, 45, 46, 48, 49, 50, 51, 53, 54, 56, 109, 212, 213, 222, 234, 254, 263, 329
human brain, 41, 46, 48, 51, 56, 329
human subjects, 48
Hunter, 227, 233
hydrogenation, 206
hygiene, 295
hyperactivity, 11, 17, 68, 71, 72
hypercholesterolemia, 143
hyperglycemia, 206, 254
hyperinsulinemia, 205, 206, 211, 330
hyperlipidemia, 205, 211
hypersomnia, 119
hypertension, 52, 148, 150, 203, 204, 216, 252, 257, 282, 311, 318
hyperthyroidism, 9, 252, 257
hypertriglyceridemia, 268, 333
hypertrophy, 149
hypoglycemia, 300
hypogonadism, 7, 8, 9
hyporeflexia, 8
hypotension, 216, 257
hypothalamus, 23, 26, 27, 29, 31, 32, 33, 39, 40, 52, 54, 55, 300, 322, 323, 324, 325, 328, 329, 330, 331, 332
hypothesis, 16, 35, 90, 99, 123, 325
hypothyroidism, 149

I

iatrogenic, 252, 258, 260
ideal, 1, 3, 77, 127, 180, 221, 226, 276
identification, 5, 14, 15, 152, 164, 174, 191, 222, 234, 239, 249, 260
identity, 183
iliac crest, 147, 148
image, 33, 65, 126, 131, 155, 175, 284
images, 34, 36, 40, 92, 247, 329
immediate gratification, 88
improvements, 159, 210, 244, 260, 293

impulses, 89
impulsive, 89, 131, 141
impulsiveness, 131, 141, 154
impulsivity, 68, 83, 87, 91, 127, 141, 144, 284
in transition, 178, 191
in vivo, 48, 209, 314, 315, 331
inattention, 68
incidence, 92, 180, 206, 232, 253, 257, 258, 260, 262, 263, 268, 275, 278, 307
income, 75, 162, 179, 193, 195, 201
independence, 315, 317
independent living, 318
independent variable, 208
induction, 251
industrial revolution, 2
industrialized countries, 177, 178, 180, 191
industry, 192
ineffectiveness, 99
inefficiency, 187, 255
inertia, 115, 117
infancy, 14, 52, 63, 65, 76, 305
infants, 30, 41, 49, 54, 61, 196
infection, 158
inferences, 33
inflammation, 257
information processing, 151
information technology, 246
informed consent, 167, 276
ingest, 97, 98, 112, 291
ingestion, 23, 24, 27, 33, 34, 35, 37, 51, 54, 96, 97, 98, 111, 115, 310
inheritance, 5, 6, 7, 8, 9
inhibition, 25, 29, 31, 35, 44, 103, 259, 281, 329, 332
inhibitor, 26, 41, 253, 255, 257, 259, 262, 281, 286
initiation, 23, 33, 38, 45, 97, 182, 299, 306
injections, 27, 327
injuries, 61, 109, 110, 111, 112
insomnia, 95, 97, 98, 111, 113, 118, 137, 253, 255, 256, 259, 281, 289, 292, 295, 301, 302
insulin, 7, 16, 20, 22, 23, 24, 25, 26, 28, 30, 39, 42, 44, 45, 47, 48, 49, 50, 52, 53, 54, 56, 57, 102, 104, 203, 204, 205, 206, 207, 209, 210, 211, 212, 213, 252, 254, 257, 258, 260, 262, 300, 308, 331
insulin resistance, 16, 20, 24, 27, 28, 42, 54, 203, 204, 206, 211, 212, 213, 252, 254, 262, 331
insulin sensitivity, 26, 30, 204, 205, 206, 207, 209, 210, 212, 254, 257
intelligence, 66
internal consistency, 133, 154
internalizing, 67
interpersonal conflict, 241
interpersonal relations, 131
interpersonal relationships, 131
intervention, 44, 71, 80, 113, 127, 128, 176, 178, 182, 184, 186, 187, 188, 192, 194, 198, 200, 211, 225, 230, 231, 232, 233, 234, 235, 240, 246, 247, 262, 263, 277, 278, 279, 282, 283, 285, 312, 314, 315, 316
intervention strategies, 71, 192, 211, 315
intestinal tract, 270
intestine, 158, 258
intravenously, 35
intrinsic motivation, 229
IQ scores, 64
Ireland, 73
iron, 273, 275
isolation, 66, 177, 179, 191
Israel, 59, 61, 63, 65, 66, 75, 76, 107, 177, 179, 180, 187, 196
issues, 2, 60, 68, 71, 160, 167, 168, 169, 177, 178, 179, 180, 182, 183, 184, 185, 187, 188, 189, 190, 191, 192, 198, 229, 231, 256, 284, 285, 290, 317
Italy, 1, 83, 95, 109, 121, 201, 203, 215, 251, 267
item response theory, 104

J

Japan, 2, 4
jejunum, 273

K

ketones, 300
kill, 318
kindergarten, 191

L

labeling, 141, 197
laboratory studies, 190
lack of control, 84, 87, 101, 136
lactic acid, 208, 253, 260
lactose, 204
landscape, 197
laparoscopy, 272
latency, 67, 113, 114
later life, 63, 64, 67, 70, 179, 185
Latin America, 65
laws, 1, 189
laxatives, 130, 131, 132, 134
LDL, 149, 205, 206, 208, 209, 258
lead, 15, 27, 28, 35, 38, 70, 128, 138, 141, 206, 221, 228, 241, 248, 306, 314, 324
lean body mass, 12, 147
learning, 9, 31, 49, 151, 238, 239, 284, 309, 314, 318, 319
learning disabilities, 9
LED, 217, 219

leisure, 211
leptin, 7, 21, 22, 26, 27, 29, 30, 40, 41, 42, 43, 44, 46, 47, 48, 49, 51, 52, 53, 54, 55, 56, 57, 102, 103, 254, 300, 301, 308, 330
lesions, 328, 329, 330, 331
level of education, 63
LIFE, 123
life changes, 168
lifestyle behaviors, 182
lifestyle changes, 5, 231, 264, 276
lifetime, 68, 69, 85, 89, 90, 100, 101, 128, 131, 160, 161, 164
light, 38, 56, 139, 168
limbic system, 31, 331
linoleic acid, 206
lipases, 257
lipid metabolism, 211, 254
lipids, 205, 207, 210, 212, 258, 275
lipodystrophy, 43
lipolysis, 11, 12, 20, 22, 26, 27, 254, 300
lipoproteins, 204, 212
liquids, 112, 168
literacy, 189, 191
lithium, 301
liver, 26, 149, 207, 252
liver disease, 252
liver profile, 149
localization, 323, 329, 332
loci, 5, 8, 9, 10, 12, 13, 14, 15, 19, 20
locomotor, 14, 18, 49
locus, 5, 12, 17, 125
longitudinal study, 78, 319

M

macronutrients, 25, 30
magnesium, 149, 205, 212
magnetic resonance, 55, 87, 147
magnetic resonance imaging, 55, 87, 147
magnitude, 6, 165
major depression, 175, 257
major depressive disorder, 101, 129, 131, 160, 163, 333
majority, 5, 6, 27, 83, 84, 87, 96, 113, 166, 167, 188, 216, 227, 244, 302, 323
malabsorption, 258, 270, 273, 275
malignancy, 43
malnutrition, 159, 271, 275
man, 50, 209, 211, 278, 308
manic, 305
manic episode, 305
manipulation, 3, 187
mapping, 46
marginalization, 79, 179
marital status, 162
marketing, 75, 178, 180, 181, 188, 189, 192, 194, 195, 199
marketplace, 75, 195
masking, 88
mass, 12, 13, 17, 18, 20, 55, 76, 147, 152, 158, 197, 207, 208, 209
masseter, 113, 114, 115, 116, 117, 118
mastoid, 114, 115, 116, 117, 118
materials, 223, 224, 225, 247, 313
media, 66, 177, 178, 180, 181, 182, 185, 188, 189, 190, 191, 196
medical, xi, xii, 15, 67, 84, 91, 97, 109, 110, 117, 119, 121, 122, 123, 137, 146, 149, 159, 162, 169, 175, 188, 190, 191, 203, 204, 210, 215, 216, 220, 225, 237, 241, 244, 245, 253, 256, 261, 267, 268, 269, 277, 282, 290
medical care, 191, 269
medical history, 117, 169
medical reason, 216
medication, 110, 137, 237, 244, 246, 281, 282, 299, 302, 305, 306, 307, 310, 314, 316, 318
medicine, 119, 193, 232
Mediterranean, 2
melanin, 54
mellitus, 20, 46, 48, 150, 252, 260, 261
membership, 283
membranes, 206
memory, 31, 42, 48, 53, 96, 112, 259, 315, 323
menopause, 51
mental disorder, 67, 90, 110, 137, 160, 165, 171, 248
mental health, 73, 129, 157, 159, 164, 166, 167, 168, 169, 171, 173, 186, 290, 317, 318
mental health professionals, 166, 171, 173
mental illness, xiii, 105, 128, 309, 310, 311, 313, 314, 315, 316, 317
mental processes, 165
mental retardation, 7, 8, 9
mental state, 64
messages, 180, 181, 183, 186, 189, 194, 216, 227, 247
meta-analysis, 5, 10, 11, 12, 18, 20, 150, 158, 173, 200, 252, 261, 264, 277, 280, 287, 312, 316
Metabolic, xii, 42, 77, 78, 104, 159, 174, 198, 201, 203, 204, 206, 210, 211, 277, 297, 300, 311, 317
metabolic changes, 50, 67, 326
metabolic disorder, 143, 203, 204, 262, 268
metabolic disorders, 143, 203, 204, 262, 268
metabolic pathways, 10
metabolic syndrome, 57, 148, 155, 203, 205, 206, 209, 210, 211, 253, 260, 263, 317, 318
metabolism, 11, 12, 22, 23, 26, 27, 29, 55, 56, 207, 273, 300, 306

metformin, 232, 256, 258, 259, 260, 262, 263, 264
mice, 12, 18, 20, 24, 52, 103, 105, 326, 329, 331
microcephaly, 9
microdialysis, 331
micronutrients, 216
midbrain, 31, 34, 38, 42, 103, 326
Millon Clinical Multiaxial Inventory, 166
Minneapolis, 96, 222, 308
minorities, 189
minority groups, 178, 179
models, 10, 88, 167, 185, 255, 284, 305, 313, 325, 328, 329
moderators, 160
Modern Age, 2
modernization, 177, 179, 191
modifications, 49, 204, 252, 253, 260, 270, 275
modules, 139
molecules, 23
monoamine oxidase inhibitors, 257
monounsaturated fatty acids, 206
monozygotic twins, 6
mood disorder, 101, 135, 164, 167, 310
mood states, 294
Moon, 78
morbidity, 69, 84, 85, 86, 89, 90, 100, 114, 115, 128, 131, 132, 267, 268, 269, 276, 322, 331
morphology, 213
mortality, 146, 158, 172, 173, 175, 204, 210, 211, 237, 244, 260, 268, 271, 272, 273, 275, 276, 278, 311, 317, 322, 331
mortality rate, 158, 272, 311, 317
motivation, 31, 43, 49, 124, 125, 126, 127, 169, 182, 216, 225, 234, 276
motor activity, 300, 301, 331
mRNA, 26, 213, 331
multidimensional, 132, 142
multi-ethnic, 194
multimedia, 247
muscle relaxation, 293, 295
muscles, 113, 114, 115, 116, 117, 118, 207
muscular mass, 207
mutation, 6, 11, 12, 17
mutations, 10, 11, 16, 17, 18, 86
myelin, 326
myocardial infarction, 155, 171, 257, 311, 323

N

narcolepsy, 303
National Institutes of Health, 152, 154, 158, 159, 174, 234, 244, 268, 278, 312
natural food, 217
nausea, 305
negative attitudes, 65, 66, 71, 187
negative consequences, 131, 239, 241, 275, 283
negative effects, 205, 235
negative emotions, 88, 102, 140
negative mood, 83, 87, 88, 92, 241
negative reinforcement, 238
neglect, 179, 198
nerve, 23, 50
nervous system, 331
neurobiology, 35
neuroendocrine system, 102
neurohormonal, 52, 53
neuroimaging, 22, 31, 32, 39, 41, 328
neuroleptics, 118
neuronal systems, 332
neurons, 17, 23, 31, 39, 42, 45, 254, 331
neuropeptides, 23, 27, 42, 332
neurophysiology, 332
neuroscience, 45
neurosurgery, 322
neurotransmission, 327
neurotransmitter, 35, 255, 328
neurotransmitters, 255
neutral, 34, 40
New England, 75, 80, 172, 175, 176, 199, 212, 232, 235
New Zealand, 197
Niemann-Pick disease, 13
nocturnal eating, 97, 98, 99, 101, 102, 104, 109, 110, 111, 113, 115, 119, 120, 127, 137, 138, 292, 296, 297, 299, 300, 301, 302, 303, 304, 305, 306, 307, 308
non-clinical population, 132
norepinephrine, 281
normal children, 47, 48
North America, 61, 74, 75, 146, 153, 159, 173, 174, 175, 176, 193, 234, 249
Norway, 202
Nuclear Magnetic Resonance, 207
nuclei, 17, 323
nucleic acid, 17
nucleus, 23, 26, 31, 34, 36, 37, 39, 40, 46, 49, 54, 199, 322, 324, 326, 327, 330, 331, 333
null, 165
null hypothesis, 165
nutrient, 22, 42, 215, 216, 251
nutrients, 22, 158, 217, 270
nutrition, 169, 176, 184, 186, 187, 189, 194, 209, 220, 223, 224, 240, 241, 275, 308, 312, 314
nutritional assessment, 282
nutritional deficiencies, 273
nutritional status, 276

O

obese children, 11, 29, 30, 36, 48, 53, 62, 64, 65, 66, 67, 71, 73, 74, 76, 77, 78, 80, 181, 182, 185, 186, 192, 198, 202
obesity in adults, 174, 222, 234, 249, 260
obesity prevention, 77, 143, 182, 184, 187, 190, 192, 193, 195, 198, 199, 200, 202
observational learning, 187
obsessive-compulsive disorder, 330
obstacles, 126, 172
obstructive sleep apnea, 114, 119, 282
OCD, 323, 328, 329
OH, 333
olanzapine, 120, 301, 307
olfaction, 9
olive oil, 144, 205, 206, 218
operant conditioning, 238, 239
operations, 27, 91
opportunities, 126, 176, 191, 253
optic chiasm, 325
optic nerve, 323, 324
optimization, 276
osteodystrophy, 9
outpatients, 100, 101, 105, 307
overlap, 85, 86, 100, 118
overweight adults, 69, 247
overweight children, 51, 60, 62, 63, 64, 65, 66, 67, 68, 69, 70, 71, 72, 74, 75, 77, 79, 80, 81, 136, 153, 181, 182, 184, 185, 186, 189, 190, 191, 195

P

Pacific, 4
pain, 237
pancreas, 22, 26
parallel, 61, 332
paranoia, 305
parathyroid, 9
parental attitudes, 79
parental consent, 198
parental criticism, 63, 71
parental pressure, 184
parenting, 184, 185, 197
parents, 6, 60, 62, 63, 66, 70, 71, 73, 77, 105, 180, 182, 183, 184, 185, 186, 187, 188, 190, 191, 193, 194, 195, 196, 198, 199, 201
paresthesias, 259, 306, 322
parietal cortex, 34
parietal lobe, 32
paroxetine, 292, 304
participants, 17, 25, 90, 99, 153, 155, 162, 166, 167, 187, 191, 224, 225, 226, 227, 228, 229, 230, 247, 290, 292, 293, 303, 311, 315
partition, 271, 273
pasta, 218
pathogenesis, 9, 99, 102, 213, 302
pathology, 73, 84, 85, 87, 91, 95, 102, 127, 132, 149, 159, 169, 193, 203, 207, 239
pathophysiological, 15, 57
pathophysiology, 10, 311, 322, 323
pathways, xi, 5, 10, 15, 22, 50, 51, 55, 122, 184
pediatric obesity, 61, 74, 188, 190, 193, 197
peer group, 231
peer relationship, 66, 72
peer support, 187, 231
penetrance, 9
peptide, 21, 22, 23, 25, 38, 42, 43, 44, 45, 46, 48, 49, 50, 51, 52, 55, 56, 57, 254, 300
peptides, 22, 23, 42, 52, 54, 325, 328
percentile, 60, 61, 269
perfectionism, 93, 99, 141
personal communication, 326
personal control, 66
personal history, 122
personal responsibility, 140, 188
personality, 3, 78, 88, 100, 101, 127, 129, 131, 140, 160, 165, 166, 171, 189, 269
personality characteristics, 140, 165
personality disorder, 88, 100, 101, 127, 131, 160, 163, 269
personality traits, 101, 129
PET, 31, 32, 33, 34, 35, 36, 38, 39
PET scan, 33, 39
pharmaceutical, 24, 25, 123, 136
pharmacological treatment, 27, 253, 261
pharmacotherapy, xiii, 53, 157, 158, 170, 176, 244, 251, 252, 253, 264, 279, 281, 287, 289, 290, 292, 297, 305, 312
phenomenology, 300
phenotype, 8, 16, 18, 19, 37, 92
phenotypes, 14, 37
phenytoin, 259
Philadelphia, 119, 277, 289, 321
phosphate, 13
phospholipids, 205, 209
phosphorylation, 212
physical education, 2
physical exercise, 130, 143, 207, 209, 220, 221
physical fitness, 3, 125, 212
physical health, 159
physical properties, 181
physical well-being, 133
physicians, 99, 109, 170, 197, 202, 292

Physiological, 22
physiology, 53, 299
pilot study, 194, 195, 230, 232, 289, 293, 295, 296, 315, 317
pioglitazone, 256, 261
pituitary gland, 28
placebo, 24, 25, 255, 256, 257, 259, 260, 261, 262, 264, 280, 281, 282, 285, 286, 287, 292, 296, 304, 305, 307
plasma levels, 57, 257, 258, 259
plasticity, 213
playing, 103, 142
pleasure, 54, 126
policy, 189, 191, 192, 194, 199
policymakers, 188, 189
polycystic ovarian syndrome, 43
polymorphism, 19, 20, 55, 86
polymorphisms, 9, 16, 20
polypeptide, 53, 55
polyunsaturated fat, 206
polyunsaturated fatty acids, 206
population, 1, 2, 4, 9, 11, 12, 16, 17, 18, 19, 20, 24, 68, 72, 77, 78, 85, 86, 91, 92, 93, 98, 100, 105, 106, 112, 115, 128, 144, 150, 153, 155, 175, 188, 189, 195, 200, 205, 208, 209, 210, 211, 249, 302, 309, 310, 311, 312, 313, 314, 315, 316, 331
Portugal, 61
positive attitudes, 191
positive correlation, 39
positron, 46, 55, 328
positron emission tomography, 46, 55, 328
potassium, 12, 149
potato, 180, 291
potential benefits, 165, 171
poultry, 218
poverty, 179
Prader-Willi syndrome, 8, 9, 16, 30, 36, 48, 49
preadolescents, 74, 78
precedent, 305
prefrontal cortex, 31, 32, 40, 52, 326
pregnancy, 8, 258
prejudice, 165, 172, 190
preoperative screening, 160
preparation, iv, xii, 109, 110, 112, 113, 125, 157, 159, 165, 168, 184, 204, 243, 301, 315
preschool, 66, 72, 73, 75, 179, 186, 190, 193, 196, 198
preschool children, 66, 72, 75, 179, 186, 190, 193, 196
preschoolers, 75, 198
preservation, 275, 282
prevention, xii, xiii, 4, 15, 68, 74, 76, 93, 177, 178, 182, 183, 187, 188, 189, 190, 191, 193, 198, 205, 209, 211, 233, 240, 243, 257, 260, 262, 264, 284, 295, 312, 313
primary school, 181, 197, 199
primate, 42
priming, 333
principles, 171, 209, 213, 229, 239
prior knowledge, 10
probability, 140
probands, 92
probe, 333
problem behavior, 202
problem solving, 223, 225, 284, 315
problem-solving, 171, 230, 318
professional development, 191
professionals, 74, 171, 173, 189, 190, 192, 289
program outcomes, 263
programming, 93, 189
project, xv, 194, 195, 325, 326, 332
proliferation, 254
protective factors, 73, 189
protective role, 28, 206
protein synthesis, 213
proteins, 204, 205
proteolysis, 26
prototype, 275
pseudohypoparathyroidism, 9
psychiatric diagnosis, 279
psychiatric disorders, 16, 31, 67, 72, 89, 90, 92, 101, 129, 131, 161, 162, 163, 174, 175
psychiatric morbidity, 67, 69, 70, 71, 179
psychiatric patients, 99, 312
psychiatric side effects, 255
psychiatrist, 168, 276
psychiatry, 119, 120, 165
psychological assessments, 122
psychological development, 64
psychological distress, 102, 104, 128, 158, 216
psychological health, 72
psychological problems, 74, 237, 268
psychological variables, 164, 165
psychological well-being, 78
psychologist, 165, 168, 244, 276
psychology, 151, 165
psychopathology, 57, 60, 64, 67, 70, 71, 76, 77, 78, 79, 84, 85, 88, 89, 90, 92, 94, 100, 105, 127, 128, 129, 132, 133, 135, 139, 150, 151, 152, 153, 154, 157, 159, 160, 163, 164, 165, 183, 189, 282
psychopharmacology, 283
psychoses, 312
psychosis, 127, 239, 252, 255, 305, 312, 313, 316
psychosocial development, 65
psychosocial factors, 179, 188
psychosocial functioning, 60, 173

psychotherapy, 136, 140, 168, 169, 249, 250, 279, 280, 281, 282, 287, 289, 290
psychotropic drugs, 115
psychotropic medications, 301
pubertal development, 7
puberty, 9, 103
public education, 189, 192
public health, 15, 41, 188, 216, 309
public policy, xii, 177, 188, 189, 191, 192
public schools, 193
Puerto Rico, 77, 199
pulmonary hypertension, 252, 257

Q

quality of life, xi, 60, 63, 64, 67, 71, 78, 80, 90, 109, 133, 134, 150, 151, 153, 158, 159, 160, 167, 170, 171, 174, 212, 221, 268, 269, 275, 277
questioning, 284
questionnaire, 38, 55, 74, 97, 112, 133, 138, 152, 154, 290

R

race, 64, 162, 164, 173
racial differences, 85
racial minorities, 85
reading, 147, 150, 165, 243
reality, 126, 130, 144
reasoning, 185, 315
recall, 111, 112, 113, 137, 138, 144
recalling, 142
receptors, 23, 24, 26, 35, 49, 54, 56, 103, 104, 118, 254, 302, 325, 328, 331, 332
recognition, 72, 80, 181, 182, 197, 267, 290
rreflux esophagitis, 119
Registry, 98, 224, 245
regression, 217, 293
regression equation, 217
regulations, 190
rehabilitation, 315, 316, 319
reinforcement, 154, 223, 315, 326
reinforcers, 328
relapses, 140, 243
relatives, 6, 14, 212
relaxation, 106, 239, 297
relevance, 14, 37, 70, 179, 190, 221, 256
REM, 110, 113, 116, 117, 308
remission, 43, 45, 268, 282, 304
renal calculus, 306
renal dysfunction, 260
replication, 10, 12, 315
requirements, 97, 167, 216, 217, 219, 229
researchers, xi, 12, 32, 63, 83, 84, 87, 95, 96, 97, 101, 117, 191, 226, 229, 247, 248, 314
resection, 275
resistance, 9, 27, 36, 41, 46, 147, 204, 205, 207, 254
resolution, 25, 30, 45, 158, 169, 171
resources, 125, 126, 168, 170, 190, 191, 295
respiratory problems, 268
response, 7, 22, 24, 28, 29, 30, 31, 32, 34, 35, 36, 38, 39, 40, 42, 45, 48, 50, 51, 52, 55, 56, 103, 115, 136, 179, 195, 206, 210, 211, 212, 242, 243, 281, 283, 284, 286, 293, 300, 309, 323, 324, 327, 328, 329, 330
responsiveness, 38, 53, 181
restaurants, 178, 179, 180, 181, 188
restless legs syndrome, 114, 119, 120
restrictions, 189, 221
restructuring, 223, 225, 240, 242, 283, 284
retardation, 8, 9
rewards, 284
rhythm, 102, 103, 105
risk factors, 5, 6, 16, 19, 61, 63, 69, 75, 85, 93, 129, 174, 182, 199, 205, 207, 211, 212, 213, 216, 232
risks, xii, 157, 158, 159, 165, 167, 169, 170, 204, 215, 220, 221, 258, 267, 276, 311
risk-taking, 67
risperidone, 118, 119, 301, 307
rodents, 56, 327

S

saccharin, 32
sadness, 87, 88, 136, 141
safety, 220, 221, 260, 261, 264, 265, 329, 330
saturated fat, 205, 211
schizophrenia, 31, 310, 311, 312, 313, 315, 316, 317, 318, 319
Schizotypal Personality Disorder, 163
school, xi, xii, 60, 61, 64, 68, 71, 72, 74, 76, 77, 79, 80, 151, 177, 186, 187, 188, 189, 191, 192, 193, 194, 196, 197, 198, 202, 290
school performance, 64
second generation, 311
second language, 50
secondary schools, 189, 199
secretion, 7, 23, 25, 28, 45, 51, 53, 103, 206, 207, 254, 270, 273, 300, 301, 308
sedative, 117, 119, 306
sedentary behavior, 178, 179, 186, 187, 189, 197
sedentary lifestyle, 2, 215
seizure, 258, 305, 306, 323
selective attention, 141
selective serotonin reuptake inhibitor, 289, 292, 296, 307
self esteem, 3, 71, 78, 105

self-awareness, 92
self-concept, 64, 73, 77, 80
self-control, 239, 284
self-efficacy, 126, 185, 190, 191, 193, 295
self-esteem, 63, 64, 65, 66, 67, 69, 71, 75, 76, 78, 79, 80, 83, 85, 87, 90, 93, 127, 131, 140, 182, 186, 196, 201, 221, 245, 253, 284
self-help sessions, 226
self-image, 126
self-monitoring, 134, 171, 187, 223, 224, 225, 226, 227, 228, 229, 239, 240, 245, 246, 247, 313
self-perceptions, 63
self-regulation, 49, 235
self-reports, 33, 85
self-worth, 66
semi-structured interviews, 89, 139
sensation, 31, 83, 84, 89, 135, 322, 327, 329
sensations, 88, 126, 141
sensitivity, 38, 44, 51, 53, 125, 205, 206, 207, 326, 328
sequencing, 315
serotonin, 19, 86, 103, 105, 257, 259, 281, 286, 295, 306, 331
serotonin syndrome, 257
sertraline, 280, 286, 292, 295, 296, 297, 304, 305, 306, 307
serum, 46, 47, 65, 103, 149, 209, 256, 259
serum bicarbonate, 259
services, iv, 143, 301
sex, 22, 29, 51, 60, 125, 207, 209, 211
sex hormones, 51
sexual abuse, 100
sexual activity, 323
sexual behavior, 47
sexual harassment, 179
sexuality, 119
SFT, 147
shame, 53, 70, 89, 98, 101, 126
shape, 62, 63, 65, 70, 85, 87, 88, 93
sheep, 329
shortage, 144
showing, 14, 33, 38, 39, 66, 146
side effects, xiii, 216, 221, 251, 252, 256, 260, 270, 275, 276, 305, 306
signaling pathway, 254
signals, 23, 25, 26, 27, 40, 43, 48, 57
signs, 127, 128, 290, 293
skeletal muscle, 208, 211, 212, 213, 254
skills training, 239, 314
skin, 7, 147, 218, 257
sleep apnea, 110, 111, 158
sleep disorders, 96, 100, 110, 111, 114, 117, 119, 120, 268, 299, 303, 306, 308
sleep disturbance, 97, 119
sleep stage, 110
sleep walking, 301
small intestine, 51, 158, 267, 270
smoking, 210, 259
smoking cessation, 259
SMS, 247
snacking, 104, 106, 184, 185, 240, 313
social class, 3, 85
social competence, 66
social exclusion, 3
social impairment, 88
social network, 66, 179, 247
social norms, 202
social organization, 71, 177, 191, 192
social problems, xi, 60, 64
social psychology, 151
social relations, 131
social relationships, 131
social rewards, 125
social skills, 64
social stigmatization, 3, 128
social stress, 71
social support, 69, 167, 223, 225, 240, 269, 282
socialization, 200
society, 3, 188, 215, 245, 247, 248
sodium, 32, 149
software, 323
solution, 37, 89, 98, 123, 271
somnolence, 110, 113, 137, 253, 259
specialists, 90, 109, 111, 123, 159, 172
stabilization, 61
starch, 211
starvation, 24, 222
state, 6, 29, 30, 32, 33, 34, 36, 38, 39, 40, 50, 102, 109, 110, 111, 119, 131, 209, 276, 312
states, 48, 84, 110, 119, 141, 187, 312, 317, 333
steatorrhea, 253, 258, 275
stigma, 66, 76, 160
stimulus, 50, 171, 223, 225, 239, 240, 242, 283, 293, 328
stoma, 158, 271
stomach, 23, 24, 27, 42, 158, 207, 217, 260, 267, 270, 271, 273
storage, 22, 26, 27, 28, 254
stress, 22, 28, 42, 45, 46, 48, 49, 53, 67, 78, 83, 87, 88, 93, 101, 102, 103, 104, 105, 106, 123, 131, 139, 170, 179, 195, 197, 241, 284, 289, 293, 295, 297, 328
stressful events, 295
stressors, 168, 295
striatum, 23, 31, 32, 33, 34, 35, 38, 39, 40, 47, 52, 53, 54, 327, 328, 333

stroke, 257, 311, 323
structurc, 42, 64, 78, 116, 133, 154, 165, 189, 224, 226, 323
structuring, 294
style, 72, 123, 144, 185, 197, 200, 230, 231, 245
Styles, 184
subcutaneous injection, 40
subgroups, 174
sub-Saharan Africa, 2
substance abuse, 137
substance use, 43, 90, 110, 129, 137, 160, 164, 167
substitution, 259
substrates, 333
sucrose, 28, 32, 204
suicidal behavior, 174
suicidal ideation, 259
suicide, 66, 67, 159, 323
sulfonamide, 258
sulfonylurea, 258
Sun, 23, 55, 264
supervision, 220
supplementation, 40, 258, 273, 275
suppression, 23, 25, 27, 44, 49, 255, 300, 301, 305, 325
surgical technique, 267, 275
surveillance, 176, 256, 276
survival, 25, 249
susceptibility, xi, 5, 6, 10, 16, 44
Sweden, 91, 106, 153, 278, 331
Switzerland, 80, 109, 155, 176
symptoms, 8, 45, 68, 70, 76, 80, 84, 97, 98, 99, 100, 106, 127, 129, 130, 131, 132, 133, 134, 136, 137, 138, 140, 144, 155, 160, 204, 221, 258, 277, 280, 281, 282, 290, 293, 301, 323, 328
synapse, 103
syndrome, 7, 9, 20, 83, 84, 86, 95, 96, 97, 98, 99, 101, 104, 105, 106, 109, 110, 111, 112, 114, 119, 120, 138, 149, 172, 203, 204, 207, 211, 212, 252, 260, 264, 289, 296, 297, 304, 307, 308, 310, 311, 317
synthesis, 42, 45, 135, 204, 316
synthetic analogues, 254

T

target, 24, 131, 139, 189, 216, 245, 280, 281, 321, 323, 326, 328
techniques, xiii, 8, 41, 70, 147, 191, 223, 225, 228, 229, 232, 238, 239, 241, 246, 267, 270, 273, 279, 282, 294, 295, 313, 314, 322, 328
technological advances, 246
technologies, 5, 10
technology, 2, 234, 250
telephone, 162, 168, 181, 216, 227, 233
television viewing, 194, 202
television watching, 68, 180, 198, 210
temperament, 91
temperature, 308, 323
tension, 101
terminals, 328
testing, 10, 16, 37, 166, 172, 184, 197, 199, 284, 292, 295
test-retest reliability, 152
text messaging, 246, 247
thalamus, 32, 33, 40, 326
therapeutic approaches, xi, xii
therapist, 122, 123, 125, 128, 232, 238, 283, 294, 295
therapy, iv, xiii, 29, 74, 97, 121, 122, 123, 125, 127, 140, 168, 171, 174, 208, 210, 213, 238, 239, 244, 246, 256, 259, 263, 264, 265, 267, 276, 278, 280, 285, 286, 290, 294, 296, 300, 305, 308, 316, 317
thiazolidinediones, 260
Third World, 177, 178, 191
thoughts, 87, 134, 140, 141, 142, 238, 239, 241, 242, 245, 283, 284, 295
threats, 215
thrombosis, 159
thyroid, 149, 252
thyrotropin, 7
tibialis anterior, 113
time frame, 239
tissue, 147, 205, 207, 208
total cholesterol, 149
total energy, 180, 216, 257, 258
toxic substances, 110, 112, 137, 138
toys, 181
trade, 88
training, 106, 132, 133, 186, 190, 191, 210, 212, 239, 240, 283, 297, 313
trait anxiety, 102
traits, 10, 12, 15, 18, 19, 44, 68, 76, 89, 127, 134, 139, 141, 183
trajectory, 323
transcription, 14
transcripts, 213
translation, xv, 15
transmission, 103, 205, 329
transplant, 234
transport, 22, 42, 213, 254
transportation, 2
trauma, 179, 194, 195
treatment of binge eating disorder, 286, 287
trial, 47, 48, 92, 99, 154, 174, 176, 192, 196, 200, 207, 222, 231, 232, 233, 234, 235, 246, 252, 257, 260, 261, 262, 263, 264, 278, 280, 281, 285, 286,

289, 292, 294, 295, 296, 297, 304, 305, 307, 316, 318
triggers, 241, 242, 245, 246, 295
triglycerides, 149, 204, 205, 207, 209, 257, 311
TSH, 149
turnover, 23, 39
twins, 6, 20, 86, 106, 107
type 2 diabetes, 9, 12, 20, 43, 46, 92, 104, 158, 174, 204, 205, 206, 207, 208, 209, 210, 211, 212, 213, 232, 234, 250, 252, 260, 261, 262, 263, 264, 268, 273
tyrosine, 57, 254

U

UK, 59, 61, 75, 193, 195, 255
UN, 149
United, 2, 4, 61, 76, 77, 85, 153, 158, 175, 176, 189, 199, 201, 216, 249, 273, 289, 311, 318
United Nations, 189, 201
United States, 2, 4, 61, 76, 77, 85, 153, 158, 175, 176, 199, 216, 249, 273, 289, 311, 318
universe, 171
unstructured interviews, 136
urban, 105, 162
urban population, 105
uric acid, 256
urinalysis, 149
USA, 5, 12, 21, 59, 61, 79, 157, 181, 187, 213, 223, 237, 279, 289, 299, 309, 321, 333

V

vagus, 22, 25, 26
vagus nerve, 22, 25, 26
validation, 61, 79, 153, 197, 211, 256
valve, 257
valvular heart disease, 264
variables, 53, 54, 86, 129, 164, 173, 208, 280, 281
variations, 9, 10, 14, 15, 308
varieties, 182
vegetable oil, 206
vegetables, 112, 144, 145, 179, 180, 183, 195, 206, 208, 217, 218, 310
ventricle, 323
victimization, xi, 60, 66, 71, 75, 78, 195
violence, 179
visceral adiposity, 209, 213
vision, 125, 142
visual processing, 31, 32
visual stimulus, 54
vitamin B1, 273
vitamin B12, 273
vitamin D, 258, 275
vitamin K, 258
vitamins, 258, 275
VLDL, 204
vocational training, 190
vomiting, 118, 131, 134
vulnerability, 8, 86, 87, 102, 103, 131

W

waking, 98, 109, 110, 138, 290
walking, 2, 111, 208, 310
Washington, 72, 77, 91, 152, 173, 198, 222, 234, 248
water, 37, 55, 147, 183, 216, 217, 218
websites, 181, 228, 230
weight changes, 219
weight control, 134, 157, 158, 168, 231, 235, 247, 248, 250, 251, 252, 259
weight gain, xi, 3, 22, 28, 29, 30, 35, 36, 37, 41, 49, 52, 54, 63, 72, 73, 74, 78, 79, 87, 98, 105, 113, 118, 122, 123, 124, 127, 128, 129, 145, 149, 150, 155, 167, 184, 186, 201, 233, 239, 241, 258, 259, 260, 301, 311, 313, 316, 322, 326
weight management, xiii, 75, 216, 218, 219, 224, 232, 234, 237, 239, 241, 244, 248, 296, 312, 313, 314, 315, 316, 317
weight reduction, 56, 69, 85, 158, 182, 185, 216, 225, 247, 252, 255, 261, 281, 325, 329
weight status, 28, 66, 73, 74, 76, 77, 180, 184, 186, 188, 194, 195, 295
well-being, 60, 63, 64, 71, 79, 125, 154, 188, 201
wellness, 87, 193
Western countries, 5, 60, 61, 178, 180
WHO, 2, 67, 150, 155, 202
withdrawal, 118, 251, 252
working hours, 178
working memory, 31, 51, 54
World Health Organization, 2, 80, 146, 147, 155, 157, 176, 189, 202
World Health Organization (WHO), 2
worldwide, 3, 73, 173, 193, 271, 322, 329
worry, 63, 71, 75, 93, 130, 132, 141

Y

yield, 10, 169, 225, 226
young adults, 2, 76, 195, 200
young women, 45, 55, 91, 92, 221